A Mental Ethnography: Conclusions from Research in LSD

Niccolo Caldararo

A Mental Ethnography: Conclusions from Research in LSD

palgrave
macmillan

Niccolo Caldararo
Department of Anthropology
San Francisco State University
San Francisco, CA, USA

ISBN 978-3-031-13744-0 ISBN 978-3-031-13745-7 (eBook)
https://doi.org/10.1007/978-3-031-13745-7

This Palgrave Macmillan imprint is published by the registered company Springer Nature Switzerland AG.
The registered company address is: Gewerbestrasse 11, 6330 Cham, Switzerland

Autopsy means in Greek the act of seeing for oneself

Preface

A Beginning Note on Form

> [A]re we on the road toward a wrong-headed, super spin-out revolution of ruin, building on defiant acts in savage side-shows where THEM and US fight forever?
> —Steve Leiper, Assistant Editor, *San Francisco Oracle*, 1967

This book was influenced by two experiences, one from an article that appeared in the Weekend section of the *Financial Times* on LSD use by tech workers and CEOs (Hannah Kuchler, "How Silicon Valley discovered LSD," 12–13 August, 2017), which was a remarkable document in that it reviewed perceptions and beliefs of people using LSD today. It is of interest how the drug is being used and its effects perceived now compared to the period in the 1960s. My presence in the Haight-Ashbury in the 1960s and at the Mogar Laboratory at San Francisco State University (SFSU) is the second influence. A number of references to the 1960s and the nature of LSD that appeared in the Kuchler article (and many others since LSD became fashionable) were incorrect in my view. Interpretation is at the center of the issue; just as a reading of Leiper's quote above is seen by many as a political statement applying to the "left and right," it was read by many people at the time living in the Haight-Ashbury district of

San Francisco as referring to those who wanted to explore the potential of human consciousness and those who feared such exploration, from the Inquisition to Richard Nixon.

This problem of interpretation has many aspects. I am calling this book *A Mental Ethnography*, because like a traditional ethnography it attempts to reveal something about a time, place, and people by using an informant, me. Ethnographies became the focus of substantial criticism after the 1950s for a number of reasons, one of which was how they were seen to "speak for the Other," to define groups in a frozen manner as if change did not happen in indigenous society, or that they played a role in colonialism and the commodification of non-European people and their culture (Clifford and Marcus 1986). While I do not agree with these criticisms from my reading of the ethnographic literature, I do agree that ethnographic writing became a kind of literature and while each could be seen as a snapshot of society and culture, what was used and what was ignored reflected interests of the anthropologists in many ways (Clifford 1988). So this book is an ethnography because it relates the behavior and culture created at a time and place due to ideas surrounding the use of psychedelic experiences. I use many approaches to examine this society and culture, some from anthropology, some from medical science, and others from a variety of Native peoples' cosmologies. All these approaches attempt to provide a broad picture and a number of unique focused aspects of what many others and I experienced. Like any ethnography it cannot be comprehensive; other people saw, felt, and experienced different things, but like people in ships at sea and fish below, they are in the same place but differently.

Language, Behavior, and the Brain

This book looks back to the 1960s and forward to today. The concerns of many of my student friends and the professors I had often revolved around the crises of the time, H-Bombs, the Soviet Union, disease, and overpopulation, among many others. Often people wondered why humans seemed to recreate the crises of the past in war, population, and intolerance. There was some focus on the problem with language and my mentor, Robert Mogar, studied the problems people faced with expressing themselves and become active and effective people. His work led to a number of articles on language, and it seemed that as smart was we were, we had some central flaw that prevented humans as individuals and societies in general from coming to meaningful resolution of difficulties that often seemed simple to solve.

In the text below I often refer to "the Mogar Lab." In doing this I am including meetings and work I was involved with in the 1960s at San Francisco State University (then College) as well as locations where Dr. Mogar and his colleagues met, worked, and had patients. This includes the Psychology Department facilities at San Francisco State University, Napa, Mendocino, and Sonoma State Hospitals and the Palo Alto facilities.

The question then was to look at pathologies and try to find keys to healing mental illness and perhaps society as well. Many people began their study of LSD as part of their path to this end. My studies began there too, but then I was led by the failures in these studies to look past the clinical findings to an investigation of culture and human evolution. In my 2017 book I describe the evolution of the human brain in comparison with other mammals, both social and solitary, and with other social animals, for example, bees, ants, and termites. In that analysis we want to know why humans or animals, in general, developed complex brains.

The idea of whether other animals have cognition similar to that of humans often ends in circular arguments, what is thought, what is an abstraction, what is a symbol, and so on. Deacon's (1997) description of this problem is a typical example, and Erikson (1951) also travels the same circular trail, "What is a symbol?" "… something that stands for something else." Then there are the problems of complexity and learning. It is the contention of Flynn (2012) that this is due to education, where the type of education focuses on abstraction and complexity as opposed to learning methods to accomplish tasks. He calls this concrete thinking versus symbolic. He regards this as the main difference in IQ scores across time, with nations and between classes and ethnicities. This idea is not new; a form of it was contained in the work of Levy-Bruhl (1966), who argued that primitive people, that is, people living in non-industrial contexts, had different thought patterns and perceptions because of their lifestyles. I am perhaps being charitable to Levy-Bruhl here, as some have criticized his theory as being racist and essentialist, that is, the idea that people's abilities are tied up in their racial makeup; however, as an analysis of how people think at a particular time in human history it is useful.

One could say, routine and learning make reality. On the other hand, a more phenomenological view I sometimes play with my students looks at how commensals, like our pets or some beetles with different species of ants, come to learn to respond to the behavior of the host in ways that benefit both. Often people argue that certain animals, usually birds and mammals, can learn complex tasks, yet the idea of a consciousness that is like our cognition is denied them. Their behavior is termed simply conditioning for rewards. I have argued that this is also true of humans—only our conditioning schedule is more complex and aided by a very efficient conditioning system, language. Another aspect of interpretation that I will comment on using a variety of sources, mainly cross-cultural, is the nature of psychiatric evaluations of individuals' expression of experience, either in clinical settings or under the influence of psychedelic drugs in other settings. There is a vast literature on this and I will cite examples from time to time, but an adequate outline is presented by Alarcon (2009). Another aspect of phenomenology that dogs research into dreams, psychedelic experience, hallucinations, and visions is the question of authenticity. We cannot yet "see" or experience and record someone's dream and so on; we have to assume that what they tell us is actually lived and not a product of conscious expression and intention. Instrumentation like fMRI has made some original inroads to this problem. Some practitioners have held that the schizophrenic hallucination is a measure of authenticity, but to assume it is devoid of intention and not the product of conditioning, however tortured is perhaps incorrect (see Laing 1959 for a critique on this). The hallucinations of delirium tremens are outside our brief, as they are caused by alcohol, but the fact that they generally produce images of animals, mainly dogs, snakes, and mice (Platz et al. 1995) falls within our theory of origin, which will be presented later on. I will discuss this below in a variety of contexts.

Consciousness, Mind, Awareness, and Experience

Crick (1994) uses the terms "consciousness" and "awareness" interchangeably. This is problematic, as many neurologists refer to "varieties of awareness," one of which provides a paradox, "the waking state," and these varieties can grade into variations of coma and vegetative states (Zeman 1997). Rivers (1920) specifically finds "consciousness" and "unconsciousness" need to be separated from temporary periods of attention that we all experience from moment to moment. Cognitive scientist Jackendoff (1987) calls this attentive moment the "phenomenological mind." Animal perception has evolved to certain conditions in the environment for survival, to concentrate attention on a limited amount of stimuli, which is why awareness is limited. This was the central point of Rivers' thesis, derived from his work with Head, though Hughlings Jackson had a similar idea earlier of higher levels of the evolution of the brain "constraining" lower ones (Sacks 2012). Seth (2021) focuses his definition of reality on this limited feature of our primate perception. Uexkull (1934/2010) extends this species-specific reality to all animals, producing a multitude of phemonomenological visions. Some have divided theories of consciousness into a "central cognition hypothesis" generally associated with a brain of some kind, and other theories grouped around an "extended cognition" where the idea of brain, as in spiders and squid is not centralized and even, as in the case of Uexkull, this extension can associate with aspects of the environment (Japyassu and Laland 2017). This experiential view has been renewed recently by scientists under a general concept of the Integrated Information Theory (IIT) where experience is translated into feeling (Koch 2019). In many ways this is much as Uexkull proposed, but benefiting from the vast advances in biology and especially neurology and the instrumentation used to chart the physiology of brains. Damasio (2021) constructs an inner self or mind by the association of images of memory with the feelings of daily experience, while Rivers' and Freud's idea of repression and suppression to produce attention and awareness at any one moment is often referred to today as a self-referencing effect (SRE) and was identified by Rogers et al. in 1977. Stendardi et al. (2021) have found its processing to be in the ventral medial prefrontal cortex (vmPFC), with an upper and lower concentration of activity. They locate in the dorsal area that aspect of the conception of being, that is, "self" from non-self, or as they put it, "self from other." Experiments by McCormick et al. (2020) found that the vmPFC is influenced by hippocampal processing most of the time during autobiographical memory recall. See the illustration below for a general picture of the brain regions.

The effects of psychedelics on connections between the hippocampus/parahippocampus and other brain regions, for example, the retroplenial cortex (RSC) (results in "ego-dissolution" and so on; see Carhart-Harris et al. 2016a), may provide models for how consciousness functions in humans. De Rios (1984) argues that this phenomenon of "ego-dissolution" happens in many cultural contexts in the use of hallucinogens and, as a result, a variety of guiding methods have evolved to provide for reconstruction. I bring this up here because I am not sure that the concept of "ego-dissolution" best describes what occurs in all contexts, yet we also will find the hippocampus involved in much of what we call the LSD experience by its role in memory. And central to this is the fact that the thalamus, a part of the brain that is called the gateway to the brain because inputs to the cortex have to pass through it, has been found to have multiple interconnections vital for human memory (Aggleton et al. 2010), and Preller et al. (2019) demonstrate LSD increases brain-wide sensory, somatomotor, and thalamic connectivity. The idea that hallucinogens are necessary to these cathartic events mentioned by many physicians and scientists working with different peoples can be contrasted with the fact that there are traditions in some people where organized physical exercise achieves the same or similar outcome, as in the Sufis or the Cathars, from where the word is derived (Holmes 1925).

One problem with awareness, mind, and consciousness is the ability of awareness to be separated into segments of varying levels. This is most striking in the study of sleepwalking (parasomnias), where we descend into an analysis of levels of sleep and sleep movement (Brown 2003). People who are afflicted with this condition generally do not recall sleep-walking or events that take place during them. This informs us of a form of consciousness, though it is often referred to as a species of amnesia.

Though this may be affected by recall bias, as proposed in a large study of people with sleepwalking episodes compared with controls (Pressman 2013), nevertheless, we will be concerned in this book with all forms of human consciousness related to memory, images, and meaning. The basis for this condition was discovered by Jouvet (1999) in the 1950s when he severed the connections in the cat brain that prevented muscle atonia, reducing the ability to control body movements. The result was when sleeping, the cats behaved as if they were awake, running, stalking, and so on as if responding to dream stimuli, perhaps as memories.

Memory, Dreams, and Reality

We also find a core principle of brain function that cortical systems must interact with each other and the hippocampus to support the multidimensional nature of episodic memory (usually defined as the conscious recollection of a personal experience that contains information on what happened as well as what location and when, thus a context of related sensations, visual, auditory, and olfactory) (see Cooper and Ritchey 2019). Therefore, if the self is to be found in the processing matrix of the components of the hippocampus and parahippocampus, then disruption of the connections and processing would affect this deeply central notion of being and bring about feelings of a loss of ego, communication with the cosmos, and perhaps even spiritual "feelings." But since a number of studies have reported different areas of the brain where subjects reported spiritual feelings, it may be that the modification of processing information from the cortical regions (with self-other representations) leads to these "experiences" (Miller et al. 2019). Timothy Leary reported having the deepest religious experience of his life after consuming seven "divine mushrooms" (Leary 1964).

We will discuss the hippocampus and some of the other structures of the "mid-brain" later on. The terms for structures at the center of the mammalian brain have names that are derived from historical individuals' ideas who discovered different parts, or from their shape and size; thus, "hippocampus" means sea horse in Greek because it looked vaguely like one to an anatomist. The hippocampus and the piriform cortex and olfactory cortex are often referred to as paleocortex or archicortex due to their three-layer structure instead of the six layers found in the entorhinal cortex, neocortex, or new brain of mammals (Wright 2020). Many vertebrates lack a neocortex—thus the idea of paleo (Striedter 2005).

At this point we have reviewed the anatomical correlates, one might say, the road maps, on which psychedelic experiences take place. This seems rather straightforward. Obviously everyone is different, has different experiences growing up, is genetically varied, and may have experienced different educational milieus, producing a variety of cosmological concepts. However, taking all that into account we have an enormous variety of experiences, including images, people report under the influence of psychedelics. Masters and Houston (1966) attempted a construction of categories of these, but we will discuss the difficulty of classification later. Also, some of these experiences are similar to pathological conditions, either physical or psychological pathologies. Further, we find significant differences in images and interpretation across cultures (Al-Issa 1977; Bauer et al. 2011); these differences extend into dreamscapes (see in Tedlock 1987). Recent research into the types and variation of hallucinations in a number of cultures (Laroi et al. 2014) reinforces anthropological concepts of culture and how culture and language create patterns of attention (Kluckhohn 1944; Sapir 1921; Whorf 1946, 1956a, b). Earlier William James 1907 [1890] had produced an explanation for unconscious differences in perception and memory which was developed into a theory of schemata or generalized impressions that form basic ideas of the world and a way of seeing. Later this was utilized in explaining how people were able to hold contradictory ideas as true, referred to as cognitive dissonance, and then processes for reducing dissonance (as in unfulfilled expectations), as dissonance reduction to reduce tension (Solso 1994).

Why we find these differences in cognition is one of the reasons for the existence of this book. I have pursued answers to this question across history, religion, psychology, and anthropology. I think there is an answer which I will propose in due time. First we need to investigate antecedents, to this study, to my relation to LSD and psychedelics in general, and to the Mogar Laboratory and what was happening in the world of the twentieth century that brought LSD, psychedelics, and science together.

Yet, consciousness is the nub of the problem; for Sacks (2012) some disruption to the lower areas of the brain, pathological or drug induced, could release images of all kinds depending on the area affected, which developed from ideas of structure and function mentioned above.

In this pursuit, we saw Crick concerned with attention, and James (1907) also defined consciousness with attention. Others like Helmholtz referred to subliminal, unconscious inference. This gives people a feeling often that they have experienced something before or "know of it." These are associated with a number of pathological conditions, including the common phenomenon of fainting, but also the condition of "temporary loss of consciousness," sometimes referred to as syncope, which is caused by a temporary reduction of blood flow and oxygen in the brain. I am not sure about this, and I feel that "awareness" and "consciousness," while alike, we experience these periods of lack of attention that are significant and thus they deserve more research. I use the term "attentive presence" for a type of consciousness that penetrates daily routine in a profound fashion and is the "platform," if you will, for social invention (see below). We have to keep in mind that the activity of the body and the presence of the brain, or whole brain, vary depending on the activity, the quality of the responses, and the specific areas of the brain (when damaged) that can be lost and behavior still remain functional. In the history of the study of the structures of the brain and its functional organization, surgery of injured patients and the study of their behavior after recovery were instrumental in providing basic information. So was the use of electrical stimulation and experimental removal of the cerebral lobes or parts of the brain. The classical studies are reported in Gerhardt von Bonin's (1960) translation. In some of these we find chickens with the entire brain removed yet still capable of some forms of typical behavior. So the question of instinct, learning, and the conscious organization of responses to stimuli becomes a matter of whole brain, parts of a brain, and regional interaction of neurons, as injuries to the brain can result in both deficits and repair and normal behavior in some cases (von Bonin 1960). The problem here is that when we speak of the brain, we are often referring to the interaction of specific neurons, of axons and dendrites that send and receive impulses of a chemical and electrical nature, and these also are influenced by little processes called "spines" (Crick [1994] calls them "twigs"). This interaction is the "brain."

Most people assign the use of substances (plant, animal, or mineral, which modify life either through changes of consciousness as perception or in death, as brought about by poisons) to specialists, as Aaronson and Osmond pointed out in 1970. Such specialists often guard or monitor the worlds of the living and the spirits. A healing shaman prevents the loss of a life to the spirit world under certain conditions delineated by the science of practice and allowed by the ritual agreement of the supernatural. Today physicians using Western medicine do much the same in the former realm of practice and empiricism. More than 100 years before Aaronson and Osmond, Ernst von Bibra published his study of foods and additives and listed the variety of effects they had on most people, from coffee and tobacco to opium and alcohol. He was a trailblazer in ethnopsychopharmacology. His research led to a number of publications about the human body, its chemistry, excretions and other residues as well as those of animals and plants. His book *The Narcotic Substances of Enjoyment and The Human Being* (1855) was the conclusion of a long journey across the globe collecting substances from various people and their effect on humans.

Methods and Definitions: Hallucinations, Visions, and Thought

In this book we will examine phenomena that can be studied, hallucinations, visions, and so on, by three methods of analysis. One is that of empiricism based on scientific principles and knowledge (some people refer to this as nomological). The second is both phenomenological in an individual sense and related to religion, belief, and metaphysics. The third comprises a realm of information, perceptions, and events for which we lack adequate information for analysis or await new technologies, as when the world of single-cell organisms was discovered by the invention of the microscope.

Shortly after this Louis Lewin began a study of Kava, a plant substance used in the South Pacific for both intoxication and health. He then began a study of ethnobotany and the uses of plant substances in health and ritual, publishing his findings in 1924 as *Phantastica*. It was divided by grouping apparent effect, as in: Inebriants (like alcohol and ether), Excitantia (stimulants like Khat or amphetamine, though Khat was considered a strong hallucinogen by the ancient Egyptians), Euphorica (narcotics like heroin), Hypnotic (tranquilizers like Kava), and Phantastic (hallucinogens like peyote or ayahuasca/yage). His assistant, Arthur Heffter, consumed an extract of *Anhalonium lewinii* (the dumpling cactus or peyote) after animal experiments failed to identify its effects. He supposedly coined the term "mescal" after also consuming a distillation of the agave plant, known to the Native people as "aquardiente" or "blazing water." There is a report of him taking the extract dated 1897. This claim is unlikely, as Edward S. Curtis used the term in his 1907 book. Nevertheless, from Bibra to Heffter and vivid experiences of Havelock Ellis (1898) and his friends, reinforced by ethnographic evidence, we can say that the psychedelic (see also Shonle 1925) experience produces dramatic imagery. The question we face is where it comes from and how it is created.

Since we do not have an agreed-upon definition of what cognition is, or what mind is, as we often find one used to define the other, we cannot attribute clever behavior to animals of other species, as we have no specific criterion to do so. Macphail's (1982) gradational approach looking at how animals solve problems is useful, and recent expansion of ideas of continuities and discontinuities in human and animal capabilities has been extensive (Premack 2007), though disagreement remains, especially regarding interpretation of bird and animal cognition (Caldararo 2017). In this context, my phenomenological view proposes one look at a cat or dog. What kind of system of perception can such an animal have to interpret the existence and behavior of humans, especially their "owners." We usually resort to behaviorism and argue that from an ethological standpoint, they are conditioned to respond to humans by transferring innate patterns for conspecifics like parents, littermates, and colony members to humans. Ethologists like Konrad Lorenz and Niko Tinbergen used concepts like "imprinting" to describe the bonding of such animals as young to their substitute parents.

Certainly trying to conjure up some logical picture of animal thought is a subjective exercise, yet it does provide us with a means of trying to understand what infants experience as they develop a brain and are conditioned to respond to environmental cues in complex patterns that come to be recognized as "parent" and object. There has been a long history of experiments to determine the nature of differences and similarities between human and other animal cognition. Macphail (1982) came to the conclusion that there was a gradation in the animal world to humans. Other researchers find an unbridgeable gap. In our study where hallucinations and visions are significant features of cognition, some researchers have made inroads to discovering methods to interpret animal responses, for example, use of dopamine, to describe similar events in animals (Schmack et al. 2022). If Grof is correct and people under the influence of LSD undergo a form of relearning or, as Mogar and some other psychologists in the 1960s suggested, they re-imprint basic character structure, then we have an interesting and perhaps useful insight into the evolution of consciousness.

Misinterpretation is often dependent on perspective. The second experience began when I was typing up research notes from 1966 in a café. In conversation with a young woman in this café in San Francisco's Bernal Heights area in the summer of 2017, I was exposed to current views of people using LSD. These ideas regarding LSD use among tech workers that she shared had a common thread (Solon 2016). A book came out that year by Waldman (2017) promoting LSD as nearly a cure for everything, marriage, mood, and money, so her attitude was clearly part of a larger community of interest. She, and her associates and friends, had no concern for the history of LSD use, and little knowledge of its history. She spoke of her boyfriend's use of LSD and "microdosing." His idea was of taking a little LSD to become more creative, which is an interesting reflection on our time in contrast to that of Drs. Max Rinkel and Robert W. Hyde (1955), who were one of the first to report on its use on a human subject. Rinkel and Hyde, and others before them, had thought that psychedelics could induce a form of temporary madness similar to schizophrenia. Their work appears tied to CIA initiatives, which involved the use of at least one subject against her consent (see MKULTRA documents; Wetmore 2014).

Here history and biology collide. The idea of microdosing, for example, was well known to researchers in psychiatry in the 1960s, as reference to Stanislav Grof's work, especially his book *Realms of the Human Unconscious: Observations from LSD Research*, 1976, will demonstrate. This book summarizes much of the scientific work in LSD studies up to that date of publication, particularly with a variety of patients presenting behavioral pathologies or chronic illness like alcoholism. Grof speaks of the many ways brain chemistry can be altered, but what is the normal range of various chemical components? Variation can be seen as a toxic alteration, one brought on by organic disease or by ingestion of a substance. What is "toxic" and what is therapeutic requires investigation in terms of ideas of normal, health, and healing.

A Historical Framework of What Has Been Done

Aaronson and Osmond begin their 1970 tome on psychedelics with a discussion of how technology changes human perception of reality over time. From clubs to plows to coffee and books, these are tools that humans have invented and have utilized over time to interact with the natural and human-created environment. In this regard they also class drugs as tools, chemical implements that can enhance healing, focus attention, and bring insight. This context is instructive and useful for discussing LSD and related psychedelics in my opinion. While some of the drugs to be discussed here can have toxic effects, like forms of ergotamine (ergotism or convulsive ergotism; Eadie 2003), most are not new but discovered by Native peoples, who invented the means of using them for desired ends. For example, LSA (lysergic acid amide) derived from the morning glory seed was so used by Mesoamerican cultures (Schultes 1972; Carod-Artal 2015). According to a book by Hernando Ruiz de Alarcon, a Jesuit priest in New Mexico in 1629, the Aztec used the effects of the seeds (Ololiuhqui; also known as *Pomoea violacea*, *Turbina corymbosa* or *Rivea coryubosa*, Christmas vine, or snakeplant; see Hofmann 1971) to commune with the gods. We have to keep in mind that this priest like others, especially Duran, had as their aim the eradication of practices of Native religion they considered devil worship (Todorov 1984).

Interpreting What We See and How

I had read Herschel W. Leibowitz's book *Visual Perception* (1965) the semester before starting at San Francisco State, while I was at Humboldt. This book set out the foundations of how our body works by interpreting light (as a wave or photon particle). The mechanics of this seemed quite clear and logical. Then I started to read Aldous Huxley's *The Doors of Perception* (1963), which begins with him describing how some Native Americans viewed peyote as if it were a deity. Wade Davis relates a similar interpretation about the variety of drugs extracted from plants in the Amazon. The plants via the substances "sing" or communicate to the people who take the drugs, or one might consider that they allow the people under the influence of the drugs to focus on the communication of the plants or the deity of the forest and its manifestations of emanations. This is a common aspect of the use of psychomimetic drugs in aboriginal culture, as reported by workers like Kluver, where the plant, with its power to illuminate or transform, is considered a god. "Psychomimetic" usually means "psychosis inducing," but has largely been used also as a motion of the psyche to unnatural means. Literally the word means "psycho = mind" and "mimesis" or mimicry, expression, resembling. The definition of "god" is understood to mean an emanation or supernatural being, though the word, "supernatural" is probably contradictory here. McKenna (1992; 1993) suggests that the psychedelic transformation by mushrooms is like a UFO or alien contact experience and one might then imagine interspecies communication is implied. He describes this process as that of "exopheromones" or "chemical messengers" that act on many species, a kind of Gaia-like language, the "Transcendent Other." As long as humans were using these hallucinogenic exopheromones they were in communication with all life. But it could be just the opposite, as he places great emphasis on the hallucinogens fostering human brain evolution and language. This process could be also seen as an avenue to close out the song of life and replace it with all but the human broadcast of language. There is considerable literature where the behavior of one species is controlled by the influence of another—Trivers (1985) gives examples of some of these cases.

On another strange note, Kluver argues that the peyote cult was not widely disseminated prior to 1890 but was likely spread by settler contact and military defeat as well as missionary dogma conflicting with Native religion. We see many revitalization cults arise on contact with complex society that challenge cosmological and power relations of Native peoples. Examples in Melanesia demonstrate this in the nineteenth and early twentieth centuries (Worsley 1957), though one might also point to the mass movements of the nineteenth century of Christian sects as science and the Industrial Revolution took hold and challenged belief and status quo (e.g., see Niebuhr 1957)—the same could be said for the "Reagan Revolution" and various related forms, as in Anita Bryant's influence on the Religious Right or later Tea Party and right-wing talk radio that preceded the assault on the US Capitol by groups like the Oath keepers and QAnon (Tamney and Johnson 1983; Whitsel 2001; Cooper et al. 2021).

Blum et al. (1964) report on the creation of groups by LSD users, men only, who generally promote the use of the drug. The initial stages included former scientists like Tim Leary and Ram Das, who gather followers who they "turn on" and spread a kind of religious ideal associated with the drug experience (Ebin 1965). An offshoot of this informal setting is the establishment of formal groups, some associated with institutions, as was the Mexican LSD community at Zihuatanejo led by Leary, and then a large number of informal as well as formal non-profit organizations dedicated to the spread of the experience and what the leaders felt was the "message" behind it. I experienced a few of these informal organizations in the late 1960s and early 1970s, where a male who had taken on the role of teacher or guru controlled a group of males and usually more females. Some would work at regular jobs to support the organization in often communal arrangements, but this often acted as a central point with satellite units of independent people, some couples who routinely met with the central male leader and the core group. The fact that people were compelled to form such groups and to join them is of interest in a number of theories related to the evolution of human groups.

This is a question of origins; one in the nature of our neurological apparatus reflects stimuli from the environment into patterns that can be processed as experience. All that, the entire sentence above, is simply an effort to explain our evolutionary history and the way we have come to structure reality. That reality is incomplete; I discuss the failures of theories of mind due to their nature in my 2017 book. For some people reality takes place in sleep, in others the reality of daily life is complemented by that of dreams, and some, like the Jivaro, believe that the only reality takes place in the dreams of yage-induced experiences in the world of the souls of the banisteria vines, of ancestors (Linzer 1970). There is cultural pressure to have dreams and Jivaro who do not have yage-induced dreams are not considered real men and lacking them is a bad omen (Karsten 1935).

One note on the use of ethnographic materials; I have addressed the criticisms of this archive of human variation elsewhere (Caldararo 2004, 2014). All I will say here is that without this archive, our view of humanity is poorer and constrained. It must be used critically and in comparison if available.

The nature of the problem is trying to define something that is the process of our evolved experience. This was the central issue to Grof, who argued that LSD research opened up a new model of study of human unconsciousness, and by extension, human consciousness. But these words, consciousness and mind and neurology define much the same thing, something that becomes circular. From Freud to Luria to Kandel, the study of how humans come to respond to the stimuli of the environment relies on models. These models stand for what we cannot measure in electrical impulses as meaning, a word that is as empty as "mind." But with Hebb's (1949) concept of cellular changes in learning (the spike-timing-dependent plasticity model; see Caporale and Dan 2008) we get a foundation of the means by which schema of the environment can become integrated patterns that could be called "mind" in a very basic sense (Kandel 2007).

The Original Thesis and Proposal and Now

The core of this book was written from 1967 to 1970 and began as a thesis proposal for my BA in Anthropology at the University of California (UC), Berkeley. That never materialized, as my mentor at the time, J. Desmond Clark, a paleoanthropologist, felt that I should study the neurology of mammals first and then attempt to apply it to hominid evolution. As a result, I stopped working on the thesis as if interrupted by a war, epidemic, or asteroid. I had started the table of contents, but only progressed to a brief foreword and Chap. 2, as I decided to write a précis first and then divide it into chapters. By the time I had reached page 14, Professor Clark's pronouncement had settled in and even the last figure was not given a number in a footnote. What is remarkable to me is that the title of the first chapter was "Symbols and Language: An Inquiry into the Maze of Conditioning of *Homo sapiens* to Social Organization." I was certainly a behaviorist and yet that topic came some 40 years later to form the framework of my book *Big Brains and the Human Superorganism.* This is surprising to me, as I had completely forgotten about this false start, yet the issue of human consciousness has gnawed at me all this time.

Grof struggles with this problem in his practice and experiments with LSD; he accepts ideas of a collective unconscious (supposed events that took place in the past and inherited for the present) and is unsure if all related experiences are derived from early childhood or from symbolic products of the unconscious. (Grof 1976, 222). Yet in learning a language a person inculcates a history of symbols and the representations of meaning are relayed in the expressed demonstrations of cultural enculturation—a process discussed in tortured complexity by Deacon (1997), but where significant progress has been made in recent years (see Vilarroya 2017). Crapanzano (1981) has argued from an analysis of dreams of the Hamadsha and psychiatric interpretation in different cultural contexts that even the process of asking subjects to place dreams into words distorts their nature and meaning. But not all people seem concerned or pay attention to the expressive context of dreams as Fabian (1966) asserts with the Jamaa. Only the signs are significant as having meaning and can readily be expressed in their language. Herdt (1987) finds that dream interpretation for shamans is often "bound up" in altered states of consciousness, which is how I have proposed a mix of images utilized by the brain from different experiences and means of processing that are central to brain function (see Fig. 8.1).

Perceiving and Meaning

A book that expressly deals with this problem was touted early in my education at UC Berkeley; it is Ogden and Richards' (1923) *The Meaning of Meaning.* A very thorough examination of the history of study of the unconscious and especially those related to Freud and psychoanalysis is Henri F. Ellenberger's *The Discovery of the Unconscious*, published in 1970. This covers basic ideas of theory of mind and subjective experiences as often defined under "qualia" (Crick 1994).

I was struck in the late 1960s by the wide diversity of experience of people, both singly and in groups. People were using the same language, but the symbols seemed to diverge in meaning between individuals. Ardener (1975a) created a model for this discrepancy in various contexts, especially gender related. This was confusing, one might imagine, from Deacon's and Vygotsky's (1978) work that conditions of learning language left "signatures" or residues of the learning context that widened meaning, as in a Venn diagram, so that different people have some kind of bleeding extensions of words and the abstractions they stand for. This caused, in my interpretation and discussion with them, some subjects to be caught on specific words and get "stuck" in trying to exercise the meaning, as if they were feeling the symbol in how a blind person might do an object.

San Francisco, CA, USA Niccolo Caldararo

References

Aggleton, John P., Shane M. O'Mara, Seralynne D. Vann, Nick F. Wright, Marian Tsanov and Jonathan T. Erichsen, (2010) "Hippocampal-anterior thalamic pathways for memory: uncovering a network of direct and indirect actions," *The European Journal of Neuroscience*, June, v. 31, n. 12: 2292–2307.

Alarcon, Ranato D. (2009) "Culture, cultural factors and psychiatric diagnosis: review and projections," *World Psychiatry*, Oct., v. 8, (3):131–139.

Al-Issa, I., (1977) "Social and cultural aspects of hallucinations," *Psychological Bulletin*, v. 84, n.3, 570–587.

Ardener, Edwin (1975a) "Belief and the problem of women," in *Perceiving Women*, (ed.) Shirley Ardener, pp. 1–18.

Bauer, Susanne M, Hans Schanda, Hanna Karakula, Luiza Olajossy-Hilkesberger, Palmira Rudaleviciene, et al., (2011) "Culture and the prevalence of hallucinations in schizophrenia," *Comprehensive Psychiatry*, May-June, v. 52, n. 3, 319–325.

Blum, Richard, Eva Blum and Mary Lou Funkhouser, (1964) "The institutionalization of LSD," in Blum, Richard, Nevitt Sanford, Eva Blum, Mary Lou Funkhouser, Joseph J. Downing, et al., (eds.) *Utopiates: The Use and Users of LSD-25, A Publication of the Institute for the Study of Human Problems*, Stanford University, Atherton Press, 124–141.

Bonin, Von, (1960) *The Cerebral Cortex*, Springfield, Ohio, Charels C. Thomas.

Brown, Chip (2003) "The man who mistook his wife for a deer, and other tales from the new science of extreme sleep," *New York Times Magazine*, February, 2, pp. 35–81.

Carhart-Harris, Robin L., Suresh Muthukumaraswamy, Leor Roseman, Mendel Kaelen, Wouter Droog, et al., (2016a) "Neural correlates of the LSD experience revealed by multimodal neuroimaging," *PNAS*, April 26, v. 113, n. 17:4853–4858.

Caldararo, Niccolo (2017) *Big Brains and the Human Superorganism, Why Special Brains Appear in Hominids and Other Social Animals*, Lanham Maryland, Rowman and Littlefield.

Caldararo, Niccolo (2014) *The Psychic Unity of Mankind*, Saarbrucken, Scholars' Press.

Caldararo, Niccolo (2004) "War, Mead and the nature of criticism in Anthropology," *Anthropological Quarterly*, v. 77, n 2, Spring, 311–322.

Carod-Artal, F.J. (2015) "Hallucinogenic drugs in pre-Columbian Mesoamerican cultures," *Neurologia*, v. 30, n. 1, 42–29.

Clifford, James (1988) *The Predicament of Culture,* Cambridge, MA, Harvard University Press.

Clifford, James and George E. Marcus (1986) *Writing Culture: The Poetics and Politics of Ethnography,* Berkeley, University of California Press.

Cooper, Rose A. and Maureen Ritchey (2019) "Cortico-hippocampal network connections support multidimensional quality of episodic memory," *eLife,* March 22, 2019; 8: e45591. https://doi.org/10.7554/eLife.45591

Cooper, Stella, Ben Decker, Anjall Singhvl and Christiaan Triebert, 2021 "Tracking the Oath Keepers who attacked the Capitol," *The New York Times,* Jan 29, https://www.nytimes.com/interactive/2021/01/29/us/oath-keepers-capitol-riot.html. Accessed 3 Feb 2021.

Crick, Francis, (1994) *The Astonishing Hypothesis, The Scientific Search for the Soul,* New York, Simon and Schuster.

Crapanzano, Vincent (1981) "Text, transference, and indexicality," *Ethos,* v. 9:122–148.

Damasio, Antonio (2021) *Feeling and Knowing: Making Minds Conscious,* New York, Pantheon Books.

Deacon, Terrence W., *The Symbolic Species: The Co-evolution of Language and Brain* (New York: W.W. Norton, 1997).

de Rios, Marlene Dobkin (1984) *Hallucinogens: Cross-Cultural Perspectives,* Albuquerque, University of New Mexico Press.

Eadie, Mervyn J. (2003) "Convulsive ergotism: epidemics of the serotonin syndrome?" *Lancet Neurol.* July, v. 2, n. 7, 429–434.

Ebin, David, (1965) *The Drug Experience,* New York, Grove Press.

Ellis, Havelock (1898) "Mescal, a new artificial paradise," *Annual Rep. Smithsonian Inst.*, page 537.

Erikson, Erik (1951) "Sex differences in the play construction of pre-adolescents," *Am J. Orthopsychiat.* v. 21, : 667–692.

Fabian, Johannes (1966) "Dream and charisma, 'theories of dreams' in the Jamaa Movement (Congo)," *Anthropos,* 61, 544–560.

Flynn, James R. (2012) *Are We Getting Smarter?* Cambridge, Cambridge University Press.

Grof, Stanislav (1976) *Realms of the Human Unconscious: Observation from LSD Research,* New York, E.P. Dutton.

Hebb, Donald (1949) *The Organization of Behavior,* New York, Wiley.

Herdt, Gilbert H. (1987) "Selfhood and discourse in Sambia dream sharing," In *Dreaming: Anthropological and Psychological Interpretations,* (ed.) Barbara Tedlock, Cambridge, Cambridge University Press, 55–85.

Hofmann, Albert (1971) "Teonanacatl and Ololiuqui, two ancient magic drugs of Mexico," United Nations, Office on Drugs and Crime, January 1, https://www.unodc.org/unodc/en/data-and-analysis/bulletin/bulletin_1971-01-01_1_page003.html.

Holmes, Edmond (1925) *The Holy Heretics: The Story of the Algigensian Crusade,* London, Watts & Co.

Hyde, R.W., Max Rinkel, Hudson Hoagland and Harry Soloman (1955) "Experimental psychiatry II. Clinical and Physio-chemical observations in experimental psychosis," *Amer. J. of Psychiatry*, v. 111, 881–895.

Jackendoff, Ray (1987) *Consciousness and the Computational Mind,* Cambridge, MA, Bradford Books, MIT Press.

James, William (1907) *Psychology,* New York, Henry Holt and Co. (originally published in 1890 as the Principles of Psychology).

Japyassu, Hilton F. and Kevin N. Laland, (2017) "Extended spider cognition," *Animal Cognition*, v. 20:375–395.

Jouvet, Michel (1999) *The Paradox of Sleep*, Cambridge, MIT Press.

Kandel, Eric R. (2007) *In Search of Memory: The Emergence of a New Science of Mind,* New York, W.W. Norton.

Karsten, R. (1935) *The Head-Hunters of Western Amazonas,* Helsingfors, Sinska Zetenskaps-Societeten.

Kluckhohn, Clyde (1944) *Mirror for Man*, New York, McGraw-Hill.

Koch, Christof (2019) *The Feeling of Life Itself: Why Consciousness is Widespread,* Cambridge, MIT Press.

Laing, R.D. (1959) *The Divided Self,* Harmondsworth, Pelican Books.

Laroi, Frank, Tanya Marie Luhrmann, Vaughan Bell, William A. Christian, Jr., Smita Deshpande, et al., (2014) "Culture and hallucinations: overview and future directions," *Schizophrenia Bulletin*, v. 40, suppl, no. 4, s213–s220.

Leary, Timothy, (1964) "The religious experience: its production and interpretation," *Psychedelic Review*, n. 3, 324–346.

Levy-Bruhl, Lucien (1966) *Primitive Mentality*, (originally published in 1923) Boston, Beacon Press.

Lewin, Louis (1924) *Phanfastica, Die betaubenden und erregenden Genussmittel, Fur Arzte und Nichtarzte*, Berlin, Verlag von Georg Stike.

Linzer, Jeffrey, (1970) "Some anthropological aspects of Yage," In in Aaronson, Bernard and Humphry Osmond, (eds) (1970) *Psychedelics, The Uses and Implications of Hallucinogenic Drugs,* Garden City, Anchor Books. Pp.108–115.

Macphail, Euan M. (1982) *Brain and Intelligence in Vertebrates,* Oxford, Clarendon Press.

Masters, R.E.L. and Jean Houston (1966) *The Varieties of Psychedelic Experience*, New York, Holt, Rinehart & Winston.

McCormick, Cornelia, Daniel N. Barry, Amirhossein Jafarian, Gareth R. Barnes and Eleanor A. Maguire, (2020) "vmPFC drives hippocampal processing during autobiographical memory recall regardless of remoteness," *Cerebral Cortex*, Nov., v. 30, n. 11, 5972–5987.

McKenna, Terence (1993) *True Hallucinations, Being an Account of the Author's Extraordinary Adventures in the Devil's Paradise*, New York, HarperOne.

McKenna, Terence (1992) *Food of the Gods*, New York, Bantam Books.

Miller, Lisa, Iris M. Balodis, Clayton H. McClintok, Jiansong Xu, Cheryl M. Lacadie, et al., (2019) "Neural correlates of personalized spiritual experiences," *Cerebral Cortex*, v. 29, n. 6, 2331–2338.

Niebuhr, H. Richard (1957) *The Social Sources of Denominationalism*, New York, Henry Holt & Co.

Ogden, Charles K. and I.A. Richards, (1923) *The Meaning of Meaning: A Study of the Influence of Language Upon Thought and of the Science of Symbolism*, London, Routledge.

Platz, W.E., F.F. Oberlaender and M.L. Seidel (1995) "The phenomenology of perceptual hallucinations in alcohol-induced delirium tremens," *Psychopathology*, v. 28, n. 5, 247–255.

Preller, Katrin H., Adeel Razi, Peter Zeidman, Philipp Stampfli, Karl J. Friston, et al., (2019) "Effective connectivity changes in LSD-induced altered states of consciousness in humans," *PNAS*, 12 February, v. 116, n. 7, 2743–2748.

Premack, David (2007) "Human and animal cognition: continuity and discontinuity," *PNAS*, 28 August, v. 104, n. 35, 13861–13867.

Pressman, Mark R. (2013) "Sleepwalking, amnesia, comorbid conditions and triggers: effects of recall and other methodological biases," *Sleep*, Nov. v. 38, n. 11, 1757–1758.

Rivers, W.H.R. (1920) *Instinct and the Unconscious*, Cambridge, Cambridge University Press.

Rogers TB, Kuiper NA, Kirker WS. (1977) "Self-reference and the encoding of personal information," *J Pers Soc Psychol.*: 35: 677–688.

Sacks, Oliver (2012) *Hallucinations*, New York, Vintage Books.

Sapir, Edward, (1921) Language: An Introduction to the Study of Speech, New York, Harcourt, Brace & World.

Schmack, Katharina, O.H. Torben and Adam Kepecs, (2022) "Computational Psychiatry across species to study the biology of hallucinations," *JAMA Psychiatry*, v. 79, n. 1, 75–76.

Schultes, Richard Evans (1972) "An overview of hallucinogens in the Western Hemisphere, in Flesh of the Gods, *The Ritual Use of Hallucinogens*, Peter T. Furst (ed.) New York, Praeger Publishers: 3–54.

Seth, Anil (2021) *Being You: A New Science of Consciousness,* Faber.

Shonle, R., (1925) "Peyote: The Giver of Visions", *Amer. Anthrop*, 27, 53–75.

Solso, Robert L. (1994) *Cognition and the Visual Arts*, Cambridge, MA, MIT Press.

Solon, O. (2016) "Under pressure, Silicon Valley workers turn to LSD microdosing," *Wired UK*, 24 August. Available at: http://www.wired.co.uk/article/lsd-microdosing-drugs-silicon-valley (accessed 9 July 2018).

Stendardi, Debora, Francesca Biscotto, Elena Bertossi and Elisa Ciaramelli, (2021) "Present and future self in memory: the role of vmPFC in the self-reference effect," *Social Cognitive and Affective Neuroscience,* Dec. v. 16, n. 12, 1205–1213.

Striedter, Georg F. (2005) *Principles of Brain Evolution*, Sunderland, Mass., Sinauer Associates.

Tamney, Joseph B. and Stephen D. Johnson, 1983, "The Moral Majority in Middletown," *Journal for the Scientific Study of Religion*, v. 22, n. 2, Jun, 145–157.

Tedlock, Barbara (1987) "Dreaming and dream research," in *Dreaming: Anthropological and Psychological Interpretations,* (ed.) Barbara Tedlock, Cambridge, Cambridge University Press, 1–30.

Todorov, Tzvetan (1984) *The Conquest of America*, New York, Harper and Row.

Trivers, Robert (1985) *Social Evolution*, Menlo Park, The Benjamin/Cummings Publishing Co.

Uexkull von, Jacob, (2010) *A Foray into the Worlds of Animals and Humans*, Minneapolis, University of Minnesota Press.

Vilarroya, Oscar (2017) "Neural representation. A survey-based analysis of the notion," *Front. Psychol.* 29 August, https://doi.org/10.3389/fpsyg.2017.01458

Von Uexkull, Jacob (2010) *A Foray into the Worlds of Animals and Humans*, University of Minnesota Press edition, originally published in 1934 as, *Streifzuge durch die Umwelten von Tieren und Menschen*, Verlag von Julius Springer.

Vygotsky, L. S., (1978*) Mind in society: The development of higher psychological processes.* Cambridge, MA: Harvard University Press.

Waldman, A. (2017) *A really good day: how microdosing made a mega difference in my mood, my marriage, and my life*, Knopf, New York.

Wetmore, Karen (2014) *Surviving Evil,* Richardson Texas, Manitou.

Whitsel, B.C. 2001 "Ideological mutation and millennial belief in the American Neo-Nazi movement," *Studies in Conflict and Terrorism,* v. 24, 2, 89–106.

Whorf, B.L., (1956a), The Hopi Language, (Chicago Microfilm Collection of Manuscripts on Middle American Cultural Anthropology, 48, University of Chicago Library, manuscript date 1935).

Whorf, Benjamin Lee, (1946), "The Hopi language, Toreva Dialect," in Linguistic Structures of Native America, ed. H. Hoijer, et al., (Viking Fund Publications in Anthropology, #6), New York, pp. 158–183.

Whorf, B. L. (1956b). *Language, thought and reality.* Cambridge: Technology Press of MIT.

Worsley, Peter (1957) *The Trumpet Shall Sound,* London, Macgibbon & Rae.

Wright, Anthony (2020) "Hippocampus," Chapter 5, in *Neuroanatomy Online,* University of Texas Health, McGovern Medical School, https://nba.uth.tmc.edu/neuroscience/m/s4/index.htm

Zeman, Adam (1997) "Persistent vegetative state," *The Lancet,* 13 September, v. 350, 793–799.

Prelude to the Study

Some Background and Context

I came to be involved in LSD research as an undergraduate student in Psychology at Humboldt State College in 1965. Work there focused on the effects of sensory deprivation experiments. Later in the Bay Area I continued studies that included student participation in research at local universities and Napa State Hospital and Mendocino State Hospital, where students were given the opportunity to observe clinical treatments and conditions. In the early 1970s I came into contact with people who were engaged in guiding LSD use and medical students and physicians who wanted to help people who had difficulties with drugs. Some of these people called themselves the Psychedelic Rangers. Some were medical students or physicians like Dr. David E. Smith (I am not saying he was one), who also founded the Haight-Ashbury Free Medical Clinic. These people could be called upon through an anonymous network to come to individual addresses and attempt to adjust problems that took place during LSD "trips," often the result of the impurity of the street drug market or simply preparations that were not LSD. Their methods were imitated by many, often just speaking softly or showing images of the oceans or forests. Some claimed that they used ancient Egyptian or shamanic means as Stevens (1988) relates, but I think their methods were idiosyncratic, developed from trial and error, much like Stevens (1988) describes for Aldous Huxley's sidekick, Al Hubbard, the uranium mine owner. Leary (1968) called for the education of psychedelic guides, but his description of their role was much too intrusive and very much unlike what the Psychedelic Rangers did.

The question of purity bedevils most research of microdosing as the drug is often self-administered and obtained from illegal sources with no information of manufacturer (Kuypers et al. 2019). Before the drug was made illegal I had the opportunity to work in a scientific study of LSD use where clinical conditions controlled for a variety of environmental factors. The researchers were both PhDs in a variety of scientific disciplines and physicians and psychologists with clinical experience.

As an anthropologist I caution people against taking psychedelic drugs outside of the cultural context in which they originated and functioned. This obviously is different for new drugs like LSD, but there is a knowledge base for these drugs as they are developed. Nevertheless, the cultural milieus of traditional society drug use have developed methods for dealing with the drugs' effect and how to interpret the biological manifestations. I once had a Native American shaman discuss with me how atropine poison (see Bishop and Tallon 1999) or a modern chemical preparation called STP (2,5-Dimethoxy-4-methylamphetamine; see Snyder et al. 1968) could produce a magnificent visual landscape inhabited by entities that were both benign and dangerous (see Myerhoff 1974). His descriptions were very similar to those I heard from young people using STP, while his people had traditionally used Jimson Weed for the same effects (Guharoy et al. 1991). In both cases, atropine alkaloids were involved in the biological effects that produced the neurological underpinnings of the psychological experiences. He warned me that young Americans were in danger from the spirits they were seeing in these experiences (and neither recognizing the entities nor understanding them) and did not know how to communicate with them. In taking the drug myself I saw tall, multi-colored, electric-like shapes traversing the landscape. He had told me not to talk to them or look at them if they looked at me. If I did, the "trouble" would start. Yet I cannot be sure he said that, or if the images I experienced were not the result of his impressions or those of people I had spoken to, yet I do not recall what "troubles" meant or if it differed from being a trickster.

Experiences: Personal, Laboratory, and Clinical

Karsten (1935) reports on just this kind of difference in experience, but in this case the drug is yage (ayahuasca). The Native users and the Europeans had very similar optical experiences—rivers, beautiful birds, plants, and light, but the Europeans did not experience the spiritual beings or their presence. Here we come to the problem of suggestion, as many Europeans since the 1960s have had "spiritual" encounters, but the nature of these is curious, not in the similarities but in the context in which these take place. See the chart on ayahuasca (Fig. 2.2).

One aspect of atropine drugs is its ability to deliver the feeling of stasis or an arrest of what Sacks (2012) calls the "river of consciousness." People on the drug can have a cinematic view of life for long periods as if nothing is moving, or the intoxication effect may last seconds and they feel as if time had stopped, as when I was driving across the Bay Bridge from San Francisco with three people in my car who were experiencing this sensation and felt in danger, as they perceived the car had stopped when it was traveling at 55 mph.

The same is true for other drugs that have a cultural context, not that I do not think it possible for people to construct a new individual interpretation of their experiences, but it might help if one could first consider how any drug has affected other people and cultures. Here we have a similar problem with the South Amerindian drug ayahuasca that anthropologist Wade Davis, among others, has made famous. Unfortunately, as with ayahuasca, some people began to promote certain interpretations of the drug's effect. While the researchers I knew concerning LSD and what was reported in most of the literature found similar "global" experiences of a pleasant nature, leading to a variety of introspective opportunities, Timothy Leary and Ram Dass (Richard Alpert), while both were psychological researchers at Harvard University, began to create a format for people to understand what was happening to them. I address their methods in more detail later in this book.

Mass "trips" undertaken to the *Tibetan Book of the Dead* (Leary et al. 2000) and some elements of Eastern religions were packaged to "help" people. Thereafter, we began to find people having what I referred to at the time as "standard" interpretations based on these suggested interpretations. It is confounding that Leary, who was one of the people to first realize the power that the setting of the experience could have, should attempt to design a modal type for everyone, that is, the mass of people. Where the experience seemed clearly to be an orbit around the individual's background and personality, Leary attempted to create a uniform matrix to limit that variety. It seems to me likely from reading over Grof's "psycholytic LSD therapy" method that he also created preconceptions for his subjects based on his theories, especially the Basic Perinatal Matrices (BPM) stages. In discussions with his subjects and patients he appears to have given them expectations of what they would experience. This was the case with Jerry Richardson (1970), who was hoping LSD would answer his career decision. In this way, many researchers, I think, differed from the more scientific approach of the Mogar Lab (and others, as in the Blum 1964a, b; Blum et al. 1964a, b report), where no interpretative expectations were given, only general ideas of physiological responses, like visual, somatic, and so on. Increased suggestibility as the result of LSD has been reported in the past and recent studies have confirmed it as one reason for the therapeutic effects of the drug (Carhart-Harris et al. 2015).

It seemed to me unethical and egotistic for two professionals to "go public" with their own brand of experience for everyone else. So instead of naive individuals having the chance to explore their own consciousness, they were encumbered with the psychological baggage of these two men. In the scientific setting, a neutral environment allowed unique individual exploration, which I found most remarkable as a young scientist of human perception. And based on my earlier experience and training in sensory deprivation experiments, it provided an exciting avenue to further work, all of which was made impossible by the government action making LSD illegal. But as I had been involved in the Psychology Department's sensory deprivation experiments at Humboldt State

College a few years before, I was quite interested in the general response of people. I cannot recall if all the subjects were students or all male; I think there might have been a few females. I will discuss the problem of how female participation in research has been ignored in general, as noted by Darlington (2002), and gender as well in later sections of this book.

The response of the staff of the Mogar group and in the hospital research sections to LSD research being made illegal, ran from disbelief (this will be temporary) to anger (why are politicians telling us what to do?). I found much the same confusion when the AIDS epidemic broke in the 1980s and I heard and read how little power physicians and scientists had in America. This was amplified during the Covid-19 pandemic when the rational scientific findings and considered opinions of scientists and doctors like Anthony Fauci were treated with contempt by President Trump and his supporters. This reservoir of irrationality was apparent in my study of disease in cross-cultural context over the past 3000 years, but was writ large during the Covid pandemic (Caldararo 2020).

Stanislav Grof's findings that people could reach the same level of hallucinations and "spiritual experience" on LSD as without it but using sensory deprivation and other methods to stimulate heightened states of "awareness," as some put it, including Carl Sagan (1974), can be found in the ethnographic literature and clinical research. La Barre (1975) derives the term from the Latin, *alucinari* = "to wander in mind," a reflection on animistic concepts of being. But Grof also emphasizes the complexity of experience variation and the significance of setting and background. I should note here the contradiction in relation of drugs and context—as with sensory deprivation and LSD, it was argued early on by Pollard et al. (1965) that the sensory deprivation context seemed to nullify the LSD and other psychedelic effects, though I do not agree with their conclusions. However, though a small sample, their results do bring to mind a possible connection to origins of imagery. If the imagery is missing or blocked, is it possible that it is derived or stimulated by the human-built and natural environment?

The human child develops language in a social context; its relations to the world are formed largely by visual associations, so if cut off from these by the sensory deprivation context or set, language remains but without reference. The fact that we store visual memories in the hippocampus would indicate that we should be able to retrieve them during the drug experience. But pictures of highly familiar or novel pictures elicited activation in the parahippocampus area. A diagram from Luria (1973) shows how interrelated parts of the brain are, with pathways to different parts of the brain passing through various parts. A posterior view of the brain demonstrates some of these areas from a drawing of a section of the human brain from an illustration in Crick (1994). Later we will discuss some experiments that show that LSD seems to reduce activity in the parahippocampus and the hippocampus (Carhart-Harris et al. 2016); could this be a blocking mechanism? But serotonin receptor mRNA levels are unchanged by acute LSD accumulation in the rat brain (Nichols and Sanders-Bush 2001). Preller et al. (2019) found a disintegration of connectivity between the cortico-striato-thalamo-cortical (CSTC) regions of the brain, as if the specific routing was opened up. Luppi et al. (2019) report similar findings with general reduction of connectivity and separation of brain areas using fMRI on subjects and patients. Others, like Sacks, might call this a disorganization and a potential for reorganization.

Sacks (2012) considered the action of all psychedelic drugs was in "boosting serotonin in the brain"; perhaps we can say producing a more general conductivity. Yet it seems more is taking place, especially between effects produced by different "psychedelic" drugs. And, importantly, a blocking of memory would be contradicted by nearly all the clinical research and reported evidence of subjects on LSD. A recent report by Dell'Erba et al. (2018), on the LSD experiences of a blind musician who was active in the 1970s and used LSD, informs us that he did not experience visual images but was flooded with auditory and sensations of various types. These were referred to as auditory and tactile hallucinations (Kiyokawa and Haning 2021). He also experienced the combination (synesthesia) of auditory stimuli and tactile as well as time distortion. This distinguishes his condition from that of the Charles Bonnet Syndrome (CBS), where people whose vision has started to deteriorate see things that are not present. In these cases, the individual experiences visual perception as simple patterns or detailed images of events, people, and/or places (Sacks 2012). These are often very elaborate, as in the case of the patient Rosalie, who saw visions of masses of people, often distinguished by dress and attitude, with walls changed to gates. In one case the episodes lasted for at least 36 hours.

We cannot be dogmatic, as some people experience different sensations, and the nature of what is a hallucination is unclear, as is the generality of the individual to report or be aware of one. Although there do still seem to be unexplained cases where people do not have hallucinations on psilocybin or peyote, but La Barre's (1975) report of these is unclear if there is a cultural or pathological context. It is possible that the pathological conditions and drugs cause disruptions in the chemical functioning of the hippocampus and not only are memories from a variety of times, places, and events in a person's life (including movies, books, stories) mixed and their relations in a number of ways distorted, but also size, number, and frame of reference all blend into an illogical narrative. Is there some hidden message, maybe ... but I am not inclined to think so.

Sacks' (2012) description of his opium "trip" is a good example. It is briefly noted in our chart on Psychedelic Experiences. He first sees his coffee turn green, then blue; thinking to pay he looks at the cashiers, where a man has an elephant seal-like head, then he runs out onto the street to catch a bus, but the passengers all have egg heads with insect eyes. One missing element here is the role of sex and gender differences, especially how hormones can affect hallucinations. While very little research has been done in this area, one interesting report was of an 84-year-old woman with age-related macular degeneration and CBS who was treated with estrogen for a condition. The estrogen apparently resulted in non-threatening hallucinations, which stopped when the estrogen treatment was ended (Fernandes et al. 2000). There are other examples and Darlington (2002) reviews the differences in perception caused by hormones in men and women. We will discuss other aspects of sex and gender differences, especially how they relate to women's experiences with psychedelics later.

McAlpine et al. (2021) treated a patient with hallucinations of speaking to god and deceased relatives after infection with Covid-19. The use of intravenous immunoglobulin restored normal function, indicating again the complex conditions that produce both visual and auditory hallucinations. People who have auditory hallucinations often feel they are exterior and authoritative. Aggernaes et al. (1976) attempted to define a series of reality characteristics to differentiate such hallucinations from other experiences. When a cohort of people who had experienced LSD auditory hallucinations were tested on these values, it was found that they could discern the voices outside themselves and note the characteristics changed, while psychotic patients were unable to interpret their experiences as independent of themselves. Auditory hallucinations in patients who had a history of these reported more under conditions of restricted sound (wearing mufflers) or exposed to white noise; a history of abuse, trauma, or stress is also associated with auditory hallucinations in patients (Bentall and Varese 2013; see also Hunter et al. 2002). This parallels reports of normal volunteers when in sensory deprivation experiments (Bexton et al. 1954). Sacks (2012) reports on one study of elderly individuals, where nearly 15% had complex hallucinations, and 80% experienced simple ones.

The main problem here is, what is a hallucination and how is a complex one compared to a simple one? Sacks argues that in Charles Bonnet Syndrome (CBS), the hallucinations (of people, animals, etc.) do not usually interact or acknowledge the hallucinatory, that is, talk to them, for example. An aspect of complexity is plausibility or incredulity. Very similar hallucinations are produced in some people by opioids (Benitez Del Rosario et al. 2001). Some hallucinations in CBS seem plausible to the hallucinatory, like a person walking into a room, others are simply incredible, as in an attack of oxen or thousands of men marching outside a window followed by thousands of men on horseback. Some are fragments of faces or things; some are parts of books, paintings, or music, but non-sensical (Sacks 2012). Often these are enhanced by movement, as in a car, which Sacks' patient Zelda was driving when she saw the road split into six or seven identical roads, with a car traveling on all of them.

Often people who experienced musical hallucinations had a musical background, but not all, and such images could appear at random, as when one was reading a book, the musical score would appear in the field of vision, blocking the printed page of the book. It is ironic that people who have musical hallucinations only rarely have visual ones, and musical hallucinations are almost always limited to the elderly, and of music heard in their early years; these vary and change and are often the result of auditory deprivation (Sacks 2012). It is often exact in detail, like visual hallucinations, but also may be repetitious, a few bars of a song over and over. They can be brought on in normal individuals by prolonged silence.

While visual hallucinations can be changed and modified from experience, reduced or exaggerated, musical pieces appear as wholes, with the original unity as heard. In these conditions some people experience the same deprivations and related hallucinations, which might seem as if they confront Aggernaes' (1972) "publicness" criterion (e.g., others experience it). But the situation might be due to the powerful suggestion or status of one person. McKenna (1992) argues that ibogaine has a "deepening" and "enhancing" effect on sex and among the Fang can be suggested to counter trends in divorce. But this is dependent on context and situation. Another "quality" Aggernaes proposed is that of "involuntariness," but not all hallucinations are so controlling. This is especially true in psychedelics (notably LSD), where people can divert and modify their trip, but also in some epileptics, where the familiar signs of an oncoming seizure can allow the person to prepare, and in CBS some modification also is reported (Sacks 2012). One could say that in most cases of sleep most people report a helplessness to interact in the dream and thus experience a type of involuntariness, though some people also experience a semi-sleep dream state as they fall asleep or continuation of the dream state into wakefulness as a type of hallucination (called hypnopompic hallucination) (Sacks 2012). A similar condition can result from the loss of vision in one half of the visual field, but images can persist for hours, days, or weeks. Such visual preservation can also result from cerebral tumors or epilepsy.

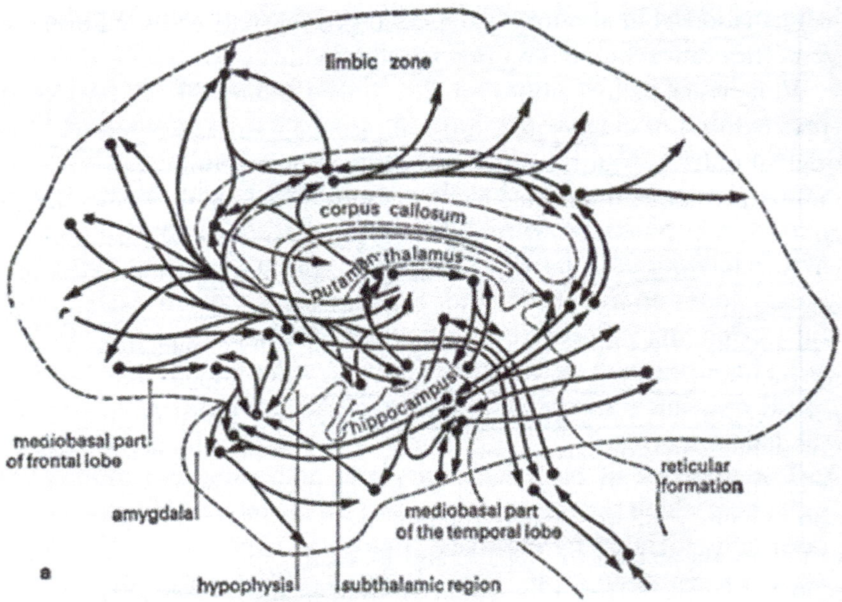

Fig. Pr.1 Pathways in the brain from the body and CNS to the primitive brain and back, from Luria (1973)

Another interesting aspect of the CBS visual hallucinations is their persistence as separate images in the visual field. On viewing a TV one of Sacks' patients noticed the images of people transferred from the screen to the side of the cabinet, yet the size of the people remained that of those on the TV screen. This would seem like an "afterimage" many people experience on closing their eyes, but here the image remains with eyes open superimposed on a second visual field. She took the drug Quetiapine and these hallucinations ended for about two years. Quetiapine is often prescribed for schizophrenia, bipolar disorder, and depression. It is a dopamine D1, D2, D3, D4, and D5 receptor antagonist, serotonin receptor partial agonist, and histamine receptor antagonist (Richelson and Souder 2000). A West African shrub's root (*Tabernanthe iboga*) has been processed by local peoples to produce a hallucinogen, ibogaine, that created vivid images. For example, it is reported to be used in initiation ceremonies by boys of the Bwiti religion (Richer 2009) and the Fang

(Furst 1972). In recent years it has been used to treat addiction to opioids and some other drugs (Lev-Ran 2020).

The process of seeing images and carrying them in time as memories is characteristic of normal individuals. Huxley (1954) argues that landscapes are "a regular feature of the visionary experience." He goes on to claim that painted landscapes are a late feature of human art and limited mainly to the West. He is wrong in this, given that we have many landscapes painted on cave walls, and that these images are evidence of the early humans' ability to carry a memory in time from outside the cave to an inner area (sometimes miles underground across underground galleries and through narrow passages and submerged rivers; Wendt 1955). This capacity and its expression appear in the earliest cave art at about 40,000 BP. Duygu Camurcuoglu (2015) has reproduced many of these images and especially the landscapes painted on the interior walls of Catalhoyuk, one of the earliest and largest Neolithic, sedentary villages. We also have examples of prehistoric art in the New World with evidence of psychedelic substances used in the caves. One was *Datura wrightii* at Pinwheel Cave in California (Robinson et al. 2020). Datura was apparently used by the Chumash to acquire a dream guide and was originally the body of an old woman, one of the original creator beings (Baker 2009). And we might have a model for a theory of the unique hallucination of a person (whether drug induced or pathologically derived) which is retold in the group and given meaning (as Luhrmann [2012] describes in our contemporary situation), becoming a social context for the foundation of a religious cosmological element of the culture. Other examples have been documented from other sites in both the New and Old World; in the Tassili Caves of Algeria we find psilocybin mushrooms used at about 7000–9000 BP (Guzman 2012; Winkelman 2019). The use of opium has been discovered in archeological context in Neolithic lake dwellings in Switzerland and Italy (Guerra-Doce 2015).

But some authorities, most notably Eliade (1964), have argued that most use of psychedelics by Native peoples is recent and that Native cultures had developed non-drug methods to reach the spirit world, like exercise, pain, hyperventilation, meditation, and so on. I, however, agree with Furst (1972), Schultes (1972), and a number of others who consider the similarities of both methods of achieving states of spiritual transcendence to be related to the search of humans and the creative discovery of the means of achieving the ends, whether by drugs or by other mechanisms.

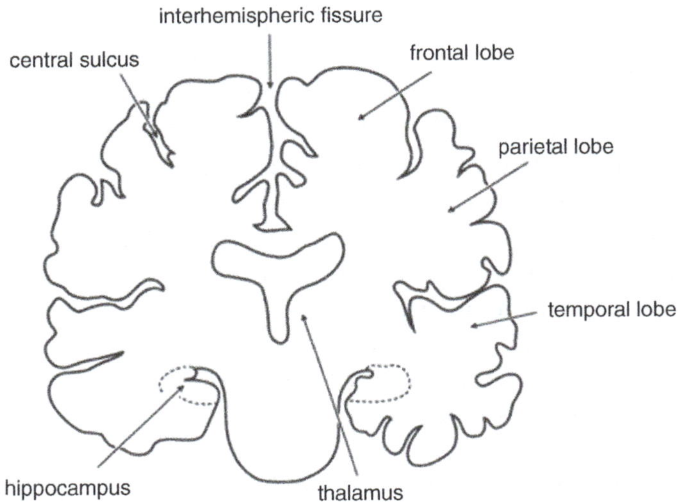

Fig. Pr.2 Posterior section of the brain. From Crick, 1994, Modified by the author

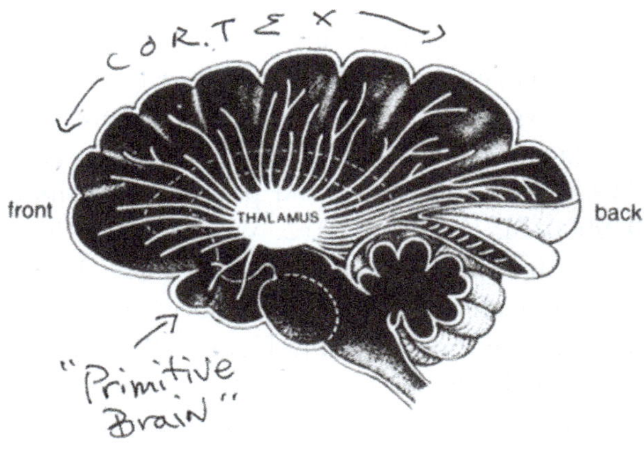

Fig. Pr.3 Sagittal view of the brain showing the central role of the thalamus. From Crick, 1994, Modified by the author

The appearance of these hallucinations (as in CBS) is not limited to immediate causes of loss of sight (damage to the eyes) but often to pathology in the visual system, including the cortical areas of visual perception, the occipital lobe. An infarction (injury or death of tissue due to inadequate blood supply) here can result in homonymous hemianopia (visual field defect involving either two right or two left halves of the visual fields of both eyes), releasing hallucinations in the regions of field defect (Flint et al. 2005). But lesions in the frontal lobe of the brain can also cause hallucinations in the temporal or occipital lobes which can be auditory, olfactory, visual, or déjà vu, or cause automatic movements (Schneider et al. 1961). Even where there is no disease in the visual apparatus there is evidence that, in many cases of visual hallucination, it is associated with reduced cholinergic function, but this does not tell us why the images appear as they do or explain their nature (O'Brien et al. 2020). However, many hallucinations are consequences of neurodegeneration (O'Brien et al. 2020). Thus, we have essentially similar, if not identical experiences, reported as images, in individuals who appear normal and healthy as well as in individuals who have illness, physical injuries due to trauma or disease, or neurodegeneration of whatever cause. The phenomenological question then is, can this conflation of outcomes be due to the opening of a door to different realities, or is it like the skewed reception of a radio, a temporary misplaced dial or physical damage to the set? Since similar images and experiences can occur in dreams and with certain drugs, we have to try and collate the origins of them all.

Barbara Tedlock (1987) has done an effective job discussing the varieties of cultural descriptions of realities and dreams. I will touch on this subject now and then in a number of contexts. But we have to keep in mind that cultures mediate personal experiences, and as we will find as we go on, interpretation is central. As in epilepsy, a subset of patients experience ecstatic seizures and wish to repeat them—they interpret many of which as spiritual (Sacks 2012). We know that some people dream of illness, and in a few documented cases, these dreams relate to actual pathological conditions they suffer from, as in sleep apnea (Fisher et al. 2011). We also have evidence that there is a comprehensive communication between the immune system and the nervous system, so some kind of neurological impressions might be expected (Dantzer

2018). I have been somewhat skeptical of theories of dream interpretation, not just because they generally contradict each other, but due to their general inconsistencies and often (as seems to me) illogical conclusions. My own dreams appear to me often so strange and devoid of reality that I am generally agnostic about their derivation and production. When compared to the vast variation and cultural influences discussed here later, it does seem that this decision is only a consequence of a lack of knowledge of the creative abilities of the mind to modify and reassemble inputs from the environment and internal physiological effects and sources.

The nature of the CBS hallucinations can change from happy to somber; they can be mixed in scale, as geometric shapes and little people or children. This is especially true where people have some vision left, and color intensity can also be a factor as well as size and misalignment and inversion of images (Sacks 2012). CBS hallucinations can move with the head or eye and are more detailed than normal images (Santhouse et al. 2000). Elaborations are common where crowds of people all dressed in similar garb appear, usually exotic in character, and incongruities are also common where a person might have a flower, for example, not in their lapel, but growing out of their face. According to Sacks (2012) the commonest hallucinations are patterns, an image filled with geometric shapes. This is often seen in LSD sessions and other psychedelic experiences. Interesting that hallucinations of "little people" as aids to shamans among the Witoto, Boras, and other tribes of Columbia have parallels (like the "paradoxical passage" Eliade describes from many shaman initiations in many people), where the shaman ingests the resin of *Virola theidora*. The resin of a variety of species of this plant is used by many tribes for access to auditory and visual hallucinations (Schultes 1972). Santhouse et al. (2000) have categorized the different kinds of hallucinations they had data on and which they have been able to associate with the anatomy of the brain. I have reproduced their chart here and associated it with my classification of types of psychedelic experiences. The number of patients that were excluded from the study was substantial and may undermine the usefulness of their categories (Santhouse et al. 2000). Using fMRI Santhouse et al. were also able to note three pathway streams of hallucinogenic stimulation: (1) one ventral, leading to the ventral temporal lobe; (2) one dorsal, leading to the parietal lobe; and (3) one projection along the superior temporal sulcus. See Illustration 6 for more detail (Fig. 1.6).

A similarity shared by CBS and LSD and mescaline users is the recognition, in most cases, of the experience as a temporary condition. Most people maintain this awareness of the moment. We might contrast this awareness with its lack, as Sacks (2012) does, in patients with dementia, Alzheimer's, or Lewy body disease (LBD). Appearance of hallucinations in Alzheimer's patients is associated with an increased risk of cognitive decline (Scarmeas et al. 2005). One potential note for interpretation could be found in the apparent frequency of multiple images of small people, things, and their seeming lack in non-Western reports and pre-industrial experiences. This is relative to a certain extent, as "small" in many reports is tiny, while among some indigenous people like the Witoto, it is interpreted by Mckenna (1993) to mean "little men." That could include in other contexts, dwarves, elves, leprechauns, imps, fairies, and so on. A study of leprechauns and the elderly found seeing leprechauns were associated with Lewy body disease (Foy 2011), so there may be a link between disruption of certain drugs and pathologies. Sacks (2012) notes that in some epileptic patients, multiple images and changes in size or shape of parts of the body occur just before seizures. Therefore, we can see that many of the features of psychedelics are produced in pathological conditions, but are not seen in all cross-cultural settings. The explanation for this might be that our information for non-Western hallucinations and pathologies is not comprehensive.

I have witnessed these (usually) terrifying delusions and hallucinations in patients both when working at Sonoma State Hospital and in the 1990s, when my mother was a patient at a private institution. About 80% of LBD patients experience hallucinations, though not all are frightening according to the National Institute on Aging (https://www.nia.nih.gov/health/what-lewy-body-dementia-causes-symptoms-and-treatments). Individuals with dementia often "see" animals, children, or changes in their environment that enlarge or contract real conditions (Sacks 2012). Such people are often surprised when real visitors do not see the same images. While some hallucinate companions who may watch a program on TV with them, some also see specific characters in odd dress that can be tiny and far off, or can become gigantic and hover. In almost all cases the apparitions do not interact with the individual affected, but seem to ignore them. To the affected individual, the duration and nature of the hallucination can be disturbing, as when food appears drastically changed on one's plate or, as in Zelda's case, ghostly people jump on the hood of her car as she drives and then disappear. The appearance and context can inform the affected individual that it is a hallucination, but the immediate effect is startling and can be dangerous. To some people the images can be entertaining and diverting, birds with shoes that turn into medieval men and women and in some cases even actors and theater entirely by hallucinogenation (Sacks 2012).

It is curious that when images seen in dreams of non-Western people are studied, as in Lincoln's (1935) works or Levy-Bruhl's (1966), we do not often see the same types of images, as in little people with hats, but of a different kind, typical of their environment, people, animals desired in the hunt, and so on. Also there is a wide variation in the origination of the dream images (who produces them) and their meaning. For example, in some cases the variation of images is theoretically limited among the Yolngu of Arnhem Land, Australia (Keen 2003), as the religious symbols arose in Wangarr ancestors in a remote time. Since among many Australian people the "Dream Time" or Alcheringa literally means "belonging to the dream," it reflects what Spencer and Gillen (1927) meant by a distinction of the creative ancestral period when the creator beings manifested the world and the production of everyday dreams—or as Stanner (1953) put it, the "everwhen," a narrative of things once happened and a charter of things still happening. The myths and tales become a kind of philosophical framework of reality, posing a "key" (Stanner's term) to how things happen. So the process of dreaming becomes a living link between today and creation, thus as Nancy Munn (1973) puts it, is the efficacy of the dream. But we cannot imagine that dreams remain static, nor does dream interpretation or elements of Native theory. We also have some information that hallucinations and delusions change over time (Mitchell and Vierkant 1989), but what this means, especially in an adaptive perspective and evolutionary one, is obscure. Thus, as I explain later in this book, the images in dream, as in visions, are expected and interpreted from what is known. Native Theory also defines the hallucinations and visions of psychedelics, as in the privilege of communication with spirits, is a right of the shaman and the power of healing is his or hers to exercise. When this privilege or access to the psychedelic agent is compromised and other group members have the experiences, as occurred with the Mescalero Apache (Harner 1972) group ceremonies where the drug used caused a breakdown, "shamanic rivalries and witchcraft flourished." Though it must be kept in mind that peyote was introduced from outside the culture, and came to be regarded as an evil power by traditional individuals, its hallucinations cloud and confuse the shaman's access to the spirits.

The specific nature of the role of the individual in the creation of and interpretation of dreams varies significantly between cultures and groups and may well reflect recent outside influences, including trade, colonial, and religious (Hollan 2003). Tedlock (1991) argues that dreams are social performances that have functional value within groups and between individuals. The new focus of anthropologists is to concentrate on the communicative context of dream retelling and interpretation, especially where the interpretation takes on a mechanism of social involvement in discovering meaning and use.

Image Origins, Distortions, and Derivations

Where do these images come from, memory? And what parts of the brain are involved? Areas of the brain activated in many hallucinations were mainly in the visual cortex and were associated with areas of normal processing, as in hallucinations of dismembered faces showed activation in areas normally stimulated in the superior temporal sulcus. Interestingly, Small et al. (2001) found that subjects viewing faces and names independently activated separate areas within the hippocampus. Viewing names and faces in combination activated a distinct area bridging between the separate face and name areas. But there was a clear distinction between visual imagination and hallucinations, indicating that hallucinations were more like perceptions (Santhouse et al. 2000). Thus, Sacks (2012) thought that there was a depository of generic images in memory that could be sorted and modified into complex hallucinations, yet these seemed to be based on memory, as he had no evidence that images without experience could be produced. His main example was musical notation—people who had never seen it did not produce hallucinations with such images.

Text images are similar in this regard, as text when it appears in hallucinations is unreadable or nonsense and this is also true of musical scores—unreadable (including blurry) and not actual music. People suffering from delirium also have musical hallucinations and "see" musical scores (Sacks 2012). One might theorize that in processing memories, the brain creates these generic types during a means of sorting. The CBS hallucinations, unlike most dreams, resist any interpretation of meaning (Sacks 2012). Studies of non-European populations found a lower rate of frequency of Charles Bonnet Syndrome, but with similar types of hallucinations. One study included 938 Chinese, 70 Indian, 52 Malay, and 17 from other Asia locations (Tan et al. 2004). An Indian clinic screening for CBS found that in 218 patients with visual impairment, about 6. 7 to 8.1 % reported experiences typical of CBS hallucinations, some with combined auditory input that was related or coordinated (Satgunam et al. 2019). Other auditory hallucinations result from specific pathology, as in a stroke to the ventroanterior thalamus reported in a 19-year-old female (Mittal and Khan 2010). This case was associated with starvation, but starvation alone, like lack of sleep, can bring on hallucinations. Considerable research, especially in recent years with a variety of new instruments (e.g., fMRI), has been directed to understanding the mechanisms of the imagination ("mind's eye" or "eye's mind") and its evolutionary history (MacKisack et al. 2016). Some studies have suggested that the inner voice or covert speech functions "all the time" in an individual's consciousness (Baars 2003).

Areas of the brain activated during mental imaging are nearly the same as those involved in visual perception, except they are more anterior, frontal, and parietal, areas involved in executive functions and attention, though visual perception and imaging differ in the excitation of neurons of the occipital lobes. This is a most interesting subject that is central to our understanding of what takes place when people use psychedelics. What triggers hallucinations is also essential to understand, and we will investigate some of the theories as we go along, but early ideas like Freud's of redirected internal drives or release theory seem to be less useful than they seemed 50 years ago, as it is argued that there is little evidence the imagery of hallucinations is linked to experience (ffytche 2013). In fact, some forms appear to be linked to specific areas, as in CBS, where patterns are notable and related to the loss of neural input to the visual cortex, whereas in ascending brain stem neurotransmitter dysfunction, patterns are lacking but images of figures and animals are typical (ffytche 2013).

Yet Hyde (1960) found that context and attitudes subjects encountered during drug use were substantial determinants of how their experience was formed, positively or negatively. This finding, referred to by many researchers as "the set and setting" of the administration of drugs (often credited to Leary et al. 1964), was reviewed by Hartogsohn (2017) validating the concept. The set and setting of the physician or researchers can have substantial effects on how the subject experiences a drug, which introduces the placebo effect. Yet there is always an element of intersubjectivity, as Taussig argues, between healer and patient. To Lévi-Strauss (1963) this could be explained as a consequence of the structural nature of culture and learning that promotes expectations:

First, the sorcerer's belief in the effectiveness of his techniques; second, the patient's or victim's belief in the sorcerer's power; and, finally, the faith and expectations of the group, which constantly acts as a sort of gravitational field within which the relationship between sorcerer and bewitched is located and defined. (1963, 168)

Levi-Strauss (1966) regards the perceptions of dreams to involve complex features of social life, in contradiction to views of Freud.

Also sensory deprivation, especially visual, could provide some blocking of initiation of visual cues that recall memories of imagery. Related to this are reports of people gaining some form of color perception during and after use of psychedelics. The mechanism here seems to be a form of synesthesia, where form or color essence is produced by tactile or auditory sensation (Anthony et al. 2020). In other cases, some interaction of the visual center and color receptors may be responsible, as some individuals with red-dichromacy/protanopia, a partial color-blindness, report experiencing vivid hues of a variety of normal color perception. Likewise, the variety of color and images reported in hallucinations of people subject to sensory deprivation appears parallel to some produced by psychedelics, and using fMRI machines it has been shown that there was an increase in excitability of the visual cortex when subjects were deprived visual stimulation. One subject during 22 days of fMRI study was found to show activation of the entire visual system in the brain, including the occipital cortex and the inferotemporal cortex, during hallucinations. However, when she was asked to recall the images of the hallucinations, only the prefrontal cortex was stimulated. This was interpreted by Sacks (2012) to indicate that the hallucinations originated from the deprivation of simulation of normal sensory input.

It is of interest that most people dream in black and white most of the time, some never have dreams in color, and only a third of dreams are reported in color and usually that in drab, almost faded tones (Hall and Van de Castle 1966). Afterimages can be negative or positive in form, vague and blurry, but eidetic imagery (also known as photographic memory) consists of vivid afterimages seen in the same colors as the original stimulus (ffytche 2013) while hallucinations often are hyperintense. The condition of afterimages is explained by the failure of receptor cells to adapt to illumination changes regarding the chemical opsin that flows out of the cell during deactivation (Ritschel 2016). PTSD images appear in the mind's eye as vivid and often referred to as all-enveloping perceptions (ffytche 2013).

The collection of data on subjects' response to psychedelics by Pollard et al. (1965) was of special interest to me as they tape-recorded sessions and then later played the tapes to students to clarify reactions. Of special interest to me was that they had been doing experiments using sensory deprivation prior to their work in psychedelics, using sensory deprivation as a stress test. In their use of psychedelics they introduced a uniform series of sounds or other stimuli to each student subject and recorded the sessions. The experimenters were also interested in the outcome of psychedelics especially, as there had been reports in the media that people had "bad trips" from using the drugs or, after the use, sometimes weeks or months, had shown pathological symptoms. In their work, they considered these events not induced by the drugs but that the drugs had elicited hidden or covert illness. This is consonant with the work they were doing with stress tests.

Some experimenters (Cohen 1960) reported using antipsychotic drugs like Thorazine (chlorpromazine) when subjects had significant difficulties. This type of drug had proved effective in limiting subject's problems and aborting the experience (Killam 1956; Murphree 1962). I had never seen them used, however, in either the Mogar Lab or private settings, but that is not to say they were not used. Leary argued (Stevens 1988) that some cases of difficulty by subjects were induced by the experimental methods used by experimenters, as in the flashing lights on Harry Asher. The question of "bad trips" is a subjective one, yet as later came to be recognized, the attitude of the setting was a strong influence. One of Leary's early associates in the Harvard Psilocybin Project, Michael Kahn, is quoted as saying that no one had bad trips, "We didn't know what a bad trip was in hundreds of psilocybin trips, I never saw one." (Stevens 1988, 130). Of one experiment recorded from that project, 175 people, mostly male and young (average age 29.5 years), over 50% reported positive results that improved their lives and 90% wanted to do it again (Stevens 1988). Then again, it appears some people like the Merry Pranksters felt "freaking out" was a good thing, but the definition of that is also vague (Stevens 1988). Of the initial reports of people requiring hospitalization after LSD use in 1965 and 1966, especially reported by Dr. William Frosch of Bellevue Hospital, most had previous histories of psychiatric problems (Stevens 1988). These news reports eventually proved almost entirely false or distorted. Also, the formula and purity of the supposed drug were unknown. Restudies like that by de Rios and Janiger (2003) 40 years later found that the idea spread by Leary and Kesey and friends that LSD would produce life-altering radical transformations was not born out. In some controlled studies and with later restudies, as in that by Pahnke (1963) with psilocybin, a more consistent idea of life change and positive effects of a long-term nature are reported. This work by Pshnke will be discussed again later. One important point made by Harner (1972) is that the purpose of psychedelics for indigenous people and their shaman is to achieve certain goals, and that the use of the drugs is framed in training. Thus the drug experience may be "unpleasant" but necessary in order to achieve goals, as is noted among the Cashinahua (Kensinger 1972). The struggles of the shaman often seem difficult if not terrifying. Dealing with the spirit world may be trying and dangerous. Thus the definition of "bad trip" has to be drawn within limits that are contextual and informed culturally. Of course, LSD had no ritual knowledge or scientifically defined maps for its use when it was discovered. By the time it was made illegal to study it and fashion such maps, a body of data had been collected. Since then more information along these lines has accrued, and perhaps some time in a more dispassionate future these filaments of directions for its use may come together.

It is remarkable how friendly and fun the events were like the acid tests or the dances at the Fillmore Auditorium and other venues. For a mass of strangers to participate in the effects of LSD or other drugs in a public and multi-sensory event like these seems incredible to me now. It seems to indicate that humans have an ability to come together in expectation of communal benefit and enlightenment and are willing to enter states of liminality (uncertain status and transformation) across social, familial, and religious identity and inculcation. While in certain situations we find similar trans-tribal unions of varying sort in sodalities, they are usually well defined in purpose and ritual. In the case of these psychedelic gatherings we find an approach to Victor Turner's (1969) idea of communitas, where individuals move outside their normal roles and engage in a milieu of equality. However, these are usually found in special circumstances, and while in certain cases they were spontaneous, the presence of strangers (in the majority) is quite interesting and unusual in the contemporary scene. The light shows, loud music, and general human contact of all kinds were unbelievable and strange as well as inviting. I had tried to produce a theory about it linking such events to pre-Christian, Neolithic societies, but like many others, such comparisons lacked some essentially biological foundation. The mesmerizing effect of the music and light could be seen as a possible unifier, as it seems Kesey and some of his group believed possible (Stevens 1988), which is strange given that the CIA thought it could cause disorientation and madness. One could argue that the anticipation and expectation that people had of what was to occur and the effects of LSD and other psychedelics resulted in the reduction of boundaries and the creation of a unifying sense among those attending. This is one explanation that Hudson (2000) provides, though generally for a more recent phenomenon, the "rave." While descriptions of some of Leary's events on the East Coast and in Mexico report a variety of responses, those of Ken Kesey's associates seem more uniform due to how they were organized and directed (Stevens 1988). This was my impression (though I did not attend all of them) and it seems to be generally consistent with other reports.

Ungerleider and Fisher (1967) reported that they considered from their subject database that those individuals who do "particularly poorly in the L.S.D. experience are those with strongly systematic and organizational structure in their lives." This seemed to be the case in my experience at the Mogar Lab, and with the subjects that Mr. Rinker worked with, that the perceptual set, the typical "character armor" (a defensive system of an individual, a term coined by Wilhelm Reich in 1970 and ranging from minor to a kind of paralysis or dogmatic fog seen today in some populists) of the individual's personality attitude, was key to their type of experience. I would suggest that the word they use, "poorly," would be highly relative, as it must also be based on the expectations of the individual and their background. I mentioned this in my report to the Mogar Lab staff (Caldararo 1967). One individual from the subjects I surveyed claimed never to have been affected in any way by any drug, stimulant, or depressant. In test situations I noted he did seem unchanged in any way, but I could not say if that meant that he had so mastered the physiological effects as to be immune psychologically, as if he was a *fakir* or *sadhu* of some sort. When I mentioned this to a friend of mine outside of the Lab who was an enthusiastic user of psychedelics, he said, "Man, he took LSD and nothing happened? Bad trip!" A different interpretation of "bad." All subjects at the Mogar Lab took the Minnesota multiphasic personality inventory (MMPI) and were given a daily interview by one of the psychologists. The nonresponsive individual's scores did not produce anything noticeable, as I recall, and the test was not infallible. This was borne out by the tragedy of one subject at Humboldt State in the deprivation experiments who had also taken the MMPI and attempted suicide after one session.

The conditions of the sessions Pollard et al. (1965) created did have some significant intrusive aspects in the use of LSD, psilocybin, and sernyl. Subjects were restrained with straps on their hands and legs and wore a white dome on their heads to limit visual sensory information. Nevertheless, the reports of the subjects were quite limited compared with most. The most common effects were sensory, visual sensations and images, auditory, body sensations of moving, sense of humor, laughing, and so on. The images were also limited and this is expected, as the cues from the human-constructed environment (walls, doors, people, windows, etc.) are all absent. But one would expect more engagement of memory in this case. "Jane" in the experiment sees a goat head briefly and some transient colors. She believes she is recalling memories of the day, but then cannot be sure. Without an anchor in real time that is visually structured, perhaps an individual's disorientation becomes more general. Some reactions are typical of sensory deprivation conditions, especially with a dome and earphones, so "Jane" in one time feels pressure and difficulty breathing. This is often reported by people in sensory deprivation experiments without drug stimulation, and was common in the Humboldt State laboratory setting. Of course, hallucinations are reported by airplane pilots, people moving across uniform landscapes like deserts, ice fields, or doing boring routine work as in watching a radar screen. Sacks (2012) refers to Donald Heeb's experiments in the 1950s (and some others; see Solomon et al. 1961) with these phenomenon as the "Prisoner's Cinema." In recent years, Heeb's work has been associated with brainwashing techniques and CIA funding, though he was Canadian (McCoy 2007).

The third drug used in these experiments was sernyl (or sertraline, sold also as Zoloft), a serotonin reuptake inhibitor (SSRI); it increases levels of serotonin and is used as a treatment for depression, PTSD, panic and anxiety, and PMS. "Jane" experienced numbness, sleepiness, bodily abnormalities, and depersonalization. "Frank's" experiences on this drug are similar; he has rapid mood changes and sensations. The subject in the experiment referred to as "Tim" has many visual sensations on mescaline, but also many bodily feelings as well as auditory, with some he characterizes as "being in a blanket" being giddy, then on a joy ride. In most of his sensations he imagines himself a child or recalls sensations as a child. In all these subjects the typical LSD elaborations are missing or very restrained. What is similar in terms of the LSD responses of "Jane," "Frank," and "Bill" is a parallel experience of personal reflection and greater variation in analysis of what they were experiencing than with the other drugs administered in the experiment. "Bill" gave a number of sexual descriptions of events of engagement with another who was not present, so this "hallucination," seemingly without visual input, is also parallel to what many people report on LSD. Even with this restrained context, we see wide variations as between "Tom" and "Carl"—one described as dull and the other shows significant "odd" and very elaborate perceptions. The amount of drugs administered was: 150 milligrams (mg) of LSD, 20 mg of psilocybin, and 10 mg of Sernyl. The overall assessment of the authors is that the use of LSD and psilocybin results in positive experiences for their subjects. One of the few long-term studies of LSD use by Schmid and Liechti (2018) found similar positive outcomes from the use of the drug, with a 12-month follow-up, using 200 mg and 16 volunteer, normal subjects (8 male and 8 female). Screening was done by psychiatric interview.

I should mention here also something about the milieu in which LSD is situated in San Francisco. A number of writers like Stevens (1988) describe the Haight-Ashbury in 1966–1967 as a kind of circus or mental ward without walls. This picture is entirely foreign to me and I will describe later in this book other examples of contradiction. The "Haight," as many people who lived in San Francisco at the time called it, was like a little village. But the majority of people I met and knew were students, students with jobs, or people with jobs. Another central problem is the way the time and events like the Human Be-In and the Trips Festival were considered at the time and the relevance they had. These events often take center stage in a morality play, devised by journalists and a few participants, as an effort to change humanity or at least human perspective. Many people regarded these events as hedonistic and this was one charge made against the 1960s in general, as America and many developed societies fear hedonism in general, and find pleasure seeking as demoralizing and corrupting. Aaronson and Osmond (1970) discuss the effect of this attitude on LSD use (see also Louria 1966).

This is a wild exaggeration in my opinion, and descriptions of psychedelic users in the media were extreme and unreal, as in William Braden's book *The Private Sea*, which opens with a man eating a kitten. Few people I knew had any idea of participating in a great scheme to revolutionize America or mankind. Sahlins (2004) has criticized the theories of history as the result of special people, the "times," and certain places occupied with extraordinary combinations of people. I do think the Haight had a special combination of immigrants, especially Russians, African Americans, Beatniks, and young students. Peter Coyote describes it in the *Digger Archives* as "really free turf. It was kind of a non-descript university." I think, from my experience, it was as many things as there were people there, but as more came to be part of "it," the place changed dramatically. It seems to me that there were many perspectives, like the Russian immigrant families who ran Andy's Coffee Shop on Haight St. or the African Americans who had been displaced from the Fillmore District's destruction. But psychological history was once popular, as in Erikson's (1975), both for people and for times. Of the serious students of society and culture who were concerned with the future of the planet and who had tried LSD or peyote among a number of other methods supposed to give one new light on reality, they were unmoved. Joining a great drug crusade to change the world seemed as wrong as being a Christian or Buddhist missionary among aborigines or a soldier in Vietnam to stop Communism. In my experience, they rejected such exploits as myopic, primitive, egotistical, and doomed. Change to them was more complicated—changing themselves and, by example, changing others if successful. That caveat, "if successful," was vague, the goal was a better world, but by "world" often the meaning was the Haight, San Francisco, their family or families, and so on.

Among the anthropologists I knew the response was generally horror, "What do they expect the outcome to be?" asked John Ames, who had used peyote among Native Americans and saw its value as a means of social integration and individual adaptation. He was reminded of La Barre's (1975, 12) experience that after using peyote many people reported a long period of pleasure for days after. For John Collier, who had spent his life studying the Native people in America, he predicted a mindless mass of rodent-like behavior, untutored and supported by no cultural foundations that could act as a rudder. Dr. Luis Kemnitzer had brought me to a meeting with Ames and Collier and other professors of the Anthropology and Psychology departments after the Human Be-In. The question before me (since I had been there and was young) was, "What happened in terms of a social phenomenon?" My answer was, in general, nothing. I had seen a lot of young people enjoying each other or trying to, many eating, dancing, and basically enjoying themselves. The Trips Festival seemed similar, a hedonistic event. As for something special, other than the individual who parachuted into the event, the music, the chanting and the general chaos, and lack of focus seemed pointless. It could be seen as a huge market event, promoting a certain product, LSD, Leary and Ram Dass' books, and so on. As for promulgating the means to save humanity from itself, no, "nothing." I did have an observation and a question, "Why would people like Leary and Ram Das, on arriving in the "Other World," want to clothe it in the oppressive ideology of the Caste System (India) on the one hand, and that of Tibetan Buddhism (a rigid theocracy) on the other?" Dr. Ames then remarked, "Because either they did not understand what they found or were disappointed." Ames and the others were disappointed by the conversation. But then so was I.

Many of us who had been watching the organizers of these events saw their efforts as directing an incipient movement, perhaps what they hoped, a change in consciousness, into their own vision of what life should be or should be seen as. It was depressing to watch, as it seemed to many of my friends that what was unformed and free, coming into existence by accident, was being stomped on and having a massive cookie cutter placed on it. The idea that the world was vast and pointless was experienced by many who took LSD or mescaline, as described, for example, by Gerald Heard in Stevens (1988). But for many this "realization" or perception was a starting point to the freedom of redefining themselves as described by Jerry Richardson (1970).

Changes people reported in one of the early studies of LSD users produced a number of outcomes seen in Table I from Blum et al. (1964, 24). The chart reflects the experiences of the "professional members" of their test population (some of who began to experiment with LSD as early as 1956) and not all of the other 92 subjects. Their Chart II shows the answers of 24 of their subjects of the professional staff, but their responses are broken down into more detail, as in "bored," "satisfied," and so on. With the same results, the before and after attitudes reflect a positive outcome after LSD treatment. After the LSD session the majority felt "closer to people" and would like to take it again. Fifteen of their "non-professional" subjects were also asked the same questions with similar results—many of these had used other drugs like peyote before, and some had used LSD as early as 1950. Of their psychiatric patients (21 patients), divided between private and clinic, those in private practice had more philosophical/religious feelings, and many in the clinical group took the drug in a clinical setting. Most of both groups felt they benefited from the experience, but some in the clinical group had negative or unpleasant effects.

I found that people often used the term "wisdom" for what they took away from the LSD experience, but it has also been common for people to say this of peyote, as in the case of Huxley (Stevens 1988). Nevertheless, Blum et al. had a small group of "black market" users, people who had used LSD and a wide variety of other drugs. Their responses to LSD were difficult for the researchers to separate from their attitudes about other drugs. A final group, the "religious-medical-center sample," was made up of volunteers who were interested in LSD as a philosophical, religious, or medical experience that was associated with ideas of bettering themselves and the world. Most described the experience as both pleasant and unpleasant, but an underlying theme seemed to be that through some

Blum, et al., 1964 TABLE I

REPORTED CHANGES BY PERSONS TAKING LSD: INFORMAL PROFESSIONAL GROUP (N = 24)

Internal psychological changes for the better	13
Improvement in interpersonal relationships	6
New and more satisfactory persona! goals	2
Greater realism about goals and abilities	2
Reduced ambition, satisfaction over reduced goals	6
Satisfying changes in interests and perspectives	4
Enhanced aesthetic values or interests	3
Desirable changes in interests centering around the self; interest in growth and expansion	6
Desirable changes in interests sought in or about other persons or in oneself in relationship to them	3
Enhancement of religious values	3
Desirable changes in values about work and career	3
Desirable changes in philosophical-emotional values	2
Increased interest in physical activities, sports	2
Intensification, deepening of values already held	4
New interest in ESP, the occult	3

Fig. Pr.4 Blum et al.'s table of reported changes after LSD suffering people became better. That was how many in this group saw negative aspects of their experience. The results were similar to those reported by other researchers, including Mogar and Grof. It is also of interest that the sample of people taking psilocybin under Leary and Clark (1963), reported that the greatest change they experienced was in the feeling of security (80%) and ability to trust others (60%) and themselves (Downing and Wygant 1964). This is astounding given that one setting was a prison with male prisoners (Clark 1970).

It is also interesting that few of the early reports break their subjects into gender categories, though Blum et al. (1964) reported that fewer women were interested in the experiments, fewer wanted to "turn others on" to the drug, and many of the women who were acceptors (positively oriented to taking the drug) and were married before the experiment divorced after it. Also, among the control women who refused to take the drug, divorce followed the experiment.

The setting for the Blum et al. experiments was uniform and might be called clinical. When we compare the argument concerning set and setting by Leary in his early psychedelic work to the Human Be-In, the result is tremendous. Leary, Ram Dass, and others chanting was really the last straw. How could a religion from India, a country with one of the most repressive and racist social organizations, the caste system, be progressive or new? It was absurd. Many people looked into the Tibetan connection of their performance and talks and also found it wanting. Why a religious context of a hierarchic and rigid, male-oriented reference? It made no sense. But many of us continued on, but elsewhere.

Yet mass gatherings have appeared at various times in human history, from the Black Plague in the Middle Ages, the Cathars before, and the barnstorming preachers in the first and second Great Awakening in America (see Heimert and Miller 1967). And group behavior has had a central role in the strengthening of values and mental health in traditional societies, as Radcliffe-Brown (1932) put it from his observations, "We have seen that the dance is the expression of the unity and harmony of the society, and by permitting at the dance the free expression of personal vanity the society ensures that the individual shall learn to feel, even if only subconsciously, that his personal value depends upon the harmony between himself and his fellows." Myron Stolaroff, J.N. Sherwood, and W.W. Harman began a foundation for the study of LSD in Menlo Park in 1961 and had acquired the aid of Mogar to teach their staff the use of the MMPI and other analytical tools; they were interested in the use of the drug as a therapeutic aid and developed a protocol focused on the setting of drug use that included music. They published some results in 1968 (Sherwood et al. 1968). They titled their work "The Psychedelic Experience" when it was first submitted for publication in 1961. Two years later Leary, Metzner, and Alpert used the same title for their book. A larger group was operating in Palo Alto as the Palo Alto Mental Research Institute, founded by Don D. Jackson, but due to some negative experiences they came to view the drug with less zeal than others. In a report of two years of study they concluded the response to LSD was quite variable and required further study (Terrill 1964).

The house I lived in became a refuge for homeless and was raided by the police. Luckily I was not there and moved to Berkeley to continue my studies in Anthropology and Psychology. Psychology led me to study spider monkeys under Louis Klein, but working at night at the Post Office to pay my way was taking its toll. I moved to the Castro District and saw the blossoming of the gay movement, then to the Mission District, where the Latino community was resetting cultural identities, then to the Fillmore in the midst of the redevelopment struggle, where the Japanese American and African American communities were fighting for survival (Caldararo 2019). Then I moved to the South of Market District with the artist movement and finally to Fairfax to accidentally join a new environmental vision. The trip goes on, as Jerry Garcia might have said, but it has to be reborn each moment, in a way, as Bob Dylan (in a 1965 song) put it, "Those who are not busy being born are busy dying." One might say that the Human Be-In and the depictions of it, especially the Haight-Ashbury of 1966–1967, are a type of mirage or hallucination.

We will return to the question of what is a "hallucination" later. I was not sure that was what was happening. Seeing people explore their own conditioning, positive or negative, that made them who they were was an extraordinary scientific boon for research, especially into the development of possible therapies. Many people were able to benefit from the drug as a means of correcting and understanding the foundations of their personalities and how their character structure had been built by whatever childhood environment they had experienced. Some of this work was associated with growth and development, as presented in Montagu's book (1986) on the skin and touching and experiments in tactile deprivation. One might recall Vygotsky's idea of a zone of proximal development (ZPD), where up to a point an individual can achieve progress on their own and then there comes a break where they need facilitation by someone more knowledgeable—this could be another child or an adult (Van der Veer and Vaisiner 1994).

In today's context, as in the 1960s and 1970s, the use of psychomimetic or psychotomimetic drugs should be approached with a significant degree of care. While many people self-administered these drugs, more took them in group settings or with friends. What is most important, in my opinion, is that people do so in a safe and secure environment. This is certainly a subjective statement, but often when people hallucinate they appear not just different to others, but troubled or threatening, when really they are seldom a threat to anyone and are rarely experiencing negative events themselves. It is the response of others, often people who want to help but are unprepared, that creates the negative outcome, whether it is a "bad trip," harmful intervention, or serious injury. It is unfortunate that people often respond to someone who is acting differently in a fearful manner. We want to experience the miraculous, but only if we understand it; if not we call the police and the "shaman," "prophet," and so on is arrested and taken away.

As early as Blum et al. (1964) many subjects had already heard of "bizarre" effects of the drug and were ready to experience strange perceptions and the unexpected. Yet the desire for some new experience for self-knowledge and growth was a motive for many of the volunteers, as reported by Blum et al. (1964) and Aaronson and Osmond (1970). It is interesting that Blum et al. (1964) report that their different groups (not really representative of the American population then) generally could be said to have basically similar experiences, which indicates prior expectations, group background, and conditions of experiment. For example, the religious-medical-center people went through an "initial horror," a pattern of psychic unpleasantness, while the private patients suffered "raw fear of madness, of loss of control, of the unknown," while among the "black market" group a general feeling was the failure of the LSD administered to meet their expectations. One wonders if the type of LSD they had received before the experiment was different or mixed with other drugs. Despite these group generalities, there were marked individual differences in experience. What was of interest was that those who went on to repeated LSD use were mainly those who had their initial drug experience outside of any institutional setting (Blum et al. 1964, 44).

It is unfortunate that we have made the drugs illegal that for most traditional people opened the "doors of perception" to the spirit world of the gods. And we fear to cross that threshold that our brains are prepared to conceive, in so many unimaginable ways. I am not being factious—one's conception of god can be quite diverse, and as an anthropologist and an empiricist, god can be as vague as life or the universe. While "bad trip" is poorly defined in most of the literature, the use of LSD and psilocybin seems to not be associated with abuse or harmful effects (Amsterdam et al. 2011; Halpern and Pope 1999; Johnson et al. 2018; Krebs and Johansen 2013). Though a syndrome of long-lasting perceptual effects has been described, Hallucinogen Persisting Perception Disorder (HPPD), by Martinotti et al. (2018), it is apparently not common.

One conceit we have to deal with is the idea of normality. When I was born the *Diagnostic and Statistical Manual of Mental Disorders* (now the DSM-5) was less than a half-inch thick; today it is over 5 inches thick. One might wonder if we as a species have become crazier since the end of the Second World War, or we have discovered a myriad number of ways of performing our cognitive apparatus. Some have suggested the idea of increased mental pathology (Torrey and Miller 2001). Oliver Sacks (1985; 2013) has given a wide view of human consciousness; Luria (1973) and a number of other neurophysiologists and psychologists have considered a realm of conditions brought on by birth defects, trauma, genetic mutations, and chemical agency. Some like Korsakoff's Syndrome (e.g., loss of ability to form new memories among other symptoms and the creation of false histories) appear in different form and from a variety of causes (Brion 1969), but how can we define normality? Is it the ability to conform, to be "domesticated," as Darwin suggested? Ruth Benedict and other anthropologists gave normality a very wide definition (see Hsu 1972).

What takes place between stimulation of nerves and the process by which the brain associates outside-body and inside-body information is still unclear. Typically, neuroscientists often use the term "representations" or "neural representations," but while the events characterized by these terms can be generally agreed upon, the exact means is not, or as Dietrich (2007) put it, "no scientist knows how representations represent." It is well established that patterns of neural activity by a variety of neurons can be recorded and seen as "mapping markers," as stimuli features, and that methods like multivariate pattern analysis (MVPA) can be used to characterize responses with stimuli (Vilarroya 2017). It is also clear that as different parts of the brain are activated in these patterns, we can talk of "ideas" and "concepts" being displayed and "memories" being activated. The hippocampus seems central to this process. It appears that in the hippocampus value is assigned to features of memories in what is called "multi-featural conjunctive representations." These joined features of images and events can be shuffled and rejoined in the hippocampus as values of the features change (Ballard et al. 2019). We will look at the hippocampus again later, but it is well known that recognition of associations of memory features is impaired, while single items may be spared in some amnesic patients (Eichenbaum 2004). Therefore, any variety of influences on the hippocampus and its ability to communicate with other areas of the brain may unleash a series of attempted connections that appear as a shuffling imagery or merging of memories; the result can then be dreams, visions, or hallucinations.

The mechanism of these processes, as they combine into the individual, is based on a number of theories and assumptions that are widely debated. It is, I think, confusing to then say that neural representations are the brain's model of the world or reality. They may be more effectively described as dynamic systems of neurons reflecting patterns of nerve cell activity that can be associated with general classes of events, including objects (Thomson and Piccinini 2018). Recently Bernardi et al. (2020) have demonstrated these kinds of associations with monkeys. A central problem is that of disentangling the "curse of dimensionality," or classes of neuron firing during an event to identity operational events as an acceptable concept of "abstraction." They work from "decoding" subjects who generalize stimuli to form what Bernardi et al. consider abstractions.

Thus, while some decode methods seem to produce "geometry reflecting abstractions" from "neural representation," the complexity of context and variation seem to indicate a considerable degree of vague association (Bernardi et al. 2020).

Nevertheless, this is in line with my view of building conditioning on simple levels to more complex and to Rivers' (1920) concept of suppression (taken from his work with Head and Riddoch 1917) of simple operations to allow for more complex patterns of response. This idea of suppression of background or redundant sensory input was later developed into a theory of "release" for hallucinations by L. Jolyon West (1976). In this scheme the normal state is a constant stream of processing sensory input that is kept out of the sphere of consciousness. Loss of input, to West, results in a release of redundant information that then appears in the conscious realm if there is sufficient cortical arousal. While some neurologists consider the theory faulty (Eysel et al. 1999), it is considered generally useful and correct (ffytche 2013). It is similar to that presented by Sacks (2012), which I discuss, but Sacks also notes that often it seems that damage to or chemical influence on the lower brain regions (e.g., hippocampus) results in the release of memories and images from the higher areas (neocortex), yet often these go from simple patterns to images and then multiple images and back again and disappear. It is easy to suggest that this represents the brain attempting to heal or compensate for the interference or damage.

One can imagine that disruption of neurological processing, by restricting neurotransmitters, for example, like the anti-cholinergic agents (atropine, Ditran, etc.), could produce such conditions. We will discuss these agents as we go along. Ralph Metzner (1968) argued then that such agents should be called consciousness-altering (psychotomimetic) and not included in the class as psychedelic or consciousness-expanding drugs like LSD and psilocybin. It seems to me this is a real distinction in terms of how the brain is affected, in one case reducing processing and in another enhancing it. Yet how humans respond to these seemingly different and distinct conditions does overlap, not only in cultural interpretation (see Laroi et al. 2014), but also in individual experience and perception. Human variation, both genetic and physiological, tends to confuse and abort general theories. For example, size distortions (things looking bigger than they are or changing size in an instant) are commonly reported for atropine and related drugs (Metzner 1970) and are often experienced in people who smoke marijuana (Sacks 2012), or in my experience, when present among those who use LSD and peyote but also due to a number of other conditions, as in delirium.

It seems likely that such neural representations are related to engagement of the hippocampus, and that types of memory, especially context-rich episodic memories, are drawn to external stimuli as exposure occurs, creating sequential organization, and the time factors involved are related, in a normal case, to present a "mental replay" (Eichenbaum 2004). Such a description of memory and external stimulation can be seen as a complex type of conditioning and association. This being based on "declarative memory," that is, long-term memories and the conscious recollection of facts associated. What is a neural representation is more explanatory than using a term like "abstraction" or "symbol" due to its encompassing of networks of discrete event actions or elements. Such concepts seem to be constructed from connectivity, and the connections of episodic memories at any one time present awareness. But how this awareness is maintained from minute to minute in a context of life challenges is the great problem of a model of consciousness (Eichenbaum 2004). Where this connectivity is interrupted, as in macular degeneration and spontaneous hallucinations in color, there has been found degeneration throughout the ventral color pathway in the post-mortem study of patients (Clarke 1994). This is similar to Rivers' (1920) discussion of Head and Riddoch's (1917) experiments of nerve damage in his suggestions on consciousness.

TABLE III
After Blum, et al. 1964

CONTROLS AND LSD ACCEPTERS COMPARED ON BACKGROUND CHARACTERISTICS

	Controls (N = 47)	Accepters (N = 71)
Education		
High school diploma or less	11%	9%
Some college or bachelor's degree	29	36
Master's, law, or doctoral degree	60	55
Age		
21-30	15	31
31-40	51	43
41-50	28	17
51-60	6	7
61—over	o	1
Religious preference		
None	51*	35*
Protestant	38	43
Jewish	9	10
Catholic	1	6
Mystic-private-universal	o	6
Derivation of surname (in the case of wives, of husband's surname)		
Anglo-Saxon	75	61
Race		
White	100	100
Maritai status		
Married	85	58
Divorced or separated	13	21
Single	2	1
Widowed	o	0
Sex	6	4
Male	43	36
Female	57	19

* Most professed agnostics, atheists, and religious non-practitioners in both samples came from Protestant backgrounds.

Fig. Pr.5 After Blum et al., background on users and controls

References

Aaronson, Bernard and Humphry Osmond, (eds) (1970) *Psychedelics, The Uses and Implications of Hallucinogenic Drugs,* Garden City, Anchor Books.

Aggernaes, A. R. Haugstedd, A. Myschetzky, H. Paikin, and J. Vitger, (1976) "A reliable clinical technique for investigation of the experienced reality and unreality qualities connected with everyday life experiences in psychotic and non-psychotic persons," *Acta Psychiatrica Scandinavica*, v. 53, 241–257.

Aggernaes, A. (1972) "The experienced reality of hallucinations and other psychological phenomena," *Acta Psychiatrica Scandinavica*, v. 48, 220–238.

Anthony, J.E.C., A. Winstock, J.A. Ferris and D.J. Nutt, (2020) "Improved colour blindness symptoms associated with recreational psychedelic use: results from the Global Drug Survey, 2017)," *Drug Science, Policy and Law*, January 1, v. 6: https://doi.org/10.1177/2050324520942345.

Baars, B.J. (2003) "How brain reveals mind: neural studies support the fundamental role of conscious experience," *Journal of Consciousness Studies*, v. 10, 100–114.

Baker, John R. (2009) "The old woman and her gifts: pharmacological bases of the Chumash use of Datura," In Warms, Richard, James Garber and R. Jon McGee, (2009) *Sacred Realms: Readings in the Anthropology of Religion*, Oxford, Oxford University Press, 207–216.

Ballard, Ian C., Anthony D. Wagner and Samuel M. McClure, (2019) "Hippocampal pattern separation supports reinforcement learning," *Nature Communications*, v. 10, 1073, https://doi.org/10.1038/s41467-019-08998-1

Bentall, R.P. and F. Varese, (2013) "Psychotic hallucinations," in *Hallucination: Philosophy and Psychology*, (eds.) Fiona Macpherson and Dimitris Platchias, Cambridge, MA, MIT Press, pp. 65–86.

Benitez, Del Rosario, Fernando Monton Antonio Salinas, Jose J. Martin and Maunel Feria (2001) "Charles Bonnet Syndrome and opioids," *Journal of the American Geriatrics Society*, 21 Dec. v. 49, n. 2: 235–236.

Bernardi, Silvia, Marcus K. Benna, Mattia Rigotti, Jerome Munuera, Stefano Fusi and C. Daniel Salzman, (2020) "The geometry of abstraction in the hippocampus and prefrontal cortex," *Cell*, November, 12, v. 183, 954–967.

Bexton, William H., Woodburn Heron and T.H. Scott (1954) "Effects of decreased variation in the sensory environment," *Canadian Journal of Psychology*, v. 8 (2): 70–76.

Bishop, A.G. and J.M. Tallon, (1999) "Anticholinergic visual hallucinosis from atropine eye drops," *Canadian J. Emergency Med.*, July, v. 1, n. 2, 115–116.

Blum, Richard, Eva Blum and Mary Lou Funkhouser, (1964a) "The institutionalization of LSD," in Blum, Richard, Nevitt Sanford, Eva Blum, Mary Lou Funkhouser, Joseph J. Downing, et al., (eds.) *Utopiates: The Use and Users of LSD-25, A Publication of the Institute for the Study of Human Problems*, Stanford University, Atherton Press, 124–141.

Blum, Richard, Nevitt Sanford, Eva Blum, Mary Lou Funkhouser, Joseph J. Downing, et al., (1964b) Utopiates: The Use and Users of LSD-25, A Publication of the Institute for the Study of Human Problems Stanford University, Atherton Press.

Blum, Richard, (1964a) "Background considerations," in Blum, Richard, Nevitt Sanford, Eva Blum, Mary Lou Funkhouser, Joseph J. Downing, et al., (eds) Utopiates: The Use and Users of LSD-25, A Publication of the Institute for the Study of Human Problems Stanford University, Atherton Press, 1–9.

Blum, Richard, (1964b) "Conclusions and commentary," in Blum, Richard, Nevitt Sanford, Eva Blum, Mary Lou Funkhouser, Joseph J. Downing, et al., (eds.) Utopiates: The Use and Users of LSD-25, A Publication of the Institute for the Study of Human Problems Stanford University, Atherton Press, 265–294.

Brion, S. (1969) "Korsakoff" Syndrome: Clinico-Anatomical and Physiopathological considerations," in George A. Talland and Nancy C. Waugh (eds), *The Pathology of Memory*, New York, Academic Press.

Caldararo, Niccolo (1967) A *Mental Ethnography, Perception, Understanding, Reality, and Need in Language: Conclusions from Research in LSD*, Xerox copy presented to Dr. Mogar and staff as a summary of field work and laboratory observations, San Francisco State University.

Caldararo, Niccolo (2019) *An Ethnography of the Goodman Building, The Longest Rent Strike*, New York, Palgrave/Macmillan.

Caldararo, Niccolo (2020) "Social Complexity, Pathogen Adaptation and Covid-19: History of Disease Avoidance, Social Spacing and Work/Home Matrix," in, *City Life and Beyond in Times of Pandemic*, Special Issue — Edited by G. B. Prato, Urbanities, Vol. 10 · Supplement 4 · September 2020.

Camurcuoglu, Duygu Secil, (2015*) The Wall Paintings of Catalhoyuk (Turkey): Materials, Technologies and Artists*, Dissertation, Institute of Archaeology, University College London.

Carhart-Harris, R.L., M. Kaelen, M.G. Whalley, M. Bolstridge, A. Feilding and D.J Nutt, (2015) "LSD enhances suggestibility in healthy volunteers," *Psychopharmacology*, 232, (4), 785–794.

Clark, Jonathan (1970) "The use of psilocybin in a prison setting," in Aaronson, Bernard and Humphry Osmond, (eds) (1970) *Psychedelics, The Uses and Implications of Hallucinogenic Drugs*, Garden City, Anchor Books: 40–44.

Clarke, S. (1994) "Modular organization of human extrastriate visual cortex: evidence from cytochrome oxidase pattern in normal and macular degeneration cases," *Eur J. Neurosci.* 6: 725–736.

Cohen, S. (1960) Lysergic acid diethylamide: Side effects and complications. *J. Nerv. Ment. Dis.* 130: 30–40.

Crick, Francis, (1994) *The Astonishing Hypothesis, The Scientific Search for the Soul*, New York, Simon and Schuster.

Dantzer, Robert (2018) "Neuroimmune interactions: from the brain to the immune system and vice versa," *Physiol. Rev.* Jan 1, v. 98, n 1, 477–504.

Darlington, Cynthia (2002) *The Female Brain*, London, Taylor and Francis.

de Rios, Marlene Dobkin (1984) *Hallucinogens: Cross-Cultural Perspectives*, Albuquerque, University of New Mexico Press.

de Rios, Dobkin and Oscar Janiger (2003) *LSD, Spirituality, and the Creative Process: Based on the Groundbreaking Research of Oscar Janiger*, Rochester, Vermont, Inner Traditions/Bear & Co.

Dell'Erba, Sara, David J. Brown and Michael J. Proulx, (2018) "Synesthetic hallucinations induced by psychedelic drugs in a congenitally blind man," *Consciousness and Cognition*, v. 60, April, 27–132.

Dietrich, E. (2007). "Representation," in *Philosophy of Psychology and Cognitive Science* ed. P. Thagard (Amsterdam: Elsevier), 1–29.

Downing, Joseph J. and William Wygant, Jr. (1964) "Psychedelic experience and religious belief," in Blum, Richard, Nevitt Sanford, Eva Blum, Mary Lou Funkhouser, Joseph J. Downing, et al., (eds.) *Utopiates: The Use and Users of LSD-25*, A Publication of the Institute for the Study of Human Problems Stanford University, Atherton Press, 187–198.

Eichenbaum, Howard (2004) "Hippocampus: cognitive processes and neural representations that underlie declarative memory," *Neuron*, Sept 30, v. 44: 109–120.

Eliade, Mircea (1964) *Shamanism*, Bolligen Foundation, Princeton, Princeton University Press.

Erikson, Erik (1975) *Life History and the Historical Moment*, New York, W.W. Norton.

Eysel, U.T., G. Schweigart, T. Mittmann, D. Eyding, Y. Qu, et al., (1999) "Reorganization in the visual cortex after retinal and cortical damage," *Restorative Neurology and Neuroscience*, v. 15: 153–164.

Fernandes, L.H., B. Scassellati-Sforzolini and R.F. Spaide (2000) "Estrogen and visual hallucinations in a woman with Charles Bonnet Syndrome," Am J. Ophthalmol., March, v. 129, n 3, 407.

Ffytche, Dominic H. (2013) "The hallucinating brain: neurobiological insights into the nature of hallucinations," Chapter 3, in *Hallucination: Philosophy and Psychology*, (eds.) Fiona Macpherson and Dimitris Platchias, Cambridge, MA, MIT Press, pp. 45–64.

Fisher, Samantha, Keir E. Lewis, Iona Bartle, Robin Ghosal, Lois Davies and Mark Blagrove, (2011) "Emotional content of dreams in obstructive sleep apnea hypopnea syndrome patients and sleepy snorers attending a sleep-disordered breathing clinic," *J. Clin. Sleep Med.*, v. 7, n. 1, 69–74.

Flint, Alexander C., John P Loh and John C.M. Brust, (2005) "Vivid visual hallucinations from occipital lobe infarction," *Neurology,* v. 65, n. 5, Sept., 12, https://doi.org/10.1212/01.wnl.0000180350.58985.5f

Foy, Kevin (2011) "Leprchauns and Lewy body disease," *Transcltural Psychiatry,* v. 48, n. 3, 362–364.

Furst, Peter T. (1972) *Flesh of the Gods, the Ritual Use of Hallucinogens,* New York, Praeger.

Guerra-Doce, Elisa (2015) "Psychoactive substances in prehistoric times: examining the archaeological evidence," *The Journal of Archaeology, Consciousness and Culture,* v. 8, n 1, https://doi.org/10.1080/1751696X.2014.993244

Guharoy, S.R., M. Barajas, et al., (1991) "Atropine intoxication from the ingestion and smoking of jimson weed (Datura stramonium)" *Vet. Hum. Toxicol.* Dec. v. 33, 6, 588–9.

Guzman, Gaston, (2012) "Nuevas observaciones taxonomicas y etnomicologicas en Psilocybe s.s. (Fungi, Basidiomycota, Agaricomycetidae, Agaricales, Strophariaceae) de Mexico, Africa y Espana," *Acta Botanica Mexicana* (100):79–106.

Halpern JH, Pope HG (1999) "Do hallucinogens cause residual neuropsychological toxicity?" *Drug Alcohol Depend* 53(3):247–256. https://doi.org/10.1016/S0376-8716(98)00129-X.

Hall, C. and R. Van de Castle (1966) *The Content Analysis of Dreams,* New York, Appleton-Centurn-Crofts.

Harner, Michael (1972) *Jivaro: People of the Sacred Waterfalls,* New York, Doubleday.

Hartogsohn, Ido (2017) "Constructing drug effects: a history of set and setting," *Drug Science,* Jan. 1, v. 3: https://doi.org/10.1177/2050324516683325

Head, H. and G. Riddoch, (1917) "The automatic bladder, excessive sweating and some other reflex conditions in gross injuries of the spinal cord," *Brain,* v. 40, 188.

Heimert, Alan and Perry Miller, (1967) (eds.) *The Great Awakening, Documents Illustrating the Crisis and Its Consequences,* Indianapolis, The Bobbs-Merrill Co.

Hollan, Douglas (2003) "The cultural and intersubjective context of dream remembrance and reporting," Chapter 9 in *Dream Travelers: Sleep Experiences and Culture in the Western Pacific*, (ed) Roger Ivar Lohmann, New York, Palgrave Macmillan,169–188.

Hsu, Francis L.K. (1972) (ed.) *Psychological Anthropology,* Cambridge, Schenkman Publishing Co.

Hsu, F.L.K., (1973), "Prejudice and its Intellectual Effect on American Anthropology: An Ethnographic Report", *American Anthropologist*, 75: 1–19, Washington: American Anthropological Association.

Hsu, Francis, (1964) "Rethinking the concept, 'Primitive,'" *Current Anthropology*, v. 5, n. 3, 169–178.

Hudson, Scott R. (2000) "The Rave: Spiritual healing in modern Western subcultures, "*Anthropological Quarterly,* v. 73, 35–49.

Hunter, Michael D., Timothy D. Griffiths, Tom F.D. Farrow, Ying Zheng, Iain D. Wilkinson, et al. (2002) "A neural basis for the perception of voices in external auditory space," *Brain*, Jan. 126, 1, 161–169.

Huxley, Aldous (1954) *The Doors of Perception, and Heaven and Hell*, New York, Harper Colophon Books.

Hyde, R.W. (1960) "Psychological and social determinants of drug action," in G.J. Sarwer-Foner (ed.) *The Dynamics of Psychiatric Drug Therapy*, Springfield, Thomas, 297–315.

Johnson MW, Griffiths RR, Hendricks PS, Henningfield JE (2018) "The abuse potential of medical psilocybin according to the 8 factors of the Controlled Substances Act," *Neuropharmacology*. https://doi.org/10.1016/j.neuropharm.2018.05.012.

Karsten, R. (1935) *The Head-Hunters of Western Amazonas,* Helsingfors, Sinska Zetenskaps-Societeten.

Keen, Ian (2003) "Dreams, agency and traditional authority in Northeast Arnhem Land," Chapter 7, in *Dream Travelers: Sleep Experiences and Culture in the Western Pacific*, (ed) Roger Ivar Lohmann, New York, Palgrave Macmillan, 127–148.

Kensinger, K., (1972) "Banisteriopsis usage among the Peruvian Cashinahua," in *Hallucinogens and Shaman*, Michael Harner (ed.), Oxford, Oxford University Press, 9–14.

Killam, K.F. (1956) "Studies of LSD and Chlorpromazine," Psychatr. Res. Rep Am Psyhiatr Asso, Oc. V. 6:35–45.

Kiyokawa, Miki and William F. Haning, (2021) "Hydromorphone-induced tactile hallucinations: rare opioid side effect," *Cureus*, v. 13, n. 2, Feb 28: https://doi.org/10.7759/cureus.13622.

Krebs TS, Johansen P-Ø (2013) "Psychedelics and mental health: a population study," *PLoS One* 8(8): e63972. https://doi.org/10.1371/journal.pone.0063972.

Kuypers, K.P., L. Ng, D. Erritzoe, G.M. Knudsen, C.D. Nichols, et al., (2019) Microdosing psychedelics: more questions than answers? An overview and suggestions for future research," *J. of Psychopharmacology*, v. 33, 1039–1957.

La Barre, Weston (1975) "Anthropological perspectives on hallucination and hallucinogens," in *Hallucinations: Behavior, Experience and Theory*, (eds.) R. K. Siegel and L.J. West, New York, John Wiley, & Sons, 9–52.

Laroi, Frank, Tanya Marie Luhrmann, Vaughan Bell, William A. Christian, Jr., Smita Deshpande, et al., (2014) "Culture and hallucinations: overview and future directions," *Schizophrenia Bulletin*, v. 40, suppl, no. 4, s213–s220.

Leary, Timothy (1968) *The Politics of Ecstasy*, New York, Putnam.

Leary, Timothy and Walter Houston Clark, (1963) "Religious implications of consciousness expanding drugs," *Religious Education*, v. 58, 251–256.

Leary, Timothy, Metzner, Ralph, Alpert, Richard, *The Psychedelic Experience*, New York, 1964.

Leary, Timothy, Ralph Metzner and Richard Alpert, (2000) *The Psychedelic Experience: A Manual Based on the Tibetan Book of the Dead*, Citadel.

Lev-Ran, Shaul, (2020) "Serotonergic hallucinogens," In *Addiction Medicine: Science and Practice*, (ed.) Bankole A. Johnson, 2nd edition, Elsevier, 434–445.

Levy-Bruhl, Lucien (1966) *Primitive Mentality*, (originally published in 1923) Boston, Beacon Press.

Lévi-Strauss, C. (1963) *Structural Anthropology*. New York, Basic Books.

Levi-Strauss, C. (1966) *The Savage Mind*, Chicago, Unuversity of Chicago Press.

Lincoln, J. S. (1935) *The Dream in Primitive Cultures*, London, Cressett Press.

Louria, D.B. (1966) *Nightmare Drugs*, New York, Pocket Books.

Luhrmann, T.M. (2012) *When God Talks Back, Understanding the American Evangelical Relation with God*, New York, Knopf.

Luppi, Andrea I., Michael M. Craig, Ionnis Pappas, Paola Finoia, Guy B. Williams, et al. (2019) "Consciousness-specific dynamic interactions of brain integration and functional diversity," *Nature Communications*, 10, 4616, Oct, 10, https://doi.org/10.1038/s41467-19-12658-9

Luria, A.R. (1973) *The Working Brain*, London, Harmondsworth.

MacKisack, Matthew, Susan Aldworth, Fiona Macpherson, John Onians, Crawford Winlove and Adam Zeman, (2016) "On picturing a candle: the prehistory of imagery science," *Front. Psychol.* 19 April,

Martinotti, Giovanni, Rita Santacroce, Mauro Pettorruso, Chiara Montemitro, Maria Chiara Spano, et al., (2018) "Hallucinogen persisting perception disorder: etiology, clinical features, and therapeutic perspectives, " *Brain Science*, March, v. 8, n. 3, https://doi.org/10.3390/brainsci8030047

McAlpine, Lindsay S., Brooke Lifland, Joseph R. Check, Gustavo A. Angarita, Thomas T. Ngo, et al., (2021) "Remission of subacute psychosis in a Covid-19 patient with an antineuronal autoantibody after treatment with intravenous immunoglobulin," *Biol. Psychiatry*, Aug, 15, v. 90 (4) e23–26.

McCoy, Alfred W. (2007) "Science in Dachau's Shadow: Hebb, Beecher, and the Development of CIA Psychological Torture and Modern Medical Ethics." *Journal of the History of the Behavioral Sciences*. **43** (4): 401–417.

McKenna, Terence (1993) *True Hallucinations, Being an Account of the Author's Extraordinary Adventures in the Devil's Paradise*, New York, HarperOne.

Metzner, Ralph, (1968) *The Ecstatic Adventure*, New York, Macmillan.

Mitchell, J. and Vierkant, A.D. (1989) "Delusions and hallucinations as a reflection of the subcultural milieu among psychotic patients of the 1930s and 1980s. *J. Psychol.*, v. 123, 269–274.

Mittal, Manoj and Saud Khan, (2010) "Starvation causes acute psychosis due to anterior thalamic infarction," South Med. J. July, v. 103, n. 7:701–703.

Montagu, Ashley (1986) *Touching: The Human Significance of the Skin*, New York, Harper & Row.

Munn, Nancy D. (1973) *Wlbiri Iconography: Graphic Representations and Cultural Symbolism in a Central Australian Society*, Ithaca, Cornell University Press.

Murphree, Henry B. (1962) "Quantitative studies in humans on the antagonism of lysergic acid diethylamide by chlorparomazine and phenoxybenzamine," *Clinical Pharmacology & Therapeutics*, v. 3, n. 3, 314–320.

Myerhoff, Barbara G. (1974) *Peyote Hunt: The Sacred Journey of the Huichol Indians*, Ithaca, Cornell University Press.

Nichols, Charles D. and Elaine Sanders-Bush (2001) "A single dose of Lysergic Acid Diethylamide influences gene expression patterns within the mammalian brain," *Neuropsychopharmacology*, 26, 634–642.

O'Brien J., J.P. Taylor, C. Ballard, Roger A. Barker, Clare Bradley, et al. Visual hallucinations in neurological and ophthalmological disease: pathophysiology and management. *Journal of Neurology, Neurosurgery & Psychiatry* 2020;**91**:512–519.

Pahnke, Walter (1963) *Drugs and Mysticism: An Analysis of the Relationship Between Psychedelic Drugs and the Mystical Consciousness*, Thesis, Harvard University, https://maps.org/images/pdf/books/pahnke/walter_pahnke_drugs_and_mysticism.pdf.

Pollard, J.C., L. Uhr and E. Stern (1965) *Drugs and Phantasy, The Effects of LSD, Psilocybin and Sernyl on College Students*, Boston, Little, Brown.

Preller, Katrin H., Adeel Razi, Peter Zeidman, Philipp Stampfli, Karl J. Friston, et al., (2019) "Effective connectivity changes in LSD-induced altered states of consciousness in humans," *PNAS*, 12 February, v. 116, n. 7, 2743–2748.

Radcliffe-Brown, A.R. (1932) *The Andaman Islanders,* Reprint edition, New York, The Free Press of Glencoe, 1964.

Reich, Wilhelm (1970) *The Mass Psychology of Fascism*, New York, Farrar, Straus and Giroux.

Richardson, Jerry (1970) "Who am I, and so what if I am," in Aaronson, Bernard and Humphry Osmond, (eds) (1970) *Psychedelics, The Uses and Implications of Hallucinogenic Drugs,* Garden City, Anchor Books, 50–58.

Richelson E, Souder T (2000). "Binding of antipsychotic drugs to human brain receptors focus on newer generation compounds." *Life Sciences.* **68** (1): 29–39.

Richer, Emily J. (2009) "Ibogaine and the treatment of Opiate addiction," *In Complementary and Alternative Therapies and the Aging Population,* (ed) Ronald Ross Watson, San Diego, Mendeley, 393–401.

Ritschel, T. (2016) "Using simulated visual illusions and perceptual anomalies to convey dynamic range," In H*igh Dynamic Range Video* (Eds.) Dufaux, Frederic, Patrick Le Callet, Marta Mrak, et al., Oxford, Academic Press.

Rivers, W.H.R. (1920) *Instinct and the Unconscious*, Cambridge, Cambridge University Press.

Robinson, David W., Kelly Brown, Moira McMenemy, Lynn Dennany, Matthew J. Baker, et al., (2020) "Datura quids at Pinwheel Cave, California, provide unambiguous confirmation of the ingestion of hallucinogens at a rock art site," *PNAS*, December 8, v. 227, (49): 31026–31037.

Sacks, Oliver (1985) *The Man Who Mistook His Wife for a Hat*, New York, Harper & Row, Perennial Library Edition.

Sacks, Oliver (2012) *Hallucinations*, New York, Vintage Books.

Sagan, Carl (1974) *Broca's Brain,* New York, Random House, 359.

Sahlins, Marshall (2004) *Apologies to Thucydides, Understanding History and Culture and Vice Versa*, Chicago, University of Chicago Press.

Santhouse, A.M., R.J. Howard and D.H. Ffytche, (2000) "Visual hallucinatory syndromes and the anatomy of the visual brain," *Brain*, v. 123, 2055–2064.

Satgunam, PremNandhini, Rebecca Sumalini, Gayathri Chittapu and Gunasree Pamarthi, (2019) "Screening for Charles Bonnet Syndrome, should the definition be reconsidered?," *Indian Journal of Ophthalmology,* v. 67, (7) 1127–1132.

Scarmeas, Nikolaos, Jason Brandt, Marilyn Albert, Georgios Hadjigeorgiou, Alexandros Papadimitriou, et al., (2005) "Delusions and hllucinations are associated with worse outcome in Alzheimer Disease," *Arch. Neurol.*, v. 62, 1601–1608.

Schneider, Richard C., Elizabeth C. Crosby, Basu K. Bgchi, Hazel D. Calhoun, (1961) "Temporal or occipital lobe hallucinations triggered from frontal lobe lesions," *Neurology*, Feb., v. 11, n. 2, https://doi.org/10.1212/WNL.11.2.172

Schultes, Richard Evans (1972) "An overview of hallucinogens

Schmid, Yasmin and Matthias E. Liechti, (2018) "Long-lasting subjective effects of LSD in normal subjects," *Psychopharacology (Berl)*, v. 235 (2):535–545.

Sherwood, J.N., M.J. Stolaroff and W.W. Harman (1968) "The Psychedelic Experience – a new concept in psychotherapy," *Journal of Neuropsychiatr.* Nov. – Dec, v. 4: 69–80.

Small, S.A., A.S. Hava, G.M. Perera, R. DeLaPaz, R. Mayeux and Stern, Y. (2001) Circuit mechanisms underlying memory encoding and retrieval in the long axis of the hippocampal formation," Nat. Neurosci. V. 4, 442–449.

Snyder, S.H., L. Faillace, L. Hollister, (1968) "2,5,Dimethoxy-4-methylamphetamine: a new hallucinogenic drug," *Science*, Mar 29, v. 159 (3822), 1492.

Solomon, P., Kubzansky, Philip E., Leiderman, P. Herbert, Mendelson, Jack H., Trumbull, Richard, & Wexler, Donald, Eds. (1961) *Sensory Deprivation: A Symposium Held at Harvard Medical School.* Cambridge, MA, Harvard University Press.

Spencer, F.J. and Baldwin Gillen (1927) *The Arunta: A Study of a Stone Age People,* New York, Macmillan Co.

Stanner, W.E.H. (1953) *The Dreaming and Other Essays,* Collingwood, VIC, Black, Inc.

Stevens, Jay (1988) *Storming Heaven: LSD and the American Dream*, New York, Harper and Row.

Tan, C.S.H., V.S.Y. Lim, D.Y.M. Ho, E. Yeo, et al., (2004) "Charles Bonnet syndrome in Asian patients in a tertiary ophthalmic center," *Br. J. Ophthalmol.*, Oct., v. 88 (10) 1325–1329.

Tedlock, Barbara (1991) "The new anthropology of dreaming," Dreaming, v. 1, n. 2, https://www.asdreams.org/journal/articles/1-2tedlock1991.htm.

Tedlock, Barbara (1987) "Dreaming and dream research," in *Dreaming: Anthropological and Psychological Interpretations,* (ed.) Barbara Tedlock, Cambridge, Cambridge University Press, 1–30.

Terrill, James, (1964) "The nature of the LSD experience," in *LSD, the Consciousness—Expanding Drug,* (ed.) David Solomon,

Thomson, Eric and Gualtiero Piccinini (2018) "Neural Representations," *Minds and Machines,* v. 28, 191–235.

Torrey, E. Fuller and Judy Miller (2001) *The Invisible Plague: The Rise of Mental Illness from 1780 to the Present,* Brunswick, NJ, Rutgers University Press.

Turner, Victor (1969) *The Ritual Process: Structure and Anti-Structure,* Ithaca, Cornell University Press.

Ungerleider, J. T. and D.D. Fisher, (1967) "The problems of L.S.D. 25 and emotional disorder," *California Medicine,* v. 106, 49–55.

West, Jolyon L. (1962) *Hallucinations,* New York, Grune and Stratton.

van Amsterdam J, Opperhuizen A, van den Brink W (2011) "Harm potential of magic mushroom use: a review," *Regul Toxicol Pharmacol* 59(3):423–429. https://doi.org/10.1016/j.yrtph.2011.01.006

Van der Veer, R. and J. Vaisiner, (Eds.) (1994) *The Vygotsky Reader,* Oxford, Blackwell.

Vilarroya, Oscar (2017) "Neural representation. A survey-based analysis of the notion," *Front. Psychol.* 29 August, https://doi.org/10.3389/fpsyg.2017.01458

Wendt, Herbert (1955) *In Search of Adam,* New York, Collier Books.

Winkelman, Michael (2019) "Introduction: evidence for entheogen use in prehistory and world religions," *Journal of Psychedelic Studies,* v. 3, n. 2, https://doi.org/10.1556/2054.2019.024

Abstract

In the 1960s and 1970s Lysergic Acid Diethylamide (LSD) began to be used as a potential therapeutic agent by a number of researchers. The author participated in a number of studies of perception, including sensory deprivation and psychotropic drugs, some of recent manufacture or discovery and some of primitive or traditional societies. This book summarizes the experiences and research of the author from that time and a re-evaluation in light of recent scientific work and social use of such drugs. This is placed in context by an analysis of the physiological aspects of hallucinations, delusions, visions, and dreams, as well as cross-cultural data on dreams, dreaming, and drug use and the social value of hallucinations, dreams, and visions. Some of the material used in this book is derived from unpublished scientific research from Dr. Robert Mogar's laboratory and related field research by the author.

Keywords LSD; Sensory deprivation; Perception; Language; Psychotropic drugs, Psychomimetic drugs, Microdosing

A Note on Terms Used in the Ethnographic Literature

In this text I use a number of terms for the people I am referring to—in some cases, these are groups that are considered original to an area either by the people themselves or by national governments, or to give ideas of cultural difference from state or global cultures of assimilation. In other cases, we have ethnohistorical data that indicates their migration movements, either in the past several hundred years or more recent. Some may enjoy relative independence, though this is rare; usually they suffer some kind of contact with encroaching states or corporations.

Often terms like *peasant* have been used for some, others have been considered original inhabitants and called *indigenous* or *aboriginal.* This term is usually employed only for the original inhabitants of Australia. It is also found in the social science literature interchangeably with "autochthonous" or "native." Both these latter terms are vague and usually misunderstood. Use of the term "primitive" has often in the past been applied to denote less complexity of technology and/or institutions, but in racist or nationalist literature it has meant demeaning qualities. I have only used this term in the sense of less complexity, while the term "traditional" is utilized to give the idea of the preservation of culture. Often in other texts people use the term "conservative," but today this term is tainted with political implication. I have avoided the term "tribal," as it denotes a certain kind of social organization and is often misused.

The terms "non-European" and "non-Western" are used specifically to note cultural or geographic location or culture, since the spread of Europeans has complicated the nature of local cultures and created confused results of acculturation. However, the qualities of local peoples need to be distinguished and in that effort I have applied these terms. The term "archaic" is sometimes used for "primitive" but this also distorts the meaning of the word and has usually been applied to pre-Christian or Bronze and Iron Age civilizations. In some of the literature today we find terms like "amoderns" or "non-moderns" and "extra-moderns." This is very confusing, as we find in biological anthropology the term included in "Anatomically Modern Humans" for contemporary people as opposed to extinct human populations that are not considered to be in our species. The term "pre-modern" is also used, as is "Archaic Humans." Some multiple terms used recently like "modern/contemporary stone age society" are even more confusing for people, as is "contemporary stone age," which is often inaccurate, as the people it is applied to are not using only a stone age technology.

It is a conundrum. Survival International and the British Association of Social Anthropologists (ASA) debated this issue in 2007, with Survival International claiming the term "indigenous" was both actuate and descriptive without being demeaning. The ASA disagreed and used the term "tribal," which was condemned by Survival International. The African Policy Information Center (November 1997) condemned the use of "tribe" as promoting timelessness and meaningless references to organization. Francis L.K. Hsu (1964) criticized the use of "primitive" but also "small" and "simple" as being interpreted as inferior. Terms like "rural" versus "urban" also are distorting, as they illustrate little as to any distinction and rural also often has a demeaning connotation. The same is true of "advanced" and "developed," as Steward noted in his theory of multilinear evolution, where the terms "stable" and "sustainable" value a certain level of orientation of a society to its ecological context and complex societies are not seen as either stable or sustainable, but short term and destructive.

I think it should be clear from this little note that I am using terms carefully to arrive at descriptions and comparisons that are based in knowledge and information of society in general and human endeavor in a long view.

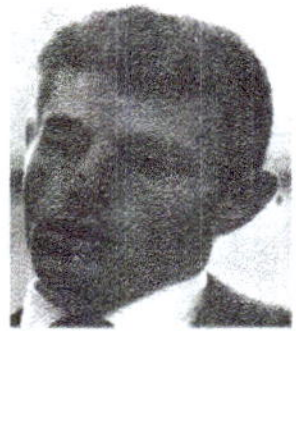

Fig. P.1 Photo of Robert Mogar

Reference

Hsu, Francis, (1964) "Rethinking the concept, 'Primitive,'" *Current Anthropology*, v. 5, n. 3, 169–178.

Contents

1 Introduction 1

2 A Question of Dose and Context: LSD, Peyote and Chemical Interactions, Human Variation, and Interpretation 33

3 Pursuit of the Miraculous or Just Piling up Confusion 135

4 A Thesis on LSD Research in the Laboratory and the Street: Sensory Deprivation, Surveys and the Mogar Laboratory, Creating Cures 213

5 The Indigenous View and Categories of Normality 249

6 A View of Possible Identities, Realities, and Futures 287

7 The Female Exception (in Research) and Gendered Experiences 305

8 Conclusion and Strange Threads 327

Appendix A: Genetics and LSD by Niccolo Caldararo 1967 337

Appendix B: Survey Questionnaire from 1966–1967 339

References 341

Index 351

List of Figures

Fig. 2.1	Grof's transpersonal experiences scheme parts I and II	59
Fig. 2.2	Chart of patterns reported for peyote by investigator	66
Fig. 2.3	Types of psychedelic experience	73
Fig. 2.4	Location of hallucination in the brain	80
Fig. 2.5	Chart on relation of trance, dreams, and other forms . From Bourguignon, 1972, reprinted with permission by Schenkman Publishing Company, Inc.	112
Fig. 2.6	From ffytche (2013), showing a number of intricate relationships between types of experience from hallucinations to visions as they are reported or tested. Reproduced with permission by MIT Press	113
Fig. 3.1	Table 1 of trance use in seeking to control supernatural powers from Bourguignon. Reprinted with permission by Schenkman Publishing Company, Inc.	140
Fig. 3.2	Ayahuasca archetypes or vision categories. *note, "fluorescent liquid" is a substance reported by Harner (1968, 1973) and called "the hyperdimensional trypamine" by the McKenna brothers, see McKenna (1993). Shannon, Benny (1997) "A cognitive-psychological study of ayahuasca," *MAPS Newsletter*, https://maps.org/news-letters/v07n3/07313sha.html. Based on Dr. Shannon's personal experiences and those of 19 subjects. Also his more comprehensive analysis of indigenous	

experiences and interpretation in Shannon, Benney (2002) *The Antipodes of the Mind*, Oxford University Press. Psychedelic Times Staff, (2017) "Universal archetypes of Ayahuasca dreams and making sense of your own visions," *Psychedelic Times*, March 14, https://psychedelictimes.com/the-universal- archetypes-of-ayahuasca-dreams-and-making-sense-of-your-own-visions/ 161

Fig. 4.1 Theodor Billroth during an operation 231

Fig. 5.1 Many voices with each person are set in the torso of the figure below; figurines from pre-Columbian Mesoamerica 272

Fig. 5.2 Within the self are held the voices of ancestors, spirits, and knowledge 272

Fig. 8.1 Chart of relation of segments of hallucinations, dreams, and so on and origins 330

List of Tables

Table 2.1 Blum et al. (1964) attributed the differences in outcome to expectation 50
Table 2.2 Summary of Native theory from Bourguignon (1972) and Laughlin (1976) 51
Table 6.1 Prevalence or appearance by gender of dream type 295
Table 7.1 Table of settings 1965–1967 318

1

Introduction

Some Contemporary Ideas About Getting High

As mentioned in the prelude, interpretation is central to understanding both the macro-level role of the use of mind-altering drugs in various societies and the individual's decision to take such drugs and the individual experience that then takes place. Recently I came across someone's experience with the drug ayahuasca. While Wade Davis and others have made its substances and preparation mysterious, others have argued that the active ingredient is DMT (Olson 2018). According to Schultes (1963) it is a decoction or infusion prepared from species of *Banisteriopsis*, mainly *B. caapi*, *B. inebrians*, and *B. rusbyana*. Since it is produced aboriginally over a wide area it is difficult to argue that a specific recipe produces the same active agency of compounds. The plant material is known to vary in concentration and is both collected from natural sources and grown in agricultural contexts (Linzer 1970). Lewin (1924) found that samples contained the chemical harmine, an alkaloid (also derived from the seeds of wild rue). An argument has also been made that some preparations contain the indole nucleus found in serotonin and LSD (Linzer 1970), while Hochstein & Paradies (1957) suggested the

N. Caldararo, *A Mental Ethnography: Conclusions From Research in LSD*,
https://doi.org/10.1007/978-3-031-13745-7_1

additional agent d-tetrahydroharmine (Evans and Evans 2009). Another complication is the interpretation of effects in two contexts, to some indigenous users in Peru the drug separates the soul and body and some experience this separation as a death, to some people of Columbia they experience a return to the womb, while others die and are reborn (Schultes 1972). Since these reports come from a variety of sources there may be translation or interpretation problems.

One can appreciate the desperation many people feel today in a world as disconnected as ours. The desire for community and meaning has caused many to search for these among Native peoples of the world. There is a central and important problem here, however, one that impinges on the survival of Native peoples and their cultures. In this regard, an article in the Pacific *Sun* newspaper by Mr. "Bill Smith" ("Visions of Moderation," April, 17–23, 2019) is a particular example of this problem.

Mr. Smith tells a common tale of personal distress and lack of orientation in our modern atomized society. It is a standard narrative of loss, suffering, and discovery, then personal triumph. He has had a history with drugs and alcohol and seeks to reorient his life with a Native practice centered around the ingestion of the combination of Amazonian plant extracts called generally ayahuasca. He refers to having just finished journalist Michael Pollan's book on his experiments with LSD as a contexting reference to his journey to join a group of similarly inclined Americans to now try ayahuasca. I think that the documentary film by Terry Macy and Daniel Hart, *White Shamans and Plastic Medicine Men* (1996), captures the feelings of many Native American people regarding the non-Native use of aspects of their culture and religion. The film showcases a number of Euro-Americans who have found salvation in Native American culture and religion. Goodison (1995) describes in a number of cases people interpreting their dreams in ethnographic meaning, that this is a search for authenticity that overlooks the nature of individual experience and background.

Ayahuasca has been found to produce "beneficial mindfulness" and self-acceptance in some subjects as well as act as a therapeutic agent for some disorders in patients (Domingue-Clave et al. 2016). It is now part of a considerable mass movement. There are some aspects of neural plasticity that have been associated in recent years with therapeutic effects.

The idea of psychoplastogens has become associated with treatments for some disorders, for example, PTSD (Olson 2021). These are claimed to "rewire neural circuitry," especially pyramidal neurons in the prefrontal cortex (PFC). Ketamine is one of these chemicals. It began use in Belgium in the 1960s as an anesthesia for animals and was approved for humans by the FDA in 1970. It is a short-acting drug with hallucinogenic effects sometimes described as trance-like and providing pain relief. Usually given intravenously, it was often abused in the 1970s and 1980s, called "Special K" by its street enthusiasts.

Mr. Smith sought a "message" to help him. Not finding it in cannabis he thought ayahuasca could produce one of value. Herein lies the rub. I have taken several mind-enhancing drugs, some in a scientific setting and some in aboriginal ones. In all cases my intent was entirely scientific and in that I differ both from people like Mr. Smith and from the aboriginal and indigenous people I worked with. Nevertheless, Wade Davis in his book *Light at the Edge of the World*, where many people first learn about ayahuasca, stresses the importance of the Native milieu and enculturation to a given meaning to the experience. In fact, the personal context with the plant is often described as so strong it is conceived as an entity that speaks (or sings) to the individual and people and can be seen as types of spirits like humans, as it is related by the Chukchee (Bogoras 1907, 1910; Davis 2001).

A Native American shaman once remarked when I described young San Franciscans' behavior when they took Belladonna or Datura (natural plants with atropine poison) that "they should not do that, the spirits will trick them, they will not know the harm done." Atropine is found in some other plants used for spiritual uses or healing, as in the mushroom *Amanita muscaria* (Buck 1961; Evans and Evans 2009). The drug was widely used among Native America people, often in rituals of initiation, as in the case of the Virginia Natives in contact with Jamestown, where the jimson weed was used in the puberty ordeals of boys. It induced a period of painful physical conditions related to the lack of food and this resulted in hallucinations.

The Hopi used it in medical conditions, the Zuni as an anesthetic and analgesic for wounds and broken bones, the Yokuts to induce dreams, and the Navajo for divination and prophesy. Among the Mountain Cahuilla, it was used as part of a prayer against shortage of food or water, but later changes in southern groups led to its use as an aid in initiation of boys (Gayton 1928, 29). Also, the Mauche used it as a punishment for unruly children and the Jivaro gave it as a means to have the ancestral spirits admonish such children in hallucinations (La Barre 1975, 36). Also, it was used aboriginally for healing and communicating with the spirits and was a powder of *Anadenanthera peregrine*, with archaeological evidence of its introduction into the nose via a pipe made of puma bone at the site of Inca cueva in Argentina (residue of variety, *A. colubrine cebil*, as bufotenin, a tryptamine related to serotonin, and N, N-Dimethyltryptamine or DMT [an analog to tryptamine] were found; Pochettino et al. 1999) dated to 2130 BCE, in Central Peru dating to 1200 BCE, and reported by Friar Ramon Pane used among the Taino in 1511. Another "snuff" taken by Native Americans, some in the Orinoco area, was from the Virola and Myristica species of trees (related to nutmeg), derived from the bark containing DMT-like derivatives (Schultes 1967; Holmstedt et al. 1980).

Some of these DMT-like derivative drugs are used on a daily basis by Native peoples, as argued by Chagnon et al. (1971) for the Waika groups of the Orinoco like the Yanomamo. The extent of the use in Central and South America is quite amazing, as Schultes and Hoffmann (1973) document. Chagnon (1968) reports they use it with "green tobacco." The drug is produced from the bark of the ebene tree, ground into powder, and blown into the nostrils with a pipe. It is said to induce colored visions and allows one to contact their particular miniature demons (*hekura* spirits), after which if they appear, they are invited to live in one's chest. These demons apparently can be aids in sickening enemies (Chagnon 1968, 109). Joined to a man by the drug, the two can fly into the cosmos, where the *hekura* attack enemy spirits, and at the end of the universe, in fragments they can heal friends as well.

Chagnon relates an amusing story of taking the drug with the Yanomamo to support their religion against the missionaries who condemned it. Chagnon's rather typical singing and dancing under the influence is not so remarkable, given his study of it, as his voluntary compliance with accepting the *hekura* during his hallucinations. He states it was the freedom of a new consciousness the drug gave him that was so much more pleasurable and exciting than the pain of the process. He emphasizes the important role of the social group in the use of the drug as does Harner (1972) and Kensinger (1972) as well as de Rios (1984).

The similarity of Chagnon's description of the use and effects of the drug on the Yanomamo is quite parallel to the earliest historical report by Las Casas, where it seems to have been used to consider problems and build solidarity (Las Casas 1909). However, reports of the use of the pods of the yupa, which is reported to be *Anadenanthera peregrine*, indicate behavior like drunkenness, incoherent ramblings, and violent attacks, as in the description by Padre Gumilla in his *El Orinoco Illustrado* published in Madrid in 1741.

We often hear of visions but they are seldom described.

Yet the books produced by Carlos Castaneda's Don Juan adventure (real or imagined) promoted the use of this dangerous drug. And others promoted the use of a new drug: 2, 5-Dimethoxy-4-methyl-amphetamine (or *STP*). I must admit I never took ayahuasca, but never had the "authentic" opportunity or desire in research. The other possibility concerning drugs and experiences is the placebo effect. While I would not suggest that what many people report concerning their experiences under what is called "Ayahuasca," is suspect. Nor am I dismissing the claims Wade Davis has made for the preparations used in Voodoo. Nevertheless, one cannot discount the power of suggestion or of the history of the placebo as Arthur and Elaine Shapiro (1997) documented in their extensively researched book. Illusions produced through context and suggestion can also be powerful (Botvinick and Cohen 1998). Rivers' (1920) discussion and examples of one mind's control of others, whether human or non-human are also still useful here. I have provided a table of responses and experiences people have reported on what was called ayshuasca, some of these are from indigenous accounts, most are from Euro-Americans.

Traditionally, the means of distinguishing between hallucinations and illusions was that the illusion was a misperception of real objects or scenes (Bentall and Varese 2013). There is a remarkable seduction in the appeal of the Other, and many people attempt to adopt the lifeways of indigenous people, as both a balm to their dissatisfaction with life and modern culture and the assumed authenticity and power of the aboriginal. Some people use this adoption as a self-help method; others foist it on people who are seeking relief and a storm-free port of consciousness. I do not condemn their desire to seek peace or discover adventures. However, I do find it unreasonable for people to take advantage of this Native knowledge to increase their stature and wealth.

A Start to Learn the Ropes of Studying the Mind

As I mentioned, in the 1960s as a student at Humboldt State College I worked on experiments in sensory deprivation. Later, when I participated in scientific research in the use of various sensory-enhancing substances, often referred to as hallucinatory drugs, including LSD, at the San Francisco State College, then, now, university. One of the grants the scientists I worked with had received was to test such drugs on addicts and alcoholics for potential therapeutic uses. The leader of one of these inquires was Dr. Robert Mogar. Many subjects suffered from depression and other conditions. This research showed considerable interest until it was stopped by legislation making many of the drugs illegal or the research unfundable. Mogar published a summary of the nature of treatment and cures as well as the variations seen in outcome among different researchers and clinicians (Mogar 1968). Mr. Smith, described at the beginning of this section, like many of these individuals, sought relief from his suffering and states he did not have sufficient funds to go to a regular therapist. The idea of substituting a drug for the expertise of a physician seems strange, but is characteristic of the independent nature of many Americans, and yet also of the attitude of American males, especially toward seeing doctors. Taking a pill suggested by the author of a book, or some friend, carries more weight, unfortunately for some. But some people do feel they have authority to "spread the word" about one drug experience or another.

Some apparently are so filled with hubris that they believe they have something to share that is valuable to others. Michael Pollan (2021) has suggested to millions that the use of Native knowledge is the best way to experiment with drugs. This is irresponsible; he uses all the usual references, like Tim Leary's "set and setting" (which I will discuss later and is not original to him) and physician Andrew Weil's position on the subject.

Weil was an early critic of public use of psychedelics that he saw going on at Harvard between researchers like Leary and Alpert and students. He wrote a series of articles in the Harvard *Crimson*, where he states, "shoddiness of their work as scientists… less [the result] of incompetence than of a conscious rejection of scientific ways of looking at things" (Russin and Weil 1973). Weil has been the subject of the same charge, that he promotes nutrients, supplements, and treatments that are not scientifically tested or proven (MacFarquhar 1997). I found it amusing as I read through Weil, Lattin, and Stevens' reports on the Harvard researchers' scene, that compared to Berkeley, Harvard was awash in a variety of drug parties and scandal. At Berkeley, where some of the faculty I knew had taken psychedelics (mainly magic) mushrooms, they had research projects in Central America and elsewhere and were knowledgeable in the cultural background of the psychedelics. There was a quiet movement of gatherings, but mostly very private. But this comparison may be inaccurate, for if we focus our comparison with the Palo Alto/Stanford area, we get a more balanced picture—there were a number of clinicians using LSD and other psychedelics, some on a large scale as Janiger, with institutes set up to collect data and acquire grants, as Myron Stolaroff's Foundation for Advanced Study in Menlo Park, or the Multidisciplinary Association for Psychedelic Studies (MAPS), in San Jose. When LSD was made illegal, Stolaroff moved his research to other promising drugs like 2C-T-2 and 2C-T-7, which were like mescaline (Stolaroff 2005). So if we include work at northern hospitals like Napa, research in Berkeley and San Francisco as well as the Stanford area, we have more experimentation, but still, in my opinion less campus-located notoriety at least until 1967. I know Mogar did some work with Stolaroff's group, mainly I believe, to help with the Minnesota multiphasic personality inventory (MMPI) tests and seemed to be involved with patients in a variety of experiments with Willis Harman, but I do not recall ever meeting Stolaroff, though people came and went both at the Mogar Lab and at the hospitals and I was seldom introduced to visitors unless there was something I was working on (especially the private uses of drugs, as in the Haight). Mogar quit the research program in Menlo Park and dropped his work on LSD with an announcement on May 24, 1966. He was fed up with the political environment, where he felt he had to take "sides" on the nature of the drug. He was neither for nor against, but as a scientist he felt the milieu was no longer constructive and the way Leary and others were romanticizing the psychedelic experience was ruining any possibilities of clear understanding of value (Daily Gater Staff 1966). Mogar had set up an organization for the study of psychedelics at San Francisco State College in 1965, the Institute for Psychedelic Research, but all the sensational media attention in the following year caused the College to back out.

Also, as Don Lattin (2010) tells it, Weil was part of the Harvard Psychedelic Club set up by Tim Leary and Alpert, and his involvement appears to have lacked the restraint he later espouses (Weil 1972). He has become a guru to many and the creator of a million-dollar health industry as well as become a large figure in the New Age healing and food movement (Baer 2008). Weil's suggestions for drug use, as are Pollan's (and both of their promotion of food fads), fall short of science and seem more like business. There was an abundance of good intensions and solid science in Leary's PhD at UC Berkeley in Clinical Psychology. It was based on his work at Kaiser hospital in Oakland, where he studied the effects of treatment methods on admitting patients suffering from psychological pathologies versus those on waiting lists who received no treatment. He found no differences in outcomes (Greenfield 2006). The failure of the techniques of psychology to cure left him in crisis to find some alternative, especially after his wife committed suicide when his affair with another women was known (Lattin 2017).

While I would not tell anyone what to do or advise them on any medical issue (having abandoned the study of medicine for anthropology 50 years ago), there are numerous caveats to drug use, and I counsel caution. Like the Kogi who train young acolytes for years to see the world as it is to them, preparation is everything, yet naiveté and innocence are also of value (Davis 2001). Those who try and mold the experience of others in our context and transpose cultural elements, as mentioned above, like Timothy Leary and Ram Dass, who interjected the *Tibetan Book of the Dead* into others' experience, seem investing in an effort contradictory to self-discovery or invention. I should mention that Leary and many of his associates in this project had engaged in years of serious, scientific research with psychedelics (see Blum et al. 1964). The personal use of indigenous peoples' cultural materials out of context is considered by most of them to be destructive of their identities and to be a kind of theft. The Lakota have declared war on such practices, and as I advised people above who are considering the use of indigenous culture in this way, they should first see the film *White Shamans and Plastic Medicine Men*, produced by Native Americans.

We must keep in mind that we are dealing with a cultural complex that is ancient and appears widely across the globe and over time in human society. These psychedelics or hallucinogens have had important roles in human society and their use and the type of drug used have changed over time. Human society is seldom static, as La Barre (1975) notes; the Texas buckeye, *Ungnadia speciosa*, a very toxic plant, has been found in archaeological contexts, where its use was supplanted by the red bean (*Sophora secundiflora*), sometimes called "mescal beans" or "dry whiskey." Also they are referred to as the seeds of the Texas Mountain Laurel. Ingestion of these produces visions and served as a divinatory medium for a number of groups. They contain three major alkaloids: cytosine, sparteine, and methylcytisine (Bourn et al. 1979). The Beans produce similar behavior responses in rats as mescaline, DMT, and psilocybin, but not normal saline, amphetamine, pentobarbital, and THC. Use of the Red Bean drug as prepared by the Pawnee initiates resulted in a dance with "peculiar jumping movements" (Skinner 1926). La Barre (1975) theorized that a red bean cult had preceded and influenced the later peyote cult, given archaeological evidence.

The Guegue, Acroa, Pimenteira, and Atanaye of Eastern Brazil once made a "miraculous drink" from *Mimosa hostilis*, which gave them "glorious visions of the spirit land" used especially before going to war (Schultes and Hofmann 1973). It is known to contain DMT and has been used in healing (Ott 1998). It is frustrating that reports of use of plant extracts with the same active agents are reported to produce "madness" in some but visions of great complexity in others. See also regarding this the use of the hallucinogenic drug curupa by the Omagua of Brazil (Hemming 1978, 431), related by some to *A. columbria* or *A. peregrine* and what is often called ayahuasca (see also, Safford 1916). One imagines that the reporters have failed to accurately describe the condition or that there is some other factor involved, either method of preparation, additives, or differences in digestion or action (Schultes and Hofmann 1973, 182–5). But this reference to "madness" appears in much of the research in psychedelics, certainly for LSD but also mescaline. Sinnett (1970) claimed to have experienced several clinical conditions of psychosis, but his description shows he retained a presence of mind that allowed him to differentiate between illness (peyote-induced perceptions) and reality.

Rinkel's general idea, mentioned above, as in many of the researchers at Sandoz, was that the drug could induce a legitimate case of insanity so researchers could study it (Stevens 1988; Osmond and Smythies 1953; Osmond 1970). This seems reasonable from the perspective of their clinical experience; they had a trove of reports from patients and other psychiatrists of what "madness" seemed like. This is another problem we face, not only in our definitions of psychological states, but also in changes in time affected by contact. When people write that psychotic disorders are recognized across cultures with patterns of symptoms that are similar (Murphy 1976; Myers 2011), we should note that not only culture contact has produced new stresses and changes in lifeways, information, media, religion, and definitions of illness, but the very tools for diagnosis are derived from contact and Western medicine. Also, it must be recognized that these tools have undergone considerable re-evaluation and change over the past few decades (Andreasen 1989). One of these criteria is when a person hallucinates several times a day (Laroi et al. 2014), but with some new explanations of consciousness, for example, that of Seth (2021), where consciousness is defined as "controlled hallucinations," the aspect of pathology becomes more a determination of the person's interpretation or learning of controlling hallucination than that of having them. The interpretation of a cosmologically shattering event can also be considered a "hallucination" until sufficient information is present. Until that occurs, the event/hallucination may be defined in cosmological terms as when Australian miners arrived in the interior of the New Guinea highlands and were perceived as ghosts of the dead or spirits on first contact (Anderson and Connolly 1983). Levy-Bruhl (1966) reports on dozens of similar events. There is a parallel here with "epic dreaming," sometimes referred to as "excessive dreaming" that can cause an individual to have daytime fatigue (Nielsen 2011). These dreams can take place all night in the perception of the individual and, occur nightly in 90% of patients who otherwise appear normal. Such "dreaming" in the daytime might appear as a form of schizophrenia.

One wonders how much of what those using LSD and other psychedelics experienced was influenced by the assumption of psychosis production. Osmond (1970, 27) refers to his experience several times as "the psychosis." His conclusion from his experience with peyote is the same as his perception of the schizophrenic, an illness and not a window to alternative universes or spiritual ladders. Huxley (1954) seems to have been made aware of the essential difference between a person on psychedelics and one with schizophrenia, the element of knowledge (frame of reference) that it is drug-induced and will end. This was emphasized by Huxley's wife Maria Nys, in a letter to Osmond of the factor of time limit and artificiality of the drug experience (Ens 2020). From a phenomenological viewpoint, however, it seems filled with hubris, as if looking at the surface of an ocean could inform you on what was within it. It also assumed that madness did not differ from one individual to another and that the categories of psychological research and practice did produce real internal species of pathological psychic states. From an anthropological perspective I would offer this definition: madness, the inability to respond appropriately to conditioned social reality. This is derived from Wallace (1972). But he notes, "Different societies do encourage different styles of mental illness." The meaning here is that societies produce conditions of stress that people respond to differently, but that many societies value forms of what we consider "madness." Some inabilities are functional and derived from pathologies or trauma; others can be induced by charismatic or hypnotic individuals. There are many described, and practitioners like Laing (Laing and Esterson 1964) offer a variety of contexts and a multitude of pathologies (psychoses) made the entity (madness) very slippery and vague (see the DSM-5 on this variety). It seems that one difficulty with these definitions of psychosis, madness, mental illness, and other similar terms is that they are often culture bound, as Wallace (1972) points out. In this regard, it is interesting that early studies of psychopathologies found that they graded in appearance with the degree of acculturation of African populations (Doob 1957). In fact, non-European peoples' way of thinking has often been defined as illogical, prelogical, or abnormal given the values and mode of thinking of Westerners

(Levy-Bruhl 1966). But as I have shown in my 2017 book, illogical thinking or any idea of an evolution of thought in complex societies over simpler, even Neolithic or Paleolithic peoples cannot be demonstrated. People today, no matter where, act often in illogical, stupid and ignorant ways and there does not seem to be any scale on which we can measure consistencies over time or type of society.

Osmond and Abram Hoffer produced a theory that the oxidation of adrenaline (epinephrine), which produced the chemical adrenochrome, was a pathway for psychosis. Central to it was their general idea that madness could be a result of chemical imbalances or abnormalities. Osmond ingested some adrenochrome and had an experience of vibrant colors and distorted vision and feelings of disorientation that seemed to verify their theory. They suggested that by preventing oxidation with anti-oxidants in the brain they could correct schizophrenia and other mental illnesses. Attempts at using megadoses of anti-oxidants were not successful in curing mental illness (Hoffer et al. 1954; Vaughan and McConaghy 1999; but see Smythies 2010). Later it was suggested that adrenochrome was involved in the neurotoxicity related to neuromelanin (Smythies 1996). As neuromelanin is missing from the brain at birth and accumulates as we age, as is associated with Parkinson's disease (PD), recent studies have focused on the instability and degeneration of melanin-containing neurons, but a role for adrenochrome has still not been established (Haining and Achat-Mendes 2017).

Sacks (2012) relates how patients with PD were often treated with L-Dopa, but post-encephalitic patients with a form of PD given L-Dopa often had dramatic dreams, "excessively vivid" ones, or nightmares. This is certainly curious, as the drug, produced naturally by plants and animals, including humans, when lacking causes pathology as PD, but when given to some patients who suffered encephalitis gave them unusual dreams and hallucinations.

As opposed to CBS, where trauma has occurred in the visual areas and pathways, in PD, post-encephalitic parkinsonism and Lewy body disease, there is damage to the brain stem and associated structures as in peduncular hallucinosis, though neurons in the visual association cortex have been found with Lewy bodies. These conditions can produce images of animal heads on walls, people in costumes, children playing and killing other people, marching in of an army and animals nearby or faces appearing distorted, people in posters or paintings coming alive, and clothes moving about as if alive (Sacks 2012). These have been interpreted as dreams or dream fragments invading daytime perceptions. Often in Alzheimer's disease and Lewy body disease, any hallucinations appear in a complex delusion, as where the patient "sees" a loved one as an alien or imposter. The relationship between hallucination and delusion is most interesting (Morrison 2002). Separating the two is often difficult, especially where belief borders on delusion and faith (Al-Issa 1995; Stanghellini 2008; Pierre 2001; Shermer 2011). We have visited this issue with religion before, but its relation to hallucinations, visions, and delusion as well as fantasy has seldom been treated in comprehensive fashion. In his assessment, Stevens (1988) seems to imply that by their experience with psychedelics, Huxley and Leary came to the delusion that they could change the world for the better with the drugs.

In another clue to the creative and reactive aspect of some hallucinations, Sacks (2012) reports that many of his parkinsonian post-encephalitic patients experienced pleasant and often social hallucinations. He considered these as a means of their brains compensating for the lack of social interaction. Hallucinations with nature or sexual contact were frequent.

Another curious fact applies to drugs used to produce hallucinations, visions, states of pleasure, and "religious" terror, suggested by La Barre (1964). The number of plants that produce active agents used by the Natives of the Americas far outnumbers the few available in the rest of the globe. La Barre called this the "New World narcotic complex" and theorized that for some unknown reason Native Americans were "culturally programmed" to value, seek, remember, and use psychotropic plants. Schultes (1970) has given a comprehensive account of world use of hallucinogens. One might modify this theory and offer that the recent entry of Native peoples into the Americas in small groups upon two continents devoid of other humans allowed for a more concentrated botanical experience different cultural choices result from varied histories and opportunities in association with the chance availability of liable plants of use. One can reference Kroeber's (1944) "configurations of culture" or Ruth Benedict's (1934) "patterns of culture." But I think Francis Hsu's (1969) development of this idea is more apt here. One also has to keep in mind that not all drug experiences have developed as we have come to see them today. The fact that a drug might appear to make people "mad" or stupefy them might have had other utility in an aboriginal state. The Dobe use of a plant containing *Puncratium trianthum* (associated with trance) by the group is apparently a means of social healing and solidarity with and without the interpretation of visions or supernatural beings (Shostak 1983).

Diggers, Pranksters, Media, and Scientists

The performer of belief, the shaman, sorcerer, soothsayer, or priest has the responsibility of representing and transmitting information to people who depend on the cultural perceptions of their ancestors for survival. In English we have a number of interesting borrowings of words that reflect this responsibility and role. The word "sorcerer" is derived from the Latin, feminine root of the word "fate." In some ethnographic settings the sorcerer uses various means to communicate with the spirits and learn the future, or at least the shades of the future. The Anglo-Saxon root for the word "soothsayer" is "truth," for the combination with "sayer," of one who speaks the truth. The Greek word "magikos" is similar in meaning to the Old Persian Magu or priests and we often find in literature the equation of magicians with Chaldean religion or that of Zoroastrians. Some of these practitioners read the signs of the stars, others read signs as well, but also could intuit aspects of purity and light, guilt or sin, for individuals as fate. Ideas associated with magic and rites in the Middle Ages were derived from confused ideas of these religions, Greek and Roman beliefs as well as those of pre-Christian European religions. The idea of the wizard who has power to cajole spirits is derived from the Old Nose word "Viskr" or clever. This gives rise to our understanding in all religions and beliefs, whether in organized form (as today in Christianity, Buddhism, or Islam) or unorganized in animism or even the ancient "wise woman" of the pre-Christian village—that the ability to predict and give practical advice is founded on a knowledge of how people live, how they age, what works in any locality, and what usually happens in certain circumstances.

To know someone means, in this context, to have knowledge of how they act.

Phenomenology has long placed an emphasis on the problem of interpretation of experience; this is a core issue in the case of LSD. Since the 1960s renewed interest has attempted to appreciate the human potential from drugs like LSD. Amanda Feilding of the Beckley Foundation described briefly the interest the Foundation has had in this research for over 20 years (Feilding 2014), especially in the use of brain imaging (Carhart-Harris et al. 2016). But much of this reflects on Terence and Dennis McKenna's (1992) theory that hallucinogens were central to the evolution of human consciousness and cognitive abilities. Their ideas had unfolded over their period of drug experiments in the 1960s and 1970s on themselves mainly, and in various areas of the world where they could partake of indigenous local plant sources. Their ideas were not too different from many people in the 1960s who held similar views, like Leary, a few of the Diggers I met, and many in the commune movement.

But as opposed to Leary and the Merry Pranksters, the Diggers were anonymous. It appears that two New Yorkers, Emmet Grogen and Billy Murcett, formed a core of expression, putting out posters on a number of topics signed "The Diggers." David Simpson states that those involved in daily routines called these "Communication Company" papers, which Grogen (1972) states were superseded by the *Free City News*. There were also broadsides referred to as the *Digger Papers* on a variety of subjects. If Leary was encouraging people to drop out, the Diggers were calling on people to do things, get involved, and their free food program was the most obvious expression of this engagement. They played on all aspects of American hierarchical corporate culture and constructed their own activities as a mocking gaggle of decentralized and jovial conspirators (the Digger Docs 2022). There was also among the Diggers a feeling that the atmosphere of the Haight-Ashbury was being commodified. The new stores with their beads, Indian clothing, religious objects, and books on spirituality were giving a tilt to the aroma of the opportunity of new change that seemed to be dragging things into the past. The *Digger Papers* was meant to be a reaction to the San Francisco *Oracle*, an "underground paper" that Grogan considered part of the "new, hip, moneyed class" that was moving in.

The *Digger Papers* were "an attempt to antagonize the street people into an awareness of the absolute bullshit implicit in the psychedelic transcendentalism promoted by the self-proclaimed, media-fabricated shamans who espoused the tune-in, turn-on, drop-out, jerk-off ideology of Leary and Alpert" (Grogan 1972, 238). What the Diggers were trying to do, to live a free life, could be summed up by the radical conclusion of David Simpson, "More or less we were trying to promulgate a spirit of self-reliance—that is, reliance on self and friends and family—outside the system. There was a sense that we were really building something, but by the end of the summer of '67, it was clear that it was just overwhelming. Too many people." This is an aspect of Psychological Anthropology that I discuss in the Goodman Building ethnography. The process of a small group of people living together and meeting regularly produces a form of interactionalism that binds people as understanding one another, beyond the superficial level of language as Mogar and others, especially Vygotsky, argued. I am not talking of cults, though I am sure such methods work for a kind of brainwashing, but rather a process of getting to know each other in a context that becomes like a small village. People can see what each other does and can assess and criticize the motives and outcome of behavior. In the Goodman ethnography I discuss the element of group pressure and of a "tyranny of leaderlessness" where both responsibility can be amorphous and denied and at the same time manipulation can be masqueraded as consensus. For the Diggers and the Haight in 1965–1968, what started as a small group of people who used LSD as a means of understanding themselves and the cosmos they lived in got buried in a tsunami of people and media redefinition.

Like any movement, having control of your identity is important. *The Digger Papers* and other forms of their communications attempted this voice. It is clear they failed and I recall how absurd were the ideas the media extracted from their "sources" about hippies and what was "happening." Ideas like hippies wanted to build a great statue of St. Francis in the Haight, repeated by Stevens (1988), is simply the kind of imagined reporting that was going on, though putting on people was something the Diggers did do, as both a test and a reality check, as David Simpson relates with an interview of a *Ramparts* reporter (the Digger Docs). People spread rumors and fantastic ideas about what hippies did as a means of expressing the extent of the hometown Other that was present in their minds, like the bizarre images of bikers as hippies in *Easy Rider*, the confused violence of *Zabriske Point* or *Upon a Time in Hollywood.* What was interesting was that these were projections of what people wanted to see, participate in, and whether those reporting the crazy events were Americans, young people, old, or from Mars, the fact was that you could go to this place in America where it was believed that people were on LSD and other drugs continuously, all lived in communal crash pads, had unprotected sex every day, and that they were on the edge of paradise or some other strange and exotic world of the unseen walking before you in a magical world. Nonsense, but it made great copy.

But then that was the problem of source and legitimacy. Who could speak for the Haight? Many of the articles and books written about the Haight-Ashbury of the 1960s create a stereotype of long-haired males and free-love women in drug communes. I visited several hundred people in their homes in the 1960s in the Haight and a few who lived in "communes" where everything was common. Rather, the vast majority were young people living together, sharing flats and costs, but with separate incomes and savings. Some students, especially the political ones, called their living arrangements "collectives," as they shared work and rent, but this was not different. But if the Diggers were anonymous, then the voice of the crowd is the random person. Ideas about change, the future, ethics, and morals quite varied. As I recall, some people were quite ethical, no stealing, no getting drunk, no heroin, for example. These were generally the political-leaning ones, others, like the Diggers and people who listened to Abby Hoffman and his crew, saw stealing as a political act of solidarity with poor and oppressed people the world over. But to many it was a symbol that the "movement" surrounding psychedelics and the "counterculture" was defining itself as an enemy of society rather than a healer of the societal problems it objected to. The house I was living at in the Haight on Oak Street in 1967 with two other students turned into a crash pad and one night they had a party with nearly 100 people. The flat was a two-bedroom, but one student lived in what was called in San Francisco at the time a utility room that was off the kitchen and led to a very large backyard that was overgrown. During the party someone I knew came up to me and said there was a problem, as the only toilet had been occupied for nearly an hour. I went to the door of the toilet and banged on it, but there was no answer. The door, however, had a lock that could be unlocked with a piece of sheet metal, as it often happened to be locked by accident. I opened the door and found two people huddled over the sink heating up a spoon of heroin (or something) for their injection. I yelled at them that it was not allowed and grabbed their fix (apparatus), threw it in the toilet, and flushed it. I then told them to leave. Two things had happened that were characteristic of the change in atmosphere: one, the two individuals had greedily seized the bathroom against the common need. The other was that their use of the drug, though a personal choice, had been made without agreement of others and so any repercussions would require other people, myself included, to deal with the outcome. Such parasitic behavior was a common problem. The common ethos was that you should take care of people even if they were harming themselves, and while that Christian-like attitude worked on a lot of people, it camouflaged the actual process of manipulating and exploiting other people. I was told I had been "authoritarian," but as they had violated my space, I felt justified. Not everyone agreed. Yet hard drugs like heroin began to seep in everywhere and were eroding the environment. As one of the old Russian women who ran Andy's Café on Haight told me after the first mass conflicts on the street, "Revolution is chaos. The best and worst are attracted, the best killed and the worst rule."

What seemed to permeate everything in the late 1960s in the Haight was the radical spirit of the time, as Dave Simpson put it in the Digger Docs. This was framed in the Civil Rights Movement and set the tone for how people saw their relationship to African Americans and racism. One of the interesting aspects of Helen Perry's (1970) ethnography of the Haight-Ashbury in the 1960s is the results of her interviews with long-time residents and their views of "hippies" and drugs. While generally supportive, and this included the Haight-Ashbury Neighborhood Committee (HANC), they were both proud of being integrated and tolerant and yet also dismayed at the flood of people. The varied experiences people were having, even with marijuana, but mainly LSD and peyote, could be seen as responsible for the different views that came to be seen as the "Haight-Ashbury"—for some a spiritual cosmos, for others a revolution for a new society, and everything in between.

Stanislav Grof called it the "LSD effect," and its nature had been generally drawn from his experience with hundreds of patients, subjects, students, and fellow investigators over his long career. The diversity of response to the drug had given him a unique understanding of how it functioned, yet also produced a caution to its application and expectations. In 1967 the paper I wrote was produced because of popular misconceptions and fantasies concerning the nature of the LSD experience and the research concerning its use. I was seeing published articles in the media and in scientific venues that seemed to me biased and tinged with sensationalism. Also, I argued the paper was needed due to the distasteful knee-jerk response of the national and state legislature and law enforcement. However, in retrospect, while these were factors, the primary reason was to place the effects of the drug and the social response, legal, scientific, and journalistic, into a framework of human evolution and social institutional development.

The obvious question to me centered on "why this negative response? What is its purpose? And what are people afraid of?" Between 1966 and 1969 I had spent over two years digesting every article I could find on LSD, but most of this literature focused on the scientific work and I often strayed into related subjects of other drugs that had significant effects on consciousness, manifested as spiritual, therapeutic, or other forms. This research led me to a study of the Black Plague and how it was linked with the number of mass psychogenic events of the fourteenth century. This phenomenon was often referred to in the literature as an illness, and this explanation has continued to the present, with a diffuse diagnosis and vague description (Bartholomew and Wessely 2002). I eventually wrote my dissertation on the subject of the Black Death (Bubonic Plague) in 1999, and reworked it for publication in 2012. Obviously there were social consequences to the Black Plague, the upheaval has been considered the opening of the Renaissance, and Huxley and Leary considered psychedelics a cure for a modern plague as well as a new spiritual renaissance.

In my interviews with subjects and study of their MMPI results, there did seem to be the kind of searching for new answers to the problems of society. With Vietnam becoming more of an issue, the nuclear bomb, and questions of racism and inequalities rising in significance, the critiques of the time were pressing. So I began a more in-depth study of what people thought the answers might be. I lived in a house with other students and it became a "crash pad" due to one of them inviting travelers from Colorado to live with us. I met groups of communes and people with ideas of change, as in the Diggers and their free store and food feeds. I write about this in detail in my book about the Goodman Building (Caldararo 2019). And in these adventures across the Bay Area, to Colorado and Southern California and New York, I lived with, spoke to, and listened to hundreds of people's ideas. I also observed their drug experiments.

The first 14 original pages also contained my observations of people taking LSD over a five-year period from 1966 to 1970 and included living with people who took the drug, personal relationships with them, observing how drug use affected personal relationships, routines, and attitudes. Knowledge of some of the individuals dated back at least ten years and so the information contained in the report covered hundreds of conversations, dozens of interviews, formal and informal, and discussion groups, both as part of university research projects and my own work. This includes my own experience with the drug, but only prior to 1967, as I have no experience with the later street illegal versions of the drug.

As an introduction to the analysis of the experiences recorded and viewed, I undertook an investigation of linguistic symbolism as it relates to individual understanding. Contextual information, as described by E.T. Hall (1959, 1969), and the cultural bases, as described by Sapir (1921) and Whorf (Whorf 1946, 1956a, b), were also considered, but a focus was on the means of determining how one conceptualizes symbolic representation in language. I place this idea of symbol in the context of the evolution of the brain and social life in a recent work (Caldararo 2017). But my research led me to communes and "squats" (illegal occupation of buildings) in the Western Addition of San Francisco, where large African American and Japanese American neighborhoods existed. Redevelopment was in the process of evicting most of these residents, which caused considerable stress on community organizations of both ethnic groups. The use of language under such conditions often displays these stresses in either increased vernacular to promote unity and identity or increased reliance on standard terms to increase a group's social identity with the dominant ethnic group, and is also true of code switching

(Harrison 2007; Gardner-Chloros 2009). It was remarkable to me how similar were the terms used in the LSD/peyote subculture (including "hippies"). I attributed this to the rapid and substantial movement of members of this community from place to place, coast to coast, and Spain or Afghanistan to San Francisco.

Two other works produced at this time appear in this book as Chaps. 3 and 4. Chapter 3 includes the original thesis proposal, which I have modified and greatly expanded, and Chap. 4 is derived from lab notes at Humboldt and some notes from the Mogar Lab experience and my internship at Napa State Hospital in 1966–1967. This chapter has also undergone substantial expansion from later research in the anatomy and biochemistry of the brain.

Some Reflections on the Human Brain

The nature of experiential information I present here is concerned with the possible roots of generational conflict, that is, the differential experiential background and categorization of information by different age groups and/or subgroups within a traditional society. This idea can apply to complex industrial societies as well, given that we know how brain development in children and teenagers is an ongoing process until early adulthood, with a proliferation of neurons followed by a "pruning" or regional reduction and then substantial connectivity growth. Though this is not unique to humans (Herculano-Houzel et al. 2010; Hofman 2014) but is similar in primates, it has been a focus of students of human cognition for more than two decades, especially the extended process of migration of neurons and the process of learning and development (Deacon 1997).

Margaret Mead noted that there was an increasing lack of relevance between information valued by different generations in America in the post–World War Two period. She called it the Generation Gap (1970) and noted it earlier as a result of colonialism on Native peoples, as did Mair (1969), among others. This process has only increased with computers, the internet, and the explosion of devices that require new learning and methods of use.

Mead used a variety of techniques to study how change was affecting children and their view of the world, as in the Draw a Picture Test. Other people looked at the dreams of Native peoples and children to gauge the effects of technology.

Regarding children's dreams, Foulkes (1971) found the dream reports of 3- to 4-year-olds to be very brief, "not dramatic or nightmarish, but rather prosaic." They dreamed little of their parents and mostly of animals or being hungry. Applebee (1978) also found a preponderance of dreams of animals and few humans in children's dreams, but Bulkeley and Bulkley (2012) find a different interpretation, though perhaps affected by their Jungian framework. Foulkes (1971) suggested from his knowledge of the children that the animals represented people, for example, an aggressive child dreaming of an angry, barking dog in a dog house. At ages 5 and 6 he saw an increase of emotion and length in dreams as well as a gender difference. Girls dreamed of being "nicer" and happier, with parental adult in dreams; boys had an increase in adult male strangers, similar to the findings of Schredl (2007) with adults. By seven and eight years dream reports were longer, averaging 70 words for girls and 48 for boys. Troublesome dreams were reduced in boys but both genders dreamed of many adult strangers. At nine and ten years, there was an increase in pleasant happy dreams, with more participation of the dreamer in the dream (Foulkes 1971). However, more recent research (Sandor et al. 2015) contradicts this view. Sandor et al. (2015) found children dreamt of more humans than animals. Studies separated in time, as Freud to Foulkes and Sandor require a number of considerations in comparing their findings. One is methods, especially in collecting recall from children, another is difference in education, media content, and dominant symbols in family and social conduct. Among many people children's dreams are not considered important, except for nightmares (Tedlock 1987) and the dreams of shamans due to their connection with spirit familiars (Herdt 1977). Among the Quiches, everyone dreams every night, and if a child does not dream then they are told to try and "catch one" (Tedlock 1987). So, in some cultures not only are dreams accepted as normal, but children can receive sanctions for not having them.

If we then approach understanding in the context of the developing brain, then the idea of a generation gap becomes an issue of not only culture change driven by technology and complexity changes in social life, but also the differences between the developing brain and the adult "completed" brain. This was an essential part of an early theory of brain development by Ramón y Cajal (1909–1911). It explained both the process of learning and the ability of the brain to change and modify concepts over a lifetime. The more use, the more learning, the more development of the dendrites and neurons; lack of learning creates no increase in complexity. In 1967 this was a most important concern for me as I saw rock music as a part of a generational change brought about by the technological change of amplification but associated with modern industrialized separation of the generations in work, education, and life. Jomo Kenyatta (1938) noted this in his ethnographic analysis of European life and the Kikuyu. The central point being that in traditional Kikuyus' context, children often learned in the place of work of their parents, either parent could be the focus of a child's study or modeling opportunity in the daily routine of work. In industrialized European culture, experienced by Kenyatta in missionary schools, education was separated from family life and regimented in segmental learning experiences addressing a variety of skills and knowledge not associated directly with the parent's work.

Learning in many traditional societies took place also in age-grade and age-set situations when all of the children and teenagers, young adults, would participate together in group exercises designed to provide a learning experience for the entire group of individuals between a certain age at once (Van Gennep 1960). These are not unusual across time and cultures (Bernardi 1985; Butts 1955), but in some cultures these groups were maintained throughout life and thus the experiences and solidarity established in youth were carried into adulthood. Ritter (1980) discussed the theories that attempt to explain differences and functions of age-sets.

So how do we put together dreams and images from drugs like LSD? Is there anything to learn from pathological conditions that produce hallucinations? Before we address these issues in some depth, we need to look at the nature of the dose of the drug, the kind of effect produced, and the variations produced in different people, both in people deemed psychotic and in those considered normal, and human variation. It is clear that culture matters, and also variations in the substances used, context, and biology of those using it. Plants evolve and people use a variety of plant species that can differ in the products of their leaves and fruit by soil and stage of growth, as Johns (1990) has described in detail for both poisonous and hallucinogenic plant products. Tobacco is an interesting case, as Native Americans reportedly received substantial hallucinogenic effects from the species they had access to and how they prepared them. Why this has not been sustained with today's varieties is curious; Native Americas using tobacco reported many of the kinds of images of people using hallucinogens, yet tobacco is not considered one and does not work on the brain in similar fashion (de Rios 1984; Swan and Lessov-Schlaggar 2007; Johnson et al. 2014), though it does stimulate activity in the prefrontal cortex, thalamus, and visual system as well as release a number of neurotransmitters, including dopamine (Benowitz 2009).

Here we meet, I think also, the power of expectation. As Wade Davis (2009) puts it for Native Americans, I would extend to most indigenous people: "But whatever the ostensible purpose of the hallucinogenic journey, the Amerindian imbibes his plants in a highly structured manner that places a ritualistic framework of order around their use. Moreover the experience is explicitly sought for positive ends. It is not a means of escaping from an uncertain existence; rather it is perceived as a means of contribution to the welfare of all one's people." It seems remarkable in reflecting on Davis' statement that Native Americans have suffered significant disease, death, and psychological damage from the alcoholic drinks Europeans provided them. These became the poisons of escape from defeat and disaster.

References

Al-Issa I. (1995) "The illusion of reality or the reality of illusion. Hallucinations and culture. "*British Journal of Psychiatry*;166:368–373.

Anderson, Robin and Bob Connolly, (1983) *First Contact*, Highlands Trilogy, Original film shot in 1930s, follow up footage in 1970s.

Andreasen, N.C. (1989) "The American concept of schizophrenia," *Schizophr. Bull.*, v. 15, n. 4, 519–531.

Applebee, Arthur N. (1978) *The Child's Concept of Story, Ages Two to Seventeen,* Chicago, University of Chicago Press.

Baer, Hans A. (2008) "The work of Andrew Weil and Deepak Chopra—two Holistic Health/New Age gurus: a critique of the Holistic Health/New Age Movements," *Medical Anthropology Quarterly,* 8 January, v. 17, 2, 233–250.

Bartholomew, Robert; Wessely, Simon (2002). "Protean nature of mass sociogenic illness". *The British Journal of Psychiatry.* **180**: 300–306. https://doi.org/10.1192/bjp.180.4.300.

Benedict, R. (1934) *Patterns of Culture,* Boston: Houghton Mifflin.

Bentall, R.P. and F. Varese, (2013) "Psychotic hallucinations," in *Hallucination: Philosophy and Psychology,* (eds.) Fiona Macpherson and Dimitris Platchias, Cambridge, MA, MIT Press, pp. 65–86.

Benowitz, Neal L. (2009) "Pharmacology of Nicotine: addiction, smoking-induced disease, and therapeutics," *Annu. Rev. Pharmacol. Toxicol.,* v. 49, 57–71.

Bernardi, B. (1985). *Age Class Systems: Social Institutions and Polities Based on Age.* Cambridge University Press.

Blum, Richard, Eva Blum and Mary Lou Funkhouser, (1964) "The institutionalization of LSD," in Blum, Richard, Nevitt Sanford, Eva Blum, Mary Lou Funkhouser, Joseph J. Downing, et al., (eds.) *Utopiates: The Use and Users of LSD-25, A Publication of the Institute for the Study of Human Problems,* Stanford University, Atherton Press, 124–141.

Bogoras, W. (1907) "The Chuchee Religion," The Jesup North Pacific Expedition, 7, *Memoirs of the American Museum of Natural History,* 11, Pt, 3, 537–733, New York.

Bogoras, W. (1910) "The Chuchee, Mythology" Jessup North Pacific Expedition, 8, *Memoirs of the American Museum of Natural History,* v. 12, Pt. 1, 1–197, 205–7, New York.

Botvinick, Matthew and Jonathan Cohen (1998) "Rubber hands 'feel' touch that eyes see," *Nature,* v. 391, 19 Feb, 756.

Bourn, W.M., W.J. Keller and J.F. Bonfiglio, (1979) "Comparisons of mescal bean alkaloids with mescaline, Delta 9 tetrahydrocannabinol- THC and other psychotogens," *Life Sciences,* v. 25, 12, 17 September, 1043–1054.

Buck, Robert W. (1961) "Mushroom toxins—a brief review of the literature," *New England J. of Medicine,* v.265, 681–686.

Bulkeley, Kelly and Patricia M. Bulkey (2012) *Children's Dreams: Understanding the Most Memorable Dreams and Nightmares of Childhood,* Lanham, Rowman and Littlefield.

Butts, R. Freeman, (1955) *A Culture History of Western Education,* New York, McGraw-Hill.

Caldararo, Niccolo (2019) *An Ethnography of the Goodman Building, The Longest Rent Strike*, New York, Palgrave Macmillan.

Caldararo, Niccolo (2017) *Big Brains and the Human Superorganism, Why Special Brains Appear in Hominids and Other Social Animals*, Lanham Maryland, Rowman and Littlefield.

Carhart-Harris, Robin L., Suresh Muthukumaraswamy, Leor Roseman, Mendel Kaelen, Wouter Droog, et al., (2016). "Neural correlates of the LSD experience revealed by multimodal neuroimaging," *PNAS*, April 26, v. 113, n. 17:4853–4858.

Chagnon, Napoleon A (1968) *Yanomamo: The Fierce People,* New York, Holt, Rinehart and Winston.

Chagnon, Napoleon, A. P. Lequesne and A. J. Cook (1971) "Yanomamo hallucinogens: anthropological, botanical and chemical findings," *Current Anthropology*, v. 12, 72–4.

Coyote, Peter (1990) "Book Introduction to *Ringolevio: A Life Played for Keeps,* http://www.petercoyote.com/ringo.html.

Daily Gater Staff, (1966) "Mogar quits LSD study," *Daily Gater* newspaper, SFSU campus.

Davis, Wade (2009) "Hallucenogenic plants and their use in traditional societies," in Sacred Realms, *Readings in the Anthropology of Religion*, (Eds.) Richard Warms, James Garber and R. Jon McGee, 2nd edition, Oxford, Oxford University Press, 204–206.

Davis, Wade (2001) *Light at the Edge of the World*, Vancouver, Douglas & McIntyre.

Deacon, Terrence W., *The Symbolic Species: The Co-evolution of Language and Brain* (New York: W.W. Norton, 1997).

de Rios, Marlene Dobkin (1984) *Hallucinogens: Cross-Cultural Perspectives*, Albuquerque, University of New Mexico Press.

Diggerdocs, (2022) "An epic conversation with Jane Lapiner and David Simpson of the San Francisco Diggers," by Jay Babcock, March 5, https://diggersdocs.home.blog/2022/03/05/we-had-a-far-more-profound-effect/#more-1259.

Domínguez-Clavé E, Soler J, Elices M, Pascual JC, Álvarez E, de la Fuente Revenga M, Friedlander P, Feilding A, Riba J (2016) "Ayahuasca: pharmacology, neuroscience and therapeutic potential," *Brain Res Bull* 126(Pt 1):89–101. https://doi.org/10.1016/j.brainresbull.2016.03.002.

Doob, Leonard W. (1957) "An introduction to the psychology of acculturation," *J. of Social Psychology*, v. 45: 143–160.

Ens, Andrea (2020) "Another aspect of reality: Maria Nys Huxley's influence on psychedelic history," *Chacruna, Institute for Psychedelic Plan Medicines*,

November 25, https://chacruna.net/maria-nys-huxleys-influence-on-psychedelic-history/

Evans, William Charles and Daphne Evans (2009) "Hallucinogenic, allergenic, teratogenic and other toxic plants," in *Trease and Evans' Pharmacognosy*, 16th edition, Saunders/ Elevier, Edinburgh, pp. 523–532.

Feilding, Amanda (2014) "Taking an enlightened approach to psychedelic drugs as treatments," The Financial Times, 8 December.

Foulkes, D., (1971) Longitudinal studies of dreams in children," In J. Masserman (ed) *Science and Psychoanalysis*, 9, New York, Grune and Stratton.

Gardner-Chloros, Penelope (2009) *Code-Switching*, Cambridge, Cambridge University Press.

Gayton, Anna Hadwick, (1928) *The Narcotic Plant Datura in Aboriginal American Culture*, Berkeley, University of California.

Goodison, Lucy (1995) *The Dreams of Women: Exploring and Interpreting Women's Dreams*, New York, W.W. Norton.

Greenfield, Robert, (2006) *Timothy Leary, A Biography*, New York, Harcourt.

Grogan, Emmett (1972) *Ringolevio*, Boston, Little, Brown & Co.

Grogan, Emmett (1978) *Ringolevio*, Boston, Little, Brown & Co.

Haining, Robert L. and Cindy Achat-Mendes, (2017) "Neuromelanin, one of the most overlooked molecules in modern medicine," *Neural Regen Res.* Mar, v. 12, n. 3, 372–375.

Hall, E.T., *The Silent Language* (Garden City: Doubleday, 1959).

Hall, E.T., *The Hidden Dimension* (Garden City: Anchor Books, 1969).

Harrison, K. David (2007) *When languages Die*, Oxford, Oxford University Press.

Hemming, John (1978). Red Gold: The Conquest of the Brazilian Indians, Cambridge, MA, Harvard University Press.

Herculano-Houzel, Suzana, Bruno Mota, Peivan Wong, and Jon H. Kaas, "Connectivity-driven white matter scaling and folding in primate cerebral cortex," *Proceedings of the National Academy of Sciences, USA* 107, No. 44 (November 2, (2010): 19008–19013.

Herdt, Gilbert H. (1977) "The shaman's 'calling' among the Sambia of New Guinea, *Journal de la societe des Oceanistes* v 33, 153–167.

Hochstein, F. and Anita M. Paradies (1957). "Alkaloids of Banisteria caapi and Prestonia amazonicum," *Journal of the American Chemical Society*, Nov. 1, v. 79:5735–5736.

Hoffer A, Osmond H, Smithies J (1954). "Schizophrenia; a new approach. II. Result of a year's research". *The Journal of Mental Science.* **100** (418): 29–45.

Hofman, Michel A., (2014) "Evolution of the human brain: when bigger is better," *Frontiers in Neuroanatomy* 8, article 15 March: 1–12.

Holmstedt, B. and J.E. Loindgren, T. Plowman, L. Rivier, R.E. Schultes and O. Tovar, (1980) "Indole alkaloids in Amazonian Myristicaceae: Field and Laboratory Research, " *Botanical Museum Leaflets, Harvard University*, v. 28, n 3, 215–234.

Hsu, Francis L.K. (1969) *The Study of Literate Societies*, New York.

Huxley, Aldous (1954) *The Doors of Perception, and Heaven and Hell*, New York, Harper Colophon Books.

Johns, T. (1990) *With Bitter Herbs They Shall Eat It,* Tucson, University of Arizona Press.

Johnson MW, Garcia-Romeu A, Cosimano MP, Griffiths RR. (2014) Pilot study of the 5-HT2AR agonist psilocybin in the treatment of tobacco addiction. *J Psychopharmacol.* 28(11):983–992.

Kensinger, K., (1972). "Banisteriopsis usage among the Peruvian Cashinahua," in Hallucinogens and Shaman, Michael Harner (ed.), Oxford, Oxford University Press, 9–14.

Kenyatta, Jomo, *Facing Mt. Kenya* (New York: Vintage Books, 1938).

Kroeber, Alfred (1944) *Configurations of Culture Growth,* Berkeley, University of California Press; 35–39.

La Barre, Weston (1964). "Le complexe narcotique de l'amerique autochtone," Diogene, v. XLVIII, 120–134.

La Barre, Weston (1975) "Anthropological perspectives on hallucination and hallucinogens," in *Hallucinations: Behavior, Experience and Theory,* (eds.) R. K. Siegel and L.J. West, New York, John Wiley, & Sons, 9–52.

Laing, R. D. and A. Esterson, (1964) *Sanity, Madness and the Family*, Harmondsworth, Pelican Books.

Laroi, Frank, Tanya Marie Luhrmann, Vaughan Bell, William A. Christian, Jr., Smita Deshpande, et al., (2014) " Culture and hallucinations: overview and future directions," *Schizophrenia Bulletin*, v. 40, suppl, no. 4, s213–s220.

Las Casas, Bartolome de (1909) *Apologetica Historia de las Indias*, Chapter 166, pages 445–446, Madrid, Serrano y Saenz.

Lattin, Don (2010) *The Harvard Psychedelic Club*, New York, HarperCollins.

Lattin, Don (2017) "Timothy Leary's legacy and the rebirth of psychedelic research, " *Harvard Library Bulletin*, 28, (1) Spring, 65–74.

Levy-Bruhl, Lucien (1966) *Primitive Mentality*, (originally published in 1923) Boston, Beacon Press.

Lewin, Louis (1924). Phanfastica, Die betaubenden und erregenden Genussmittel, Fur Arzte und Nichtarzte, Berlin, Verlag von Georg Stike.

Linzer, Jeffrey, (1970) "Some anthropological aspects of Yage," In in Aaronson, Bernard and Humphry Osmond, (eds) (1970) *Psychedelics, The Uses and*

Implications of Hallucinogenic Drugs, Garden City, Anchor Books. Pp.108–115.

MacFarquhar, Larissa (1997) "Andrew Weil, Shaman, M.D." *The New York Times Books,* August 24th.

Mair, Lucy (1969) Anthropology and Social Change, New York, University of London and the Athlone Press.

McKenna, Terence (1992) *Food of the Gods,* New York, Bantam Books.

Mogar, Rober E. (1968) "Research in psychedelic drug therapy: a critical analysis," in J.M. Shlien (Ed.) *Research in Psychotherapy,* American Psychological Association, 500–511.

Morrison, Anthony P. (2002). "The interpretation of intrusions in psychosis: integrative cognitive approach to hallucinations and delusions," *Behavioural and Cognitive Psychotherapy,* v. 29, n. 3:257–276.

Murphy, J.M. (1976) Psychiatric labeling in cross cultural perspective," *Science,* v. 191, 1019–1028.

Myers, N.L. (2011) "Update: schizophrenia across cultures," *Curr. Psychiatry Rep.* v. 13, 305–311.

Nielsen, Tore (2011) "Disturbed dreaming as a factor in medical conditions," in Principles and Practice of Sleep Medicine, 5th In *Principles and Practice of Sleep Medicine,* (Eds.) Meir H. Kryger, Thomas Roth and William C. Dement, Chapter 98, Edition, St. Louis, Missouri, Elsevier, 1116–1127.

Osmond, Humphry, (1970). "On being mad," in Aaronson, Bernard and Humphry Osmond, (eds) (1970). *Psychedelics, The Uses and Implications of Hallucinogenic Drugs, Garden City, Anchor Books,* 21–28.

Osmond, Humphry and John R. Smythies, (1953). "*The present state of psychological medicine,*" Hibbert Journal, 133–142.

Olson, David E. (2018) "Psychoplastogens: a promising class of plasticity-promoting neurotherapeutics," *J. of Experimental Neuroscience,* v. 12, 104.

Olson, David E, (2021) "The subjective effects of psychedelics may not be necessary for their enduring therapeutic effects," *ACE Pharmacology & Translational Science,* v. 4, 563–567.

Ott, Jonathan (1998). "Pharmahuasca: Human pharmacology of oral DMT plus Harmine". *Journal of Psychoactive Drugs.* **31** (2): 171–7.

Perry, Helen (1970) *The Human Be-In,* London, Allen Lane The Penguin Press.

Pierre, J. M. (2001). "Faith or delusion: at the crossroads of religion and psychosis," *Journal of Psychiatric Practice,* v. 7, n. 3:163–172.

Pochettino, M. L.; Cortella, A. R.; Ruiz, M. (1999). "Hallucinogenic Snuff from Northwestern Argentina: Microscopical Identification of *Anadenanthera colubrina* var. *cebil* (Fabaceae) in Powdered Archaeological Material". *Economic Botany.* **53** (2): 127–132.

Pollan, Michael (2021) "How should we do drugs now?" *The New York Times*, July 11, page 4.
Ritter, Madeline Lattman, (1980) "The Conditions Favoring Age-Set Organization," Journal of Anthropological Research, Vol. 36, No. 1 (Spring, 1980), pp. 87–104.
Rivers, W.H.R. (1920) *Instinct and the Unconscious*, Cambridge, Cambridge University Press.
Russin, Joseph M. and Andrew T. Weil, (1973) "The *Crimson* takes Leary, Alpert to task," January 24, *The Harvard Crimson.*
Sacks, Oliver (2012) *Hallucinations*, New York, Vintage Books.
Sandor, Piroska, Sara Szakadat, Katinka Kertesz and Robert Bodizs, (2015) "Content analysis of 4 to 8 year-old children's dream reports," *Front. Psychol.* 30 April, | https://doi.org/10.3389/fpsyg.2015.00534
Safford, William Edwin (1916) "Identity of cohoba, the narcotic snuff of ancient Haiti," *Journal of the Washington Academy of Sciences*, v. 6, n. 15: 547=562.
Sapir, Edward, (1921) Language: An Introduction to the Study of Speech, New York, Harcourt, Brace & World.
Schredl, M. (2007) "Gender differences in dreaming," In D. Barrett & P. McNamara (Eds.), *The new science of dreaming*—Volume 2: Content, recall, and personality correlates (pp. 29–47). Westport: Praeger.
Schultes, Richard Evans (1963) "Hallocinogenic plants of the New World," *Harvard Review, 1*, 18–32.
Schultes, R. E. (1967) The botanical origins of South American snuffs. In D. Efron, B. Holmstedt, and N. S. Kline (Eds.), Ethnopharmacologic search for psychoactive drugs. Washington, D.C.: Public Health Service Publication No. 1645.
Schultes, R.E. (1970) "The botanical and chemical distribution of hallucinogens," *Annual Review of Plant Physiology*, v. 21, 571–598.
Schultes, Richard Evans (1972) "An overview of hallucinogens in the Western Hemisphere," in Flesh of the Gods, *The Ritual Use of Hallucinogens*, Peter T. Furst (ed.) New York, Praeger Publishers: 3–54.
Schultes, R. E., and Hofmann, A. (1973) *The botany and chemistry of hallucinogens*. Springfield, Ill.: Charles C Thomas.
Seth, Anil (2021) *Being You: A New Science of Consciousness*, Faber.
Shapiro, Arthur K. and Elaire Shapiro, (1997) *The Powerful Placebo*, Baltimore, Johns Hopkins Press.
Shermer, Michael (2011*) The Believing Brain, From Ghosts to Goda to Politics and Conspiracies—How We Construct Beliefs and Reinforce Them as Truths*, New York, New York Times Books.

Shostak, Marjorie (1983). *Nisa, the life and words of a !Kung woman* (1st Vintage books ed.). New York: Vintage Books.

Sinnett, E. Robert, (1970) "Mescaline: Experience and reflections," in Aaronson, Bernard and Humphry Osmond, (eds) (1970) *Psychedelics, The Uses and Implications of Hallucinogenic Drugs,* Garden City, Anchor Books, 29–34.

Skinner, Alason (1926). "Ethnology of the Iowa Indians," *Bulletin of the Public Museum of the City of Milwaukee,* Volume 5, No. 4. Milwaukee.

Smythies, John (1996) "On the function of neuromelanin," *Proc. Biol. Sci.*, Apr., v. 283, (1369) 487–9.

Smythies, John (2010) "The adrenochrome hypothesis of schizophrenia revisited," *Neurotoxicity Research,* v. 4, n. 2, 147–150.

Stanghellini, Giovanni (2008). Schizophrenic delusions, embodiment, and the background, *Philosophy, Psychiatry, and Psychology*, v. 15, bn. 4,:311–314.

Stevens, Jay (1988). *Storming Heaven: LSD and the American Dream*, New York, Harper and Row.

Stolaroff, Myron (2005) *The secret Chief Revealed: Conversations with Leo Zeff, Pioneer in the Underground Psychedelic Therapy Movement,* MAPS.

Swan, Gary E. and Christina N. Lessov-Schlaggar (2007) "The effects of tobacco smoke and nicotine on cognition and the brain," *Neuropsychol. Rev.*, Sept, v. 17, n. 3, 259–273.

Tedlock, Barbara (1987) "Dreaming and dream research," in *Dreaming: Anthropological and Psychological Interpretations,* (ed.) Barbara Tedlock, Cambridge, Cambridge University Press, 1–30.

Van Gennep, Arnold, (1960) *The Rites of Passage,* Chicago, University of Chicago Press.

Vaughan K, McConaghy N (1999). "Megavitamin and dietary treatment in schizophrenia: a randomised, controlled trial". *Australian and New Zealand Journal of Psychiatry.* **33** (1): 84–88.

Wallace, Anthony F. C. (1972) "Mental illness, biology and culture," in *Psychological Anthropology*, (ed) Francis L. Hsu, New Edition, Cambridge, Schenkman Publishing Co. pp. 363–402.

Weil, Andrew (1972) *The Natural Mind: Another Way of Looking at Drugs and the Higher Consciousness*, Boston, Houghton-Mifflin.

Whorf, B.L., (1956a), The Hopi Language, (Chicago Microfilm Collection of Manuscripts on Middle American Cultural Anthropology, 48, University of Chicago Library, manuscript date 1935).

Whorf, Benjamin Lee, (1946), "The Hopi language, Toreva Dialect," in Linguistic Structures of Native America, ed. H. Hoijer, et al., (Viking Fund Publications in Anthropology, #6), New York, pp. 158–183.

Whorf, B. L. (1956b). *Language, thought and reality.* Cambridge: Technology Press of MIT.

2

A Question of Dose and Context: LSD, Peyote and Chemical Interactions, Human Variation, and Interpretation

Most works on LSD begin or place in a prominent location in their text the experience Albert Hofmann reports of his first use of the drug (1980/2009). We often read that the amount he took was "infinitesimal" (Dyck 2008), yet he reports riding his bike on a road that seemed to be painted by Salvador Dali and that he had trouble coordinating his legs to propel the bike. In attempting to talk to his assistant he found he had no voice. So it was apparent from the beginning that a small amount could have remarkable effects. His first ingestion was accidental and apparently of unknown quantity, the second was 250 micrograms (mg) (Grof 1976, 7–8). Two hundred milligrams of mescaline was considered a "standard" effective dose by some in the 1950s (Sinnett 1970). Dyck is intrigued that as few as 25–50 mg can produce hallucinogenic effects compared to aspirin, which requires a dose of 300,000 mg for effect. What really interests her is how researchers were attracted to the drug for studies of the origins of mental disorders and consciousness. In my experiences at the Mogar Lab and in my own research in the late 1960s and early 1970s, I found it interesting that some people, when they became intoxicated by LSD, were quite interested in the process, and even after several trips, enjoyed charting their own physical mental variations as they became

N. Caldararo, *A Mental Ethnography: Conclusions From Research in LSD*,
https://doi.org/10.1007/978-3-031-13745-7_2

apparent. Just as interesting, however, was the drug tolerance of some people who after taking many LSD trips found they came to anticipate the drug's effect and came to "surf" the high as it unfolded while others claimed to "feel" nothing. A tolerance to the effects of LSD has been reported and is summarized by Buchborn et al. (2016); see also Trulson and Crisp (1983) *on microdosing and tolerance.* It appears within 24 hours and reaches a maximum effect in four days and is generalized to psilocybin and mescaline. A similar effect is reported in animals. Since the effect of drugs can be affected by a number of factors, especially human variation, the rationale for dose is a central problem. Janiger (de Rios and Janiger 2003) computed dose to body size, developing a scale, for example, 150-pound male received a dose of 136 mg, and claims that street doses in 2003 ran between 60 and 80 mg. Alpert and some of Leary's other cohorts are claimed to have taken megadoses of several thousands of micrograms, but there is no evidence for the actual amount, though this may establish some reference to claims of toxicity or increased efficacy, as Alpert reported no more effect than several hundred micrograms (Stevens 1988).

Inserra et al. (2021) found that with mice different dose to weight had different effects on the animals, with even low doses (10 mg/kg) able to reduce spontaneous firing and burst-firing in the reticular thalamus—at 40 mg/kg another population of neurons showed an increase in firing and burst-firing and was accompanied by an increase of firing and burst-firing activity of thalamocortical neurons in the mediodorsal thalamus. But LSD excited infralimbic prefrontal cortex pryramidal neurons only at the highest dose tested (160 mg/kg). The authors suggest that as the reticular thalamus is a thin sheet of "neurons that surrounds the thalamus and keeps thalamocortical relay cells under inhibitory control, selectively releasing them from inhibition to integrate and process incoming stimuli," LSD's modulation of this control may explain its effect as a source of altered states of consciousness. This must include the principal cells of the lateral geniculate nucleus (LGN) projecting to the visual cortex (Crick 1994).

Let's look at this situation by contrasting experience with a placebo. Below I will report on the use of fMRI to track changes in the brain and reported experience with LSD, but for the moment experiments with microdosing and placebo have been of interest. Lindsay Cameron (2021) summarized work done with microdosing and placebo recently. The most recent study is by Szigeti et al. (2021), who attempted to answer questions about LSD effects, microdosing, and placebo. They found little difference between microdosing LSD and placebo effect in subjects' reported experiences. Claims of increased positive mood and creativity have been reported (Anderson et al. 2019; Johnstad 2018; Malone 2016) usually in contexts without medical supervision or rigorous measurements and comparative LSD products (Fadiman 2011). Fadiman has been collecting a considerable archive of LSD user comment on their experiences and so his work reflects this diversity. Yet such reports of positive outcomes numbered over 1000 by 1979 (Grinspoon and Bakalar 1979). A study by Anderson et al. (2019) is part of a larger investigation in benefits and drawbacks of microdosing and uses a variety of metrics, including psychological effects like depression as well as creativity, applied to microdosers and non-microdosers in their study populations.

We should note that there are other limits; early researchers found that some 25% of those who took LSD reported no effect. I can recall one woman in the Mogar Lab study who was administered LSD but felt nothing after 24 hours (Stevens 1988). Also, I mention from Rinker's subjects one who never had any response to several recorded administered LSD sessions. "Acid heads," who claimed to be able to clearly and deliberately chart their LSD experience, seemed to vary in this. I did sit with several who were able to go on their "journeys" as designed in predrug itineraries, as much as I could determine from their responses. At the other extreme, Hoffman (1980/2009) reports attempts to determine the nature of a lethal dose of LSD with animals as varied as mice to elephants and to establish if the drug can induce behavior similar to that in humans in everything from chimps to spiders. This inquiry was extended by a number of people, including Ronald K. Siegel (1977), who developed methods to test whether religious experiences and hallucinations could be induced in a variety of animals. The results seem both contradictory and subjective. Pahnke (1963) argued that from his study, the most difficult part of the psychedelic experience came afterward, in the attempt (for a religious professional as himself and some of his subjects) to understand it. One can contrast this attitude with those who took the drugs under the influence of the Pranksters, where instant fun, psychic adventures, and sexual joy were expected.

As mentioned earlier, the idea that one could study the origins of organs or species by an analysis of comparative embryology dates to Haeckel (1866; see references to Haeckel's ideas in Chaps. 4 and 5). Most research oriented to origins of consciousness using psychedelics, however, seems to have been aimed in the creation of psychopharmacology, either at altering human biochemistry to relieve symptoms of disease (antihistamines) or at suppressing aspects of mental disorders to allow people to adapt or cope with underlying disease (anti-depressants), most all of which took place in the post-WWII period of the 1950s and 1960s (Dyck 2008). And as in the effects of drugs like opium that induced a state of pleasure and contentment, drugs like Thorazine (or chlorpromazine and other supposed "dream-inducing" drugs; see Trigoni 2019) seemed to indicate that the human brain was not a black box, but rather a mechanism that could be analyzed to find what was missing or blocked, which could then be identified and added to achieve cures. By 1960 more than 1000 articles had appeared in major medical publications on the possible roles LSD could play in psychiatric treatments (Dyck 2008). It is interesting that many studies were with animal models, others with experimental subjects, and some in patients and many involved self-administered experiments. The production of books and articles with references or descriptions of indigenous use of hallucinogens appeared and caused cross-fertilization of ideas of potential agents for cures. Some caution was expressed early by people like Sidney Cohen, who found that some patients experienced marked improvements (he called this "integrative experience"), but it did not last for all who took the drug (Eisner & Cohen 1958). The discovery of earlier texts relating to indigenous drug use as in Kluver's *Mescal*, which first appeared in 1928, led to their republication, in *Mescal*'s case in 1966. Kluver reports (Kluver 1928/1966, 14) from Mooney an ethnographic context of use of peyote where a child of 12 years consumed six mescal buttons and adults would consume from 12 to 20, with one man taking 90, though no information is given on age or gender related to this dose. He notes that many experimenters he had information from ate 3–7 of the dry mescal buttons, again without any information of age or gender. Others ground the buttons to a powder and "took the powder" in some way, and others drank it as a "decoction," while still others injected one or several buttons subcutaneously. The most comprehensive report on an ethnographic context for the use of peyote is in my opinion that by Furst (1972) of its use among the Huichol. Contact reports (mainly from Christian priests; see Furst, p. 143) related that those taking the drug perceived "horrible images," yet the drug was associated with important ceremonies (cleansing of mind and spirit) of the indigenous religion as well as healing rites (Myerhoff 1974). This needs to be put into perspective both regarding the variations in experience and in dose by a variety of indigenous people. Schultes (1972) points out that there are significant differences in peyote intoxication if the "buttons" are made from the dried head of the cactus with its total alkaloid content, or "mescaline" preparations that contain only one of the alkaloids.

Native Theory, Explanations, and Defining Miraculous

At the same time the phenomenological approach to mental illness developed by Karl Jaspers (1959), had formed a prerequisite to many psychiatrists for assessment and description of the pathologically modified experience of patients (Burgy 2008). Central to the problem of psychological symptoms was the question, did they arise from organic disease that had entered the body or were they the result of changes in the normal functioning of the brain brought about by endogenous factors, or from social exogenous ones? These sources were debated and defined in the nineteenth and early twentieth centuries, with important syntheses produced by Mobius in 1875 and Kraepelin and Jaspers afterward. In 1924 this was further refined by Bunke by the separation of influences and sources as exogenous and somatogenic origin. Still, we are left with the problem of classification of types of disease expression and limitation of cognition or death in the individual or even, and more to our interest, of changes in cognition. Some of this research was and still is aimed at replacing what are considered necessary agents that a patient's body does not produce in sufficient or normal amounts. Early attempts at classification were generally built on contemporary cosmologies, as in St.

Augustine's on his Greek philosophy linked to Judeo-Christian theology or Augustin Calmet, whose first class, that of apparitions of angels, demons, and souls, could be considered real (Berrios and Markova 2015). The question becomes more complicated in cultures where there are several realities, as today we have theories in cosmology of multi-universes. Ethnographically recorded drawings, both Paleolithic and contemporary, are often assumed to depict events like hunting, but for some, like the San rock paintings, they may report on dreams (Lewis-Williams 2009).

The analysis of mescaline by psychiatrists Humphry Osmond and John Smythies (1953), with the help of organic chemist John Harley-Mason, was one of these attempts at finding a biochemical answer to mental disorders. It appeared to them that the chemical structure of mescaline was similar to adrenaline and thus its effect might be a result of either a replacement of a lack or addition to a normal amount (Dyck 2008, 17). A somewhat chicken-and-egg relation can develop in this analysis, does the lesion in the brain derive from an agent introduced into the individual, a poison, a pathogenic organism, or is it the result of an endogenous development, multiple sclerosis, or cancer, for example? But we should not separate abnormalities produced by disease, psychological adaptations to social or other stress, or birth defects from those considered to be normal.

Cultural definitions of disease shape the social interpretations of unique behavior as communication (Fabrega 1997, 252–4). Also, people had interpreted abnormalities, not only visions, hallucinations, and so on, but physical deformations, as communications from the gods (Lincoln 1935; Fromm 1951). To Socrates (Plato, *Phaedo*), dreams were the voice of a person's conscience, but to Plato they are the irrational and savage expression of our nature (Fromm 1951, 119). The Roman lawyer Cicero also rejects dreams as being messages of the gods (Fromm 1951), but in general many Romans saw them as emanating from the gods, producing inspiration and direction in prophesy. Yet oracles and seers of various types were an accepted and important part of Greco-Roman religion. They varied in trustworthy regard, as that at Amphiaraus, which was considered especially skillful as a diviner of dreams in the time of Pausanias circa 180 CE (Grant 1953). Yet by the fourth century CE, a philosopher like Synesius of Cyrene could argue that divination by dreams should not be dismissed, as it shares obscurity with oracles, but it comes within a person and reflects his or her soul and is a true reflection of one's nature (3/1288). Thomas Aquinas

(1922) uses this definition also in his analysis of what he considered to be the four kinds of dreams. One originating within as a reflection of the self, another related to the body (as in the humors of some Greek medical philosophers), the effect of the external world brought by air, and the impression of a heavenly body or spiritual intervention or demon.

Voltaire (1764) and Kant (1900) and Bergson (1914) generally relegated dreams to distortions, for Kant, of the stomach, but he also thought that ideas could be made clearer in sleep through dreams. For Goethe it is rationality and creativity that comes in dreams (Goethe 1836/1898). Wondering if a person's eyes could see (if stimulating the retina affected images) in sleep and register images seen as memories, Allan Rechtschaffen had volunteers' eyes taped open, and when they were asleep he put images in front of their eyes and then woke them up. None of his subjects recalled the images, though they did have other dream images. This was true of other stimuli during sleep; dreaming images did not seem affected, for example, if the person was denied water, no dreaming of thirst, or seeing violent films before or sexual ones, though men's dreams were of sex about 12% of the time; no report on female dreams. Some studies report differences comparing female dreams to males, especially where common mythological sequences are reported, as in Kracke's (1987) discussion of dreams of the Kagwahiv in the Amazon. These differences can be assumed to result from different rites of enculturation and gender identity enforcement. Around 30–40% of dreams are achromatic in his studies (Rechtschaffen and Siegel 2000). He also developed evidence that sleep was necessary for survival in a series of experiments, describing the deleterious effects of a lack of sleep (Rechtschaffen 1983). People with narcolepsy are deficient in orexin ("wakeful hormones") and hallucinations are not uncommon, and sleep deprivation affects the orexin neurons as well, and we find hallucinations (mainly hypnagogic, i.e., just before sleep) are common in sleep-deprived individuals (Sacks 2012; Briggs et al. 2019; De la Herran-Arita et al. 2011). People who do not suffer from narcolepsy sometimes experience a waking sleep paralysis and related hallucinations (Sacks 2012). It has been reported among the Zuni, who refer to it as in the category of bad dreams, and among the Kagwahiv of Brazil, a deadly paralysis of terrifying dreams where the ghosts of the dead are seen in hallucinations to try and kill the sleeper. Similar forms have been reported among a number of other peoples, including Fijians, Zuni, and

Quiches (Tedlock 1987). It is possible that some of this, especially when the person feels a heavy weight on their chest or shortness of breath, might result from underlying health concerns, as in heart disease or apnea (Adler 2010). A similar form of "nightmare death" has appeared in recent young Hmong refugees to North America, some Laotians, and a few others (Tobin and Friedman 2009).

The reverse analysis has also appeared in history—this is where the dream exposes the beliefs and motivations that are hidden in daytime. This approach was taken by the Spanish padres during the colonization of Mexico and other areas of South and Central America. Diego Duran wrote in 1581 that in the process of extinguishing Native beliefs, it was necessary to root out and destroy every recollection of Native gods and ritual. He argued that dreams were a source rife with such information (Todorov 1984; 204–5).

In all these examples, however, what is apparent is the personal focus, as in the case of Emerson (1883), who finds a connection in daily life of "poetic integrity and truth." His description of dreams tells of a variety of wonder that can be present, perhaps not for all who dream, but then we are curious of those who do not dream, who never remember their journeys if they do dream. Sundkler (1961), working among Bantu speakers in Africa, and Burridge (1960), in New Guinea, both considered dreams to be an essential key to understanding religious life and belief, though Fabian (1966) came to less positive conclusions. What is missing is an idea of how the millions of people, not the exceptions, experience dreams. While vast libraries of dream interpretation do exist now, and I have drawn on some of this body of knowledge in this book, there is the problem of the great background of hallucinations, visions, and psychedelic experiences of people of different backgrounds, ages, gender, and cultures. Here is where I have tried to create a bridge between our knowledge of all these elements of human consciousness and mass experience in various societies over time.

For Freud, the dream is a clue and from its manifest content background information about the individual who dreams could be fashioned in his opinion. The use of a variety of methods were used to bring out this latent content. If, as he argues, the remembered dream is not "genuine material" and its elements only substitute for actual events or actions, then it is obvious some key is necessary. This sounds like cognitive scientist Ray Jackenoff's concept that what we are conscious of is the result of our brain's computations of events and not the computations themselves; thus, information structures what we consider memories (Jackendoff 1987). Fromm (1951) suggests that background and association is not necessary. He argues we can use general categories, like Freud, since dreams seem to represent wishes, rational and irrational, and according to Fromm, we often wish for things that are "rooted in our weaknesses and compensate for it." He believes that fantasies and dreams are often the beginning of many actual deeds and give inspiration. Fromm uses this idea on nightmares, contra Freud, who sees anxiety as the source of the fear wish fulfillment of nightmares. Fromm believes that like the desire generated in masochistic acts, fear and desire are unified, as are feelings of self-hate, abuse, and revulsion in immoral acts—somewhat like the psychology student's violent self-harm I describe in a later chapter.

Both Sundkler (1961) and Fabian (1966) agree that there is a standardization of symbols and experiences, with "model" dreams being imitated. As these dreams are a basis for social action we might argue that they differ from the ethnographic dreams reported by Lincoln (1935) and Laughlin (1976), and so can we argue that the ethnographic dream begins to alter under external stress? Though Tedlock (1987) criticizes Lincoln's methods and classifications, they do seem useful. We find Europeans appearing in indigenous dreams, sometimes in vague conditions, as in the Yawing initiation dream reported for a man (Kempf & Hermann 2003); in others, as threatening forces, as in Black Elk's, yet we find in his visions also ancestors in communication with him and animals (Black Elk 1932). The dream narrative appears as a potential prediction, but is in several visitations modified by his feelings and events. This dream is much like that related by a Xavante man to Laura Graham (2003), only in the Xavante case it was a public, group performance and related songs like the Yanomani and Huichol (though with a drug), while Black Elk's was private—though the Huichol differ, according to Myerhoff (1974) in that the dream is personal and not to be shared, at least that of the Sacred Journey. Though there are explanations where incoherence occurs in dreams, visions, or hallucinations due to the existence in each person of different souls or selves. Among the Kalapalo of Brazil the experience of the dream by the dreamer's self obscures its meaning to the dreamer

(Basso 1987). But they do see dreams as related to future events in waking life; thus, like the Zuni, they avoid sleeping at certain times or during certain events to prevent actualizing perceptions, as when the Zuni stay up all night when masked dancers impersonate death should they dream of joining the dancers in the land of the dead. Not all dreams are shared in some ethnographic settings. The Zuni process the dream in waking life, a good dream kept in the heart and silently performed, while a bad dream (of illness or death, for example) may be told to relatives, who will arrange for appropriate intervention by a masked deity to break the chain of causation (Tedlock 1987). Likewise, to the Mehinaku (Gregor 1981) the dream results from the travels of the soul in the nocturnal world, where invisible beings populate nearly every corner. Their dreams are related to others in the morning and can be clues to the future. This idea is not so strange as might appear at first when we consider that should we be able to see bacteria, viruses, and other life forms in the night it would be certainly a crowded space. But dreamed occurrences are symbols readily understood by tribal members who provide guidance; thus, here we have another example of a Native theory. Gregor (1981) lists these symbols, which include events like being stung by a bee, sexual behavior or desires, or killed by a monster or chased. An interesting feature of their (the Mehinaku) dreaming, which is similar to hallucinogenic visions among other people, is the transformation of figures in dreams from animals to people. Tedlock (1987) cautions that several dream theories have been found in the same group, and she references concepts of dreaming and dream sharing as a means of intergroup communication.

The process of having a dream and then sharing it is part of a process of myth and rite and demonstrates the adaptability of the spiritual aspect of the interpretation of the unseen world as an aid to the seen. The visions and trance of shamans, however, vary so greatly (some having unintelligible dreams and visions, sometimes based on personal spirit languages [Eliade 1964] and some suffering also from conditions like menerik; Radin 1937) that comparison is difficult and uniformity is elusive. Winkelman (1992, 2000; Craffert et al. 2019) has produced a counterargument to this assessment, concluding that shaman methods do produce healing. The main problem with his analysis is the definition of what is a shaman (Kehoe 2000), and that he has relied on outdated methods

(Guthrie 2004). It is clear from a number of studies that religious intervention, whether shamanistic, animistic, or derived from the major religions (e.g., Judeo-Christian-Islamic tradition, Buddhism), fails to produce more than a placebo effect (Caldararo 2020; Benson 2006)—though methods and design of such studies have attracted criticism (Andrade and Radhakrishnan 2009). Craffert et al. (2019) argue from two points: one, the assumed ubiquity of belief, ignoring largely the existence of agnostics and atheists, and second, a reliance on phenomenologist Merleau-Ponty's idea that humans are engaged in a "perceptual faith," a process where the human mind adapts to the limits of perception and knowledge. This concept is nothing more than a version of Malinowski's argument that all people have science and religion, fitting into each method that, from moment to moment, works to craft a canoe or jet plane or to satisfy the need for psychic comfort and love. What is most amazing, however, is not so much this capacity, but the strength public opinion and group consensus have on belief. Here Durkheim would be surprised, perhaps, to find his idea so dramatically proven when the Soviet Union was formed and millions conformed to an atheist state ideology.

In this context, it is most interesting that a healer, psychoanalyst Carl Jung, when in conflict over Freud's dream theory has a dream where he lies in wait with his companion, a "small, brown-skinned man, a savage." Jung "knows" they must kill Siegfried. Jung combines his intellectual feelings that this image of Germanic aggressiveness in Siegfried is incompatible with civilization, yet he is joined in this enterprise by a "savage" (Parsons 2010).

Like Freud, Fromm uses myth and fairy tales as a means of uncovering unconscious explanations for dreams (though neither were the first to publish on the unconscious—that was Eduard von Hartmann in 1869, who also opposed the idea that dreams were wish fulfillment). He compares his view on this with Freud's, for example, Oedipus Rex. This interpretation by Freud (1966) has always bothered me. The story is derived from a play by Sophocles, *Oedipus Rex*, first performed in Athens in about 429 BCE. It tells the story of a man who is born to the king of Thebes. The king is told by a seer that he will have a son who will kill him and marry his wife. To avoid this the king has a son born to his wife left on a hillside to die. This child is saved by a shepherd, who raises him, and as a young man he fulfills the prophecy, killing his father and marrying his mother, all in the wake of plague and catastrophes.

As H.D.F. Kitto (1966) has argued, the context of political and moral strife in which the play was written and performed gives us a means of understanding how Greeks, and especially Athenians, saw the play. Rational and natural philosophy had become increasingly popular in Greece at this time, especially from the followers of Thales. The questioning of morals and the influence and even existence of the gods were strong. The play emphasizes the idea that abandoning tradition and taking on new ideas can be dangerous. In the play, the tradition of infanticide, common in Greece at the time, helped regulate population (Feen 1984). It was obviously a difficult decision to make for a family to give up a child to death. But violating the tradition, sanctioned by the gods, invoked their anger. In the case of Oedipus, not only does his father suffer the fate he hoped to escape, but so does Oedipus and the entire city of Thebes. The message is clear: hold fast to belief. Nonetheless, the interpretation of the dream had individual, social, and political implications, then and since. In other cultures dreams also have implications that are seen as political as well as individual. Burridge (1960, 1969) has written of how significant dreams are to some Melanesian societies and how myth and dream function in a complex of meaning. They actively use the dream as a means of utilizing cultural signs and symbols to manipulate events in daily life (see also, Hollan 2003). Yet other groups, in the same area, for example, the Southeast Ambrymese, of Vanuatu, never seem to have significantly utilized dreams in political or social pursuits—though these people have had considerable contact since this information was gathered by Tonkinson (2003).

Much of Fromm's secret language of dreams comes down to power, and from it, authority. He argues that there has been a long struggle of the matriarchy versus the patriarchy (derived from Bachofen 1861, 1926) and that myths and fairy tales explain the conditions of life and resulting tensions between men and women as a result. It is easy to see how dreams, especially unusual dreams, can have significant social impact, as when they are interpreted in the context of crisis and social change, and can be used by a seer to validate a course of action (Radin 1937; Patai 1990).

Messages, Conversion, and Inner Voices

Sometimes such abnormalities mark a person as a messenger of the gods, a shaman or priest (Eliade 1964). Their "message" can sometimes create a new religion, or a "conversion" of one person to a different faith. This process of conversion is quite unclear in terms of what happens in a person's mind to reorder cosmological ideas. We will discuss this again later on. It might be useful to construct a typology of interpretations of hallucinations, visions, and dreams, as shown in the figure below. These terms can vary depending on the focus and perspective—for example, if we were to substitute the Ayurveda for the Western medical model below for the Complex Society context, then categories 4 and 5 would reflect aspects of the Ayurveda if applied to another society or to indigenous peoples within India (see Anderson 1996 for some comparisons). We are somewhat hampered by the difficulty some scientists and practitioners have had in defining hallucinations and abnormal perceptions. Horiguchi et al. (2009) attempted to delineate the specific nature of hallucinations and/or delusions by examining responses of normal subjects to drug-induced perceptions as opposed to clinically ill experiences of patients. They were unable to define borders or categories. Using fMRI, Howard et al. (1997) were able to "see" hallucinations versus the normal condition of a patient with Lewy bodies.

We might define hallucinations as false perceptions of a temporary nature, and delusions as false ideas or beliefs that can last a lifetime or be temporary over time—that is, a person can change their beliefs at will. However, this distinction breaks down when we consider states of mind like fanaticism, where people reject all objective evidence and maintain false beliefs while functioning normally in society. Thus, "pathological delusions" can be associated with individuals who are not functioning normally in society. This is often the textbook definition (see Munn 1961, 242).

Hallucinations and delusions will have no evident dependence on external stimuli, but other perceptions, of a similar nature, may appear in normal people as misinterpretations of known circumstances (Munn 1961, 564). The borders of such definitions have been criticized by a number of scientists, for example, Szasz (1960). Women are reported in modern settings to experience more auditory hallucinations than men (Rector and Seeman 1992; Dhossche et al. 2002; Shevlin et al. 2007; Tien 1991) and girls slightly more hallucinations than boys (Kellener et al. 2012). Since most of the data in these reports is drawn from pathological and clinical conditions, we cannot consider they cover all hallucinations or visions. A study of Japanese adolescents found a similar prevalence of auditory hallucinations in girls as opposed to boys and provides a cross-cultural example for reference. The girls' hallucinations, however, were secondary to depressive syndromes (Morokuma et al. 2017).

Sacks (2012) discusses "hallucinations in the sane," with a case of a woman who regularly heard voices, always in American English, usually when falling asleep at night, and in conversation. She was never a participant and never addressed. In 1894 the Society for Psychical Research published an International Census of Hallucinations in the Sane. Of 17,000 people surveyed, about 10% reported affirmatively, with a third of these being auditory, that is, hearing voices. One might consider the context of the study, where at the time, many educated and especially famous people attended séances and were attracted to the occult. There was probably a certain degree of acceptance of such reports in many people, given this atmosphere. At about the same time Sigmund Freud noted hearing voices calling his name while he was living in a foreign city (Freud 1901). Sacks (2012) also distinguishes between auditory hallucinations and an "inner voice" of authority or comfort, though the main difference is vague, as it seems to be an awareness of the voice being an inner, Native self. Some people have reported hearing two voices within when in a threatening situation, voices that often have different goals or attitudes. Rivers (1920) notes multiple personalities associated with trauma of soldiers as well as the ability of some individuals to experience independent temporary passages of life (fuges). In some cases individuals hearing voices or communicating with multiple personalities are aware of their existence and attempt to influence them. These are also discussed by Laing (1959).

Thalamocortical Functional Disconnections

Hearing voices for many begins in childhood and continues through life. Sacks (2012) suggests that these inner voices can also lead to disastrous ends, as in suicide. He argues that the nature of human thoughts might be mistaken for an inner voice, but another idea is activation in stress of memory of others' voices during threatening situations being activated in an immediate context. Instead, Sacks (2012) reverts to Julian Jaynes' (1976) idea that some social or biological change in human evolution is responsible. Jaynes proposed that at some point in the past all humans heard voices generated from the right hemisphere and perceived them in the left hemisphere as being external. He called this the "bicameral mind." A mutation inverted the assumed external voice of god generated in the right hemisphere of the brain, silencing this panhuman communication (Jaynes 1986). He also suggested that schizophrenics retain this state and thus explains why they hear voices. The main problem with this scenario is that we have no evidence that masses of people in 10,000 or 1000 BCE heard the voice of god as an external stimulation, and were conditioned as a group experience. This does have a parallel to paleoanthropologist Richard Klein's (1989) theory of a creative explosion (though the idea appeared earlier in Chomsky's theory of the origin of language [Berwick et al. 2013], and then in a popular version by John Pfeiffer in 1982 and a later restatement by Ian Tattersall in 1998) after a putative mutation that he thinks gave early *Homo sapiens* fully complex speech and other cognitive abilities he associates with his view of modernity. It is interesting, however, that de Rios (1984) argues that the only form of written communication the Australian Aborigines developed was the message sticks related to trade in the psychedelic plant they call pituri (apparently from *Duboisia hopwoodii*, with the active agent scopolamine but may also include *Nicotiana* species; see Ratsch et al. 2010). They also used the drug to immobilize their main prey, the emu, by lacing waterholes with it to intoxicate them for killing. Thus, the drug hallucinations and the sacrifice of the emu united the people in a kind of "you are what you eat" survival and recognition of the circle of life (Cawte 1964).

Not everyone believes there is evidence for a "creative explosion" of language and abstract abilities. Archeologists Sally McBrearty and Allison Brooks (2000) lay out a well-supported and logical critique of this idea and present an alternative view that there was a gradual increase in hominid cognitive abilities over the past million years that followed increases in brain size.

Jaynes (1976) relies on a number of aspects of conscious and unconscious behavior to build support for his theory. One of these is the Greenspoon Effect, where individual's behavior can be changed and learning can take place without the recipient being aware of the process (Dean and Hiesinger 1964). While operant conditioning is well established, several researchers found problems with Greenspoon's methods shortly after the publication of his work in 1951, for example, Spielberger and De Nike (1962). Greenspoon was a graduate student in Psychology at Indiana University when B.F. Skinner was the Chairman of the Department of Psychology there. His work was found to be useful, however, and led to the development of behavior modification therapies.

Jaynes' theory argues that as hominids evolved from hunting and gathering to food producers and urban life, it was necessary to "carry around with them the directions of the chief or king as verbal hallucinations." This allowed for efficient social control of large populations. He states that this process began in the Neanderthal stage with one mind as decision-making and one as habit and oriented to following routines (group think), and evolved with the complexity of language unification of the hemispheres (as mind, not as completely separated) and the appearance of consciousness. With consciousness comes volition, the development of identity and self (Moore 2021). He posits this happened sometime in the Bronze Age. He is referring to both visual and auditory hallucinations. A major problem here is that historic and contemporary hunters and gatherers do not display the pre-urban "bicameral mind" he suggests as the foundation of this evolutionary process.

The development of religious urbanized civilizations like the Inca and ancient Egypt is used as an example by Jaynes of how gods and kings were the constant image of control seen by all people as continuous hallucinations. So one can see that this is similar to Seth's idea and to that of Wasson and Wasson (1957), only in their idea, mushrooms are the vehicle for human consciousness. However, for Jaynes, there is a loss of these constant hallucinations due to overpopulation, disasters, chaos, and writing. Neither Seth's nor Jaynes' idea here is convincing, not least of which is Jaynes' claim that the fact that many children have invisible playmates and that this is an example of a retention of the ability, which is lost with development. Here he is relying on the connections between the two hemispheres as a process of, first, the bicameral mind and, second, its loss in the pruning of the connections and the separation or specialization of the hemispheres' functions (Jaynes 1976).

It is obvious in our culture that if a person has such visions they are likely to keep them private; this is probably true of children and teens, who are anxious about appearing different. On the other hand, if a person feels compelled to relate their visions to others, it can be interpreted as a symptom of illness (Cook 2015). This is especially true where the hallucinations are strange and foreign to daily life, as in hypnagogic visions (images "seen" with eyes closed or in darkness, just before falling asleep, reported in ethnographic context, e.g., Eskimos; see Tedlock 1987). Even Edgar Allen Poe found this not only unfamiliar but having the "absoluteness of novelty" (Sacks 2012). These kinds of visions are considered to be common to most people but are unnoticed. Hypnopompic hallucinations are reported by a few people but just upon waking and are "seen" in light or illuminated rooms as projected real objects or fantastic creatures, and may appear to recognize the newly awake person in a threatening fashion. Where do they come from? In some American subgroups, having visions or hallucinations (auditory or visual) is valued, as in some Baptist sects and in many other cultural settings (Radin 1937, 106–110; Eliade 1964; Gearing et al. 2011). Gumilla (1741) reported on diametrically different responses of two separate people when under the influence of yupa, the *Anadenanthera* snuff in the Orinico basin. The Otomac became increasingly agitated and violent, while the Saliva became more gentle and benign. Schultes (1972) suggests, however, that different components and preparation methods might also be at work, but analysis from some sources indicates the active agent is bufotenine. But significant variation appears in other areas of experience, as in Blum et al.'s (1964, 61–2) subjects and their feelings of euphoria in LSD perceptions. The results are quite different (Table 2.1).

Table 2.1 Blum et al. (1964) attributed the differences in outcome to expectation

Groups	Euphoria	None
1. Informal professional	50%	50%
2. Religious-medical center	50%	50%
3. Informal black market	75%	25%
4. Private patients	75%	25%
5. Public-clinic patients	14%	86%

The problem of definition is significant, as what one person feels is subjective and open to phenomenological interpretation by the researcher. We note that Blum et al.'s sample was heavily weighted by men over women. The fact that of 92 subjects in their study, 32 (34.7%) had taken LSD prior to the experiment is significant. Ten of their subjects were suspected of engaging in repeated use but no evidence was produced and two more expressed the intention to do so. This produces a sum of 42 (45.6%) who either had continued use or were planning to as a result of the experiment. In statements given by subjects, 54 expressed a desire to take LSD again and 12 others were interested but not sure.

Are hallucinations and visions culturally defined? Our chart on psychedelics-induced ones seems to argue that this is so, and Charles (1972, 1975) in a comprehensive analysis of the concept regarding states of consciousness and "altered" ones describes culturally biased aspects. Wittmann (2018) takes a more physiological approach from research with pathology and psychedelics, seeing altered states linked more to alterations of brain function and related to time, an approach consonant with studies of the role of the hippocampus I note here. So, what about variations? Bourguignon (1972) argues from her data collected in Haiti (Bourguignon 1954) that the Native theory influences and structures the perception and organized experience of the dreamer. She also argues that the Native theory gives us clues as to how dreams function in a culture or social setting, and what is their function for the individual and group. Perceptual experience seems related, as in North America, with the vision quest and dreams or drug-induced hallucinations (Bourguignon 1972). In this case, as in some others, the culture encourages people to have visions or hallucinations and thus one might suggest the culture primes people for the perception, though forms of sensory deprivation, exhaustion, fasting, or self-inflicted pain are used (Sacks 2012). These cases can be classed with the "Arctic hysterias" like *kayakangst* and *windigo*, where La Barre (1975) thinks the featureless Arctic landscape, white glare, isolation of the hunter, and fixing of concentration for cues of animal presence are central elements. *Windigo* is a culturally stylized form of possession and hysteria where the failed hunter returns and attempts to bite chunks of flesh off his family and friends. Similar experiences in hallucination appear to wanderers in deserts.

I think this is also true of contemporary drug experiences like peyote. For LSD I also think that prior perceptions or expectations, information people have of what the drug experience will be like, "reliving past lives," "being reborn," and so on play a similar role. Most of these events people experience lack "consensual validation" where other people have the same perceptions (e.g., in seeing an image, etc.; see Sacks 2012).

Laughlin (1976) tells us that for the Zinacantecans the Native theory also provides a number of expected responses that give the "measure of the person" and here we can see that when the dream is told to the group, the individual's response to the dream tells the group something significant about the person (Table 2.2).

We have to be careful here, for some aspects of "visions" or "seeing things" can be related to attention, opportunity, suggestion, and/or enhanced physiological response, as in the case of phosphenes. Sacks (2012) sees basic differences between hypnagogic hallucinations and dreaming. He argues that dreams have narrative and meaning and hypnagogic hallucinations do not. Hobson (1999), among others (some discussed in this book), disagrees with this division, and sees dreams as a form of delirium. I would not go so far, but I disagree with the assumption that all dreams have meaning and I think we overinterpret most of them. Hobson's theory of mind argues that it is a product of the constant

Table 2.2 Summary of Native theory from Bourguignon (1972) and Laughlin (1976)

1	Native theory (emic view)
2	Individual meaning (phenomenological view)
3	(Etic views: complex society)
4	Psychological theory (e.g., Freudian)
5	Physiological theory (biochemical, pathological)

Permission to reproduce from Schenkman Publishing Company, Inc.

reconstruction of consciousness between neurotransmitters, the physical sections of the brain, and waking/sleep. Hallucinations and dreams then are the fragmentary residue of this process.

However, there can be a crossover between dreams and visions, as in the Saulteaux reported by Hallowell (1942), where a vision acquired as part of a quest can be informed later on by a dream. So important are dreams to some people that the Zinacantecans told Laughlin (1976), "They dream to live a full life. They dream to save their lives." These people are born with a soul and an animal companion spirit. A shaman sees best in dreams and can act as a lawyer before the gods for his patient or seek the cause of illness. But for most Zinacantecans, dreams can be battlefields where witches attempt to steal their souls. When they die each is reborn in the body of the opposite sex, to begin life anew. The world they live in, and ours as they see it, is constructed of portions "on the earth" (waking time) and sleep. Without the seeing of the soul in sleep, they can understand only a part of why things happen as they do, or know what is happening (Laughlin 1976, 4).

Levy-Bruhl (1966) summarizes the reports of peoples in ethnology who believe dreams are a part of reality. Travel in dreams to converse with ancestors or other spirits is widespread, for example, in Melanesia; see Codrington (1891). But spirits met in dreams are not always what they seem, as Firth reports in Tikopia, where spirits can impersonate a sister or mother and initiate sex. This was a common act of Greek gods. The dreamer is not in violation of incest taboos, because the spirit is not really a mother or sister, but also due to the fact that the spirits can control acts and minds and determine behavior (Firth 1936, 282).

There is a psychological condition, considered a pathology, called Dream-Reality Confusion (DRC). Here the dream state seems to overtake waking life, a condition I have seen in patients with dementia. Studies have shown that many people experience varieties of this condition and some are apparently functionally active or normal people who do also engage in more fantasy (Skrzypinska et al. 2018). It is also associated with narcolepsy (Wamsley 2014). Some individuals with lucid dreaming show this confusion (Christoff et al. 2018; Voss et al. 2009), a state also called oneirophrenia (Lazzari et al. 2017) when it appears in those with dementia, first noticed in people with AIDS-dementia complex. Yet in a cross-cultural study it was found that many people today believe god speaks to them in dreams and that dreams can reveal important information about life (Morewedge and Norton 2009). There is a long history of such beliefs and many examples among indigenous people (Levy-Bruhl 1966), yet the dream state, as many people describe it, resembles that reflected in the passages of the memory in temporal lobe seizures, a twilight consciousness, and seen in "the memory of patients after bilateral lesions of the mesial temporal lobes, a vague, fragmentary, fleeting, or nonexistent" (Blumer and Walker 1969). This similarity was early noted in the field of psychology as a means of using psychedelics that induced this likeness in some individuals to study psychosis.

Generally the reality of the dream's prediction is made clear in life, as when a woman dreamt that she saw herself as a corpse, but on the earth's surface she found her sister had died (Laughlin 1976). Among the Mount Hagen Melpa people, there are two kinds of dreams, positive ones and negative (taboo dreams). The latter include divinatory objects, repositories of truth, where lying has concealed information. It also includes references to boundaries. Analysis of these dreams and their use appears to show how the dreamer and the group allow for interpretations of events in daily life, clarifying and projecting knowledge so as to produce useful conclusions (Stewart and Strathern 2003). One might say that in like manner, the psychological framework of enculturation as performed by each individual in a complex society (or bee or ant society) is made up of unseen patterns that guide and ease the interactions of daily life, modulating the desires, needs, expectations, motivations, disappointments, and yearnings of everyone into a system of rewards and punishments defined by measures of conditioning. Etzioni's (1961) monumental study of how complex societies work was one approach to this problem. My 2017 book took a different approach, but this topic is not important here.

Laughlin (1976) provides a list of 152 dream "motifs" which are not simple symbols but are like scenarios that explain if one thing occurs like this, then it means that. Also, though most people understand the meaning of these motifs, there are some private ones. Of these, only 30 have favorable import and 90 predict sickness and death, 4 predict good health, 18 signify poverty, and 8 prosperity. But though the motifs have specific meaning, it is the response by the dreamer that determines the outcome, so the motifs present provisional contexts. Men and women dream and respond to the motifs, but if a man dreams his wife comes to his aid in dreams he will not be prey to sickness and death. Dreams that cannot be interpreted are considered the soul's madness. So perhaps we can learn something about cultural expectations from dreams.

A central question to the interpretation of dreams and hallucinations or visions is the identity of the actor or actors in the scene. This is hardly acknowledged by Grof; he simply assumes the patient is the actor or is the one acted on. For Grof (1976, 178–9), this is usually taken up as ego extension or identification with other actors, a type of transcendence but where the patient retains self-identity, which Grof calls "Dual Unity." Grof (1976, 135) gives the example of women who re-experience giving birth to a child only to find that it is they who are being born, not their child. But it seems to me from experiences I have observed that this is a frequent occurrence, where people see actors who are revealed as others or themselves, and this is very similar to what the Zinacantecas experience when in a dream it is unclear if an actor is the person themselves or a god or devil in disguise (Laughlin 1976, 10). It seems similar to how the Japanese founder of Shingaku, Ishida Baigan, described the seeking of the lost heart—the highest aim of study or *Gakumon* was to achieve this lost heart of heaven and earth in what Bellah (1957, 150) describes as a mystical experience, the arrival at complete tranquility and a "great feeling of happiness." Such states are often described by religious formulators, and some definitions of the encompassing of a special individual into the godhead, the apotheosis, come close to this feeling. The term "apotheosis," as derived from Greek, usually is translated as "to deify." But an older idea can be seen in the ethnohistorical literature, where humans are seen as undergoing a syncretism with a god or hero, as in the case of Quirinus and Romulus. This had several implications for the Romans of the Early Republic, as it unified a Sabine god of community with the leader Romulus, murdered by nobles, representing an agricultural deity whose parts, like Osiris, were scattered but reborn (see Plutarch, *Lives*, chapter 28).

However, in his chapter 5, Grof (1976) introduces transpersonal experiences in LSD. He argues that "ego death" can take place at the end of sessions, or during "high-dose" sessions. In this the subject's consciousness expands beyond his ego boundaries and can encompass all time and space, or other individuals, or many or the loss of self and identity entirely. This kind of experience is typical in my view and in the subjects at the Mogar Lab that I heard or read of in discussions. Such a perception of loss of self is different from identity with others or time and space. Some subjects in the Humboldt State experiments also experienced forms of euphoria that included aspects of such transpersonal nature, and hallucinations from such deprivation are common (Latham 1972), and there are pathological conditions that can bring forms of delirium on as well (Granberg-Axèll et al. 2001). In delirium some people experience hallucinations of body changes, numbers and spheres, and others of an incoherent flood of images from memory (Sacks 2012). There is an element of creativity that has been associated with delirium, as in the case of Lord Alfred Wallace and his bouts of malarial delirium (Wallace 1905).

Mefloquine (marketed as Lariam), an anti-malarial drug, induces in many people a kind of delirium, in others extended and detailed dreams, nightmares, and ranging in others to panic attacks, personality changes, and auditory or visual hallucinations. It has been suggested that it can induce encephalitis or inflammation of the limbic system. This includes the thalamus and hippocampus as well as the amygdala, so affecting these areas would be expected to produce the kinds of symptoms noted and are involved in most other hallucinations and similar expressions we have been discussing. It has affected thousands of people from soldiers to tourists (Ritchie et al. 2013). The range of symptoms and variation in appearance and expression are remarkable, but possibly related to aspects of susceptibility, extent of inflammation, and other factors of population variation.

Grof (1976, 155) suggests that transpersonal experiences are so diverse that it is difficult to define differences between what various individuals undergo, as they range from people reporting reliving evolution to dancing with spirits to becoming others and god. Some reported memories of being a fetus and knowing their mother's feelings about being pregnant. After stating this Grof then attempts a typology with everything from birth trauma to reliving past lives, subdivided by whether they include changes in time or space. The idea of reliving past lives takes on a more complex nature when we consider aboriginal concepts.

While children are reborn ancestors to some people (e.g., the Arunta), among the Kimberly Djaru, children exist as spirit-children (*djinganara:ny*) and are not ancestors. They were placed in pools by the Kaleru, the rainbow serpent in the *narungani* or Time Long Past before there were people. They were often temporarily incarnated as birds, reptiles, fish, or other animals and wander about the country very small, the size of a walnut or small red frogs. They enter a woman for conception by food or by her foot and a dream by her husband or a totem place (Kaberry 1939). One might imagine then that such a world of images in transformation could explain a variety of dreams of one's origin, history, and relations to plants and animals. Often transformations are represented as central icons or themes; people in some pathological cases imagine themselves as god, historical figures such as Napoleon, and familiar characters. This often happens in many psychedelic conditions, but also in the process of metempsychosis, in a form of prediction of future lives as animal or plant or as a temporary transition with other spiritual entities (West 1971). A simple description of the possibilities of this process appears in Napier (1986) discussing West's comments (1971):

> [A] tenet of Orphic and Pythagoreans, "its emphasis on the genuine transformation of humans into animals in natural and supernatural life cycles underlies both the ritual sense of bestial cohabitation and the sacred nature of cyclical revivification. Thus, the nature of each person's transmigration, the character of one's future identity, is inseparable from ritual identity, since every individual embodies an ambivalence overcome only by appropriate ritual acts. The success or failure of ritual, finally, provides every reason for one's present state."

We might consider what is of great interest here is whether such experiences (including Grof's transpersonal ones) are the result of some chemical change in the brain, induced by illness, stress, or cognitive pressure brought on by voluntary "willing." In other words, the "places people go," the animals or people they become, are they figments of some neurochemical actions, especially regarding the idea that an individual could induce by one's own desire a fantasy of personal transformation that could become so compelling by its rewards or stimulation that one becomes an occupant without return? Such transformations do occur in ethnographic dreams, as among the Zinacantecans—for example, a person dreams they are a goat. Any transformation into an animal is interpreted as meaning seeing one's companion animal spirit (Laughlin 1976, 9). More often they are chased by animals like snakes, cows, and bulls (Laughlin 1976, 102, 135). Grof interprets such "autosymbolic animal transformations" in rather common terms—as when subjects change into predators, he sees this as an expression only of aggressive feelings. Grof's descriptions of these examples, like reliving birth, ontogeny, or evolutionary history, also sounded to me like Ernst Haeckel's famous dictum, "Ontogeny recapitulates Phylogeny." My biology instructor once was quick to pour negative data on this mostly from Steven J. Gould's criticism of Haeckel.

I do not deny the statements made by Grof in his interpretation or the data he collected from his subjects, but I was a bit intrigued by them. Grof relates this to subjects who experience a transcendence where their consciousness has expended to encompass all life and existence. Once in my research a subject had this experience and when someone else present objected that their consciousness was not affected, it caused a long philosophical discussion on how one would know their consciousness was encompassed by another. I find that argument today like the algorithms hunting the internet, collecting our information and predicting our next choice. Others experience the inorganic world of atoms in forms like diamonds, gold, and so on as forms of consciousness. I recall such an experience when I perceived the structure of all things as if I had a kind of micro and macroscopic vision capable of "seeing" the internal structure of all things. Several other subjects I knew had similar visions and one had a very architectural description of molecules, which Grof reports as well and relates some subjects who interpreted consciousness as a form of energy allowing all things to intermingle and for them to sort of melt across dimensions of solid and gaseous worlds and reality.

Some subjects reported to Grof (1976, 181–3) transformation into plants or identification with plant life. He attributes this to intellectual preferences for philosophies that see plants as the perfect expression of life. In ethnographic context Wade Davis argues that many Native peoples interpret their experiences with plant-derived drugs as a means of ingesting the spirit of the plant or its consciousness (Davis 2001). Flying is a very common experience reported by Graf's subjects; it is related to time travel and "traveling clairvoyance," where the individual's consciousness only moves. Flying is typical in ethnographic settings—among the Zinacantecans, they report flying but it means death. That Zinacantecans can experience events at a distance also brings us within our own culture's extrasensory perception, mind reading, and interpretation of facial expressions (clairvoyance and mediumship; see Aiken 1970). Grof (1976, 190) brings up the possibility that telepathic knowledge is an aspect of familiarity and context. What a person knows of others and how this knowledge and the patterns of life can give a "seer" a valuable insight to predict the behavior of individuals not present, a form of mind reading can be derived from this as well, though facial reading, as defined by Paul Ekman and Friesen (2003), can be used in the same way, though this has been criticized; see Lutz and White (1986) and Russell and Fernandez-Dols (1997). This use of culturally defined interpretations brings us to the topic of "culture dreams."

Another aspect of this is noted by Bourguignon (1972, 416) regarding what Lincoln and Laughlin refer to as culture dreams or dreams with social meaning. Black (1975) recounts the hallucinations (visions) people have of foxes. Foxes, like some other animals, were regarded in some districts of Japan as benevolent animal spirits. In other areas they are seen as potentially dangerous, and when people see them, it verifies claims that the houses of people they appear near are malevolent in nature. Thus, in the case she describes, the priest Taikyuji "sees" a fox, which is evidence of the evil nature of the inhabitants of a place. Black likens these visions to those in the United Kingdom where spirits appear as spectral birds, dogs, or radiant boys when a member of a family is about to die. Such a "seeing" can also be a means of justifying control and legitimizing social sanctions (Fig. 2.1).

Grof's Transpersonal Experiences Scheme Parts I and II

I. Experiential Extension within the Framework of "Objective Reality"
   A. Temporal Expansion of Consciousness
      1. Embryonal and Fetal Experiences
      2. Ancestral Experiences
      3. Collective and Racial Experiences
      4. Phylogenetic (Evolutionary) Experiences
      5. Past-Incarnation Experiences
      6. Precognition, Clairvoyance, Clairaudience, and "Time travels"

   B. Spacial Expansion of Consciousness
      1. Ego Transcendence in Interpersonal Relations and the Experience of Dual Unity
      2. Identification with Other Persons
      3. Group Identification and Group Consciousness
      4. Animal Identification
      5. Plant Identification
      6. Oneness with Life and with All Creation
      7. Consciousness of Inorganic Matter
      8. Planetary Consciousness
      9. Extraplanetary Consciousness
      10. Out-Of-Body Experiences, Traveling Clairvoyance and Clairaudience, "Space Travels," and Telepethy

   C. Spatial Construction of Consciousness
      1. Organ, Tissue, and Cellular Consciousness

II. Experimental Extension beyond the framework of "Objective Reality"
   1. Spiritistic and Mediumistic Experiences
   2. Experiences of Encounters with Superhuman Spiritual Entities
   3. Experiences of Other Universes and Encounters with Their Inhabitants
   4. Archetypal Experiences and Complex Mythological Sequences
   5. Experiences of Encounters with Various Deities
   6. Intuitive Understanding of Univeral Symbols
   7. Activation of the Chakras and Arousal of the Serpent Power) Kundalini)
   8. Consciousness of the Universal Mind
   9. The Supracosmic and Metacosmic Void

Fig. 2.1 Grof's transpersonal experiences scheme parts I and II

Grof's Transpersonal Categories

Obviously, writers of all kinds can create fictional worlds that are compelling and "real," even addicting, as in fans and stories like Star Wars, Star Trek, and Game of Thrones. The world of the internet (Jiang et al. 2013) and even cell phones can become addicting (Carbonell et al. 2013). This brings us back to Lincoln's distinction between the unsought after, spontaneous dream versus the desired or induced "culture pattern" dream. We may desire one and attempt to bring it on, or we may be subject to dreams of no interest but which can affect us dramatically. In some people fasting can bring on a desired dream state (Levy-Bruhl 1966), but some indigenous people apparently do not have general "culture pattern" dreams (as it is claimed for the Navajo) but mainly personal dreams (Spaulding 1981). It is as if we were radios walking about, subject to a spinning dial where transmissions of dream sequences of no relation to us are capable of being "picked up." However, as I have noted elsewhere, I think these "unsought for," confusing dreams are likely to be as Freud and others suggested, a means by which our brain edits contemporary events in the context of a rain of memories always present from our past as infants and children, images of incomprehensible experiences (huge parents, tubs of water, rain, etc.; see also Winson 1990). This is similar to the views of some Icelanders (Anderson 2005) and is reflected in a book by Gudjonsson (1976). Reincarnation and ghosts are a common consideration for dreams among many, especially the Icelandic geologist and spiritualist Helgi Pjeturss. His book *Nyall* [*The Discovery of the Way Out*] published in 1919–1920. The book, and several companion texts, presents ideas of dreaming, the afterlife, astrobio, and telepathy. As Anderson relates, many Icelandic people share ideas of parallel worlds and communication with dead relatives and spirits.

The method of experience combination into dream sequences is theoretical, but one can imagine the use of cartoons, photos, TV, plays, conversations, radio, and so on, all integrated as the mind chops up the memories and sorts them into segments. Cerf et al. (2010) have shown how sensory stimuli can be sorted and suppressed or used to create hybrid images that did not exist before. This can be a part of a model for dream construction, as Wamsley (2020) has described other components, especially regarding people lacking a hippocampus. See page 164 for more on this problem.

Types of Hallucinations, Visions, Archetypes, or Physical Features

Optical effects of various phenomenon associated with the eyes can produce retained images, as when one looks away from a scene but the image travels onto other visual contexts (known as visual perseveration). Or in patterns perceived by people from "seeing stars" in trauma, pressure on the eyes in different ways (as in a finger in the corner of the eye socket), or in certain chemically induced conditions, as in peyote use described by Knauer and Maloney and cited by Kluver (1928/1966, 19, 22, 32–33). Kluver relates his own experiences with mescaline and these include phosphene-like patterns that turn into a variety of objects, like a rotating wheel, screws, and a picture of god as a human male with a pale face and red cheeks. The constantly changing colors are common and his scene changes into a water scene like a Japanese painting, then sparks (again phosphenes), and then to heads, which change to a mushroom and a skeleton. These are later in the experience, reported to give way to other forms, geometric or animal. Kluver's revision (1942) suggests four general classes of form: lattices, spirals, cobwebs, and tunnels. Kluver's self-experimentation gave him a list of patterns created by psychedelically induced hallucinations, and Ermentrout and Cowan (1979) demonstrated how these were produced from the electrical activity of the first layer of the visual cortex as geometric shapes. Goldenfeld suggested that these were the "Turing Patterns" proposed by Alan Turing in 1952, which includes noise and is called a "stochastic Turing mechanism" (Karig et al. 2018).

This brings up the issue of what is perceived; here with Turing Patterns and phosphenes, we are dealing with the physical results of brain functioning—one might say its neurochemistry and effects. When we perceive objects and things, including people, planets, and rocks, for example, that are present, this is called, veridical perception—from the root, truthful, and measured in degrees of information or knowledge of an object and its context. When we are perceiving images of reality, but that are not present, this is often called "veridical hallucinations" (Macpherson 2013). We can contrast such images with those that do not exist, perhaps a chimera, like a unicorn or a mermaid, or a fly with a human head. These kinds of images are reported by people in dreams, on psychedelics and in pathological states. This touches on the phenomenal character of life experience, what is called "qualia" or the unique experience of each individual (Crick 1994). Thus, to be able to communicate a feeling, we must be able to describe it to another, yet that experience is unique to each person and must be generally expressed, as Nagel (1974) argued, to agree that there is "something that is like" what each understands. Where such a common feeling or aspect of reality can be expressed, it is sometimes called a "common-kind view of hallucination."

Where one experiences images and feelings that are in no way related to common experience (reality) and one is left with no ability to translate the experience to past experience or common-kind views, then this can be classed as a disjunctivist conception of hallucination, and finally an experience where the components of reality are so formed that the individual mistakes it for actual reality but where no other person experiences it. It may be momentary or continuous as in schizophrenic pathologies, where an individual becomes some figure, even a historical person, and lives the hallucinogenic narrative (Macpherson 2013). Such a narrative can be broken into lucid periods and some functionality of the individual can occur or become a mission in life, as in hearing the voice of god, ancestors, or spirits. These are perhaps poor classifications; they do not present the vast variety of experience people have. For example, I once had what ophthalmologists call a "floater" experience. Here the microscopic fibers in the vitreous substance of the eye clumped and tugged at the retina (as the ophthalmologist I saw described the process). What I experienced in one half of my visual field was a complete rippling of the landscape or anything I looked at. It took an instant to conceive of the condition as a physical change in my vision, and not knowing the cause I immediately phoned my doctor and was informed. In that instant, reality seemed to change inconceivably and without cause or purpose. One cannot call this a "common-kind hallucination," even though it can be explained medically, because most people do not have the experience and thus have no framework for comparison as a commonality. It could be a form of disjunctivist hallucination, but again, as with phosphenes and Turing Patterns, not everyone has the experience or recognizes it.

Alternative stripes of firing and non-firing neurons are transmitting to the striate cortex, producing patterns. And this seems logical for phosphenes and abstract patterns, but what about the marching faces and repeated patterns of CBS patients' hallucinations? Here Ernentrout and Cowan (1979; see also Ouellette 2018) argue that the brain has evolved to identify patterns and associate them with images in memory, so we might reflect on this, given the role the hippocampus has in CBS and some other pathologies (Santhouse et al. 2000). But why psychedelics produce strange images seemingly unrelated to memories may be due to the vast memories from childhood or those seen in media in a lifetime and jumbled during the LSD or other drug session. Obviously, the phosphenes, "Turing Patterns," and memories appear in individual people's psychedelic experiences in a mixed form. This is apparent even in Huxley's (1954) examples that are described in sequential form; usually such changes are so quick and so mixed it would be difficult to transcribe or recall them. From my experience and from those related to me and in the literature, there seems to be little object pattern to this alternating, though since the focus of attention can be changed in a second by a change of stimuli (images, environmental conditions, light, sound, etc.), we can, I think, fall back to a physiological explanation, that the brain is attempting to find patterns and is simply processing new stimuli with internal stimuli on a random basis of firing neurons, some inhibiting and connectivity being modifying in a chaotic stream. This then could be seen as a modified release theory, as discussed earlier. This conclusion seems consistent with some recent findings. For example, Winkelman finds that most psychedelics disrupt the normal functions of the prefrontal cortex and the default mode network (DMN), releasing thalamic and other brain discharges that stimulate the visual information representation system, releasing "the effects of innate cognitive function and operators" (Winkelman 2017; Palhano-Fontes et al. 2015).

Yet, recent comprehensive imaging and molecular studies of psychedelics, while producing findings consistent with earlier studies, reflect the difficulty of specifying effects in the brain (Cumming et al. 2021). But it is curious, as Sacks (2012) points out, that much of this information about hallucinations was gathered by F.W. H. Myers at a time when he introduced the term "hypnopompic" in 1901. It seems that little progress has been made even with the discovery of new psychedelics.

However, this does not illuminate the experiences both in history and in contemporary indigenous cultures or some specific drug combinations, as in ayahuasca, of prophetic messages or personal predictions and journeys (see the variety listed in the charts on ayahuasca archetypes and types of psychedelic experiences). These might be explained, as I will later discuss, by both cultural learning and cueing as well as expectations and personal desire (back to wish fulfillment). In both cases, the experience would demand some degree of self-discipline to maintain a thread of consciousness, at least in my opinion. Being cued in a cultural context would provide the individual to construct and reflect as the experience unfolds to produce a coherent narrative at the end, one admittedly in most cases, with degrees of ad hoc reconstruction. Harner (1972) addresses the similarity of experience and motif (flying, snakes, felines, etc.) in a number of reports where subjects were unaware of the nature of the drug or the cultural background or both (see some similarities but many differences in non-indigenous subjects who had no knowledge of yage by Naranjo 1972). While more controlled studies are needed, there are some indications that physiological responses of humans to psychedelics may provide answers to these similarities.

The phosphene study gives us another example of scientific curiosity and enthusiasm. It was discovered in the eighteenth century that if a group of people held hands in a circle and received a shock from a high-voltage electrostatic generator, it produced a certain entertainment and novel feelings. Benjamin Franklin found during one of these events that while holding his eyes shut he observed flashing lights, thus phosphenes. Alessandro Volta discovered that these flashes only appeared when making or breaking the circuit and were most easily experienced by placing the electrodes on the temples of one's skull. In 1819 physiologist Johannes Purkinje published an account of intense phosphine experience by holding one electrode on his forehead and one in his mouth (Oster 1970).

Images, as people report them, are often intriguing, as in Kluver seeing "nuns in silver dresses," an image that would be interesting to explore, but usually questions about images in the course of a "trip" causes a loss of image and no knowledge reported by the subject about it. Graf (1976) gives more information from his questioning of subjects that may reflect method, familiarity. or subject. Kluver (1928/1966, 29) states, regarding attempts to study the effects reported, "On the one hand, the investigators emphasize that the phenomena defy all description. On the other hand, the phenomena reported present such striking differences in appearance that it seems adequate to stress the diversity of these phenomena than the 'common elements.'" He quotes Havelock Ellis, "the chief character of the visions is their indescribableness." This idea of a lack of uniformity of experience or character of individual images as failing categories from person to person is repeated by other investigators summarized by Kluver and reinforces the idea that the peyote experience, and perhaps many others, can be individual if taken outside of a similar cultural context where a suggestion of what is to be expected is lacking. Some investigators do find patterns of responses; however, what Kluver produces and I have found are placed in a chart below.

Kluver (1928/1966, 57) argues also that one such "category" or type of vision is the incomplete sequence, or "Presque vu." Events or actions appear to lead to a certain end or direction. They suggest an unfinished state, there is, as noted in Gestalt, as lack of closure. This lack of completeness can be seen to represent in some cultures the ongoing circle of life, or life before death, or the lineage of a family from past into the future. The missing element can take the form of a horizon where the factor is just out of view—which in dream therapy could mean the missing spouse or solution to a problem. The subject of dreams and death is often linked in some cultures. Among the Nuer, Evans-Pritchard (1956, 134) found a horror of death, which is linked to the idea that dreams are "prognostications of death." For the Nyakyusa, Wilson (1963, 96) discovered that proof of the activity and identity of witches could be discerned in dreams as well as the defenders of villages who were believed to see and fight witches in dreams.

Another category of Kluver is the set of oppositions. One may be highly active, the other slow, one solar, the other polar. They may approximate each other as if resolving their differences, as in the case of one of Beringer's (1927) subjects, but just at the moment of resolution, all falls apart and opposition is restored (Fig. 2.2).

Some of these designs appear to transform into scenes that the individual finds himself or herself inside or climbing on. In addition to specific form, like a tunnel, transformation can result in a funnel or alleyway. A lattice can become a tree or plant with leaves. Lattices in patients with CBS have similar character to the aura in migraines and are referred to as tesselloptic grids, perhaps having a common foundation (Santhouse et al. 2000). Though Sacks (2012) states that migraines often are accompanied by a kidney-shaped blind spot that is scintillating, and he could see in his geometric structures a constant motion. A whole range of other

Investigator	type of response
Knauer	| wavy lines | mosaics | carpets | floral | land | monuments
	| ornaments | wood-carving | windmills | mausoleums |
	| men and animals | episodes connected
Rouhier	| Geometric figures | kaleidoscopically changing forms
	| landscapes faces
	| monstrous forms fabulous landscapes
H. Ellis	| visions never resembled familiar objects always novel
	|| almost familiar: fields of jewels, sparkling or glowing
	flowers change to butterfly
Beringer	| gratings | lattice | fretwork | filigree | honeycomb
	| chessboard designs | cobweb

Fig. 2.2 Chart of patterns reported for peyote by investigator

distortions in perception can also occur at the same time, as in changes of color, depth, and size perception. Some perceive objects in motion or acting as if motivated. Serko (1913) describes his legs turning into spirals. Havelock Ellis and many of the subjects quoted by Kluver note that the colors are often not true; instead they are blends, radiating variations in saturation and hue (Kluver 1928/1966, 43). Havelock Ellis sees textures in color, woven elements, and, at times, dull, but then polished and semi-transparent. Grof (1976, 116) gives this a special category of robotic nature, where the subject perceives a lack of organic life. Related to this is how the colors can disappear and yet become illumination, and this aspect of brightness and changes in it seem to be very common reports. Huxley (1954), referring to Plato's *Phaedo*, suggests the brilliant colors seen, like the quality of gems in light, reflect on an aspect of another world or that gems came to be valuable not for their stability and durable colors, but the psychedelic experiences early humans had that gems seemed a lost part of an imaged world. Beringer notes subjects seeing light coming from backgrounds of objects, or from overhead, and this idea of a directionality of light was significant to Kluver (1928/1966, 44). Localization of images is often vague, yet images do not usually move when the eyes or head do. Objects may appear larger than normal, if there are reference points in the vision, or smaller. Sometimes they speak to the dreamer or tripper—often this is incoherent, or they may ignore the subject entirely.

Intention expressed during peyote, that is, a will to see or experience certain things, was not usually achieved. Some individuals do seem, however, in Kluver's (1928/1966, 51–2) cases, to be able to control images and this parallels certain kinds of dreamers' experiences without drugs, as in eidetic memory or lucid dreaming. Some eidetic dreamers report images appear and disappear as if dream snippets (which seems contradictory, as eidetic implies the ability to recall), though others can recall dreams with apparent detail. In some cultures the telling of dreams is routine and expected. Du Bois (1945) tells how at night most families are woken by a member who has dreamed and gets up to stoke the fire and tell the dream. Lucid dreaming and organized or controlling hallucinations have become part of a popular movement in neo-shamanism (Kent 2010). Many dreamers feel limited in action (as an audience) or frozen in dreams and peyote experiences. The loss of control is the obverse of this and often people report a sense of chaos, as if witnessing a Pandora's Box or Sorceror's Apprentice experience. This involves the individual in some degree of control of interest in events, as if they were responsible for them taking place (thus a sense of guilt) but lack the ability to control or stop them.

Background to Miracles, Demons, Boredom, and Patterns of Life

It is of interest to some of the discussions here that comparisons of people who have often experienced lucid dreaming with a control population that do not show more connectivity in the lucid dreamers' brains between the prefrontal cortex, the bilateral angular gyrus, bilateral middle temporal gyrus, and right inferior frontal gyrus (Baird et al. 2018). It also appears as a hybrid state of consciousness, with differences between waking and REM (rapid eye movement) sleep in the frontal areas of the brain (Voss et al. 2009). The association of REM sleep and dreaming has been a topic of interest in dream analysis and La Barre (1975) reviews the experimental work in both cross-cultural and pathological context as well as in species comparison (cats). In a limited study Petre-Quadens et al. (1975) found that the Temiars of the Malayan peninsula, who were hunter-gatherers, had a low percentage rate of REM sleep (16%) compared to studies in urban industrial populations of between 20% and 25% (Colten and Altevogt 2006).

Siegel (2001) reexamined the nature of REM sleep both regarding memory and learning and found the evidence for memory consolidation weak and contradictory and that for learning inconsistent and not correlated with learning ability for humans. But La Barre (1975) argues from experimental foundations that when people are deprived social interaction, including deaf individuals, they can produce a form of hallucination to reproduce the lack of stimulation. To a certain extent this is true of the sensory deprivation information and it would seem to parallel ideas of Vygotsky (1978) on the development of language in a social context mentioned elsewhere in this text. La Barre (1975) associates hallucinations of this type with cultural isolation some people experience as well as that of prisoners in solitary confinement. He calls this "compensatory hallucination" for social isolation (La Barre 1975). Smith (2006) reviews the literature on this phenomenon beginning in the Middle Ages.

Another related question of what happens to the brain to subvert consciousness or create it relates to the patient under anesthesia or in coma. Anesthesiologists refer to general anesthesia as induced coma, but avoid mentioning that to patients. Yet the facts of what happens to the brain indicate this is true (Brown et al. 2011), and the changes that induce this state and coma are very different from sleep. Different anesthetic agents have produced a range of states from a complete absence of subjective experience (unconsciousness) to varying degrees of partial consciousness, with some memory of experience. Experiments with these agents appear to support concepts of between-region connectivity in the creation of consciousness (Bonhomme et al. 2019). Though some anesthesia agents like chloroform can produce hallucinations, those of a sexual nature are most noted for some newer agents like midazolam, benzodiazepines, nitrous oxide, and propofol (especially in combination with fentanyl or sufentanyl) (Balasubramaniam and Park 2003).

Solitary confinement is rather like a huge social experiment, as about 20% of all prisoners in the United States are forced into these conditions for at least 22.5 hours a day (Metzner and Fellner 2010). One individual, Albert Woodfox, spent more than 40 years in isolation. Hallucinations and mania are not uncommon under these conditions (Reiter et al. 2020). La Barre (1975) also notes the hallucinations of people for long periods, as in the case of Admiral Byrd, Captain Joshua Slocum, and Sir Ernest Shackleton and his companions in the Antarctic who had hallucinations. There are famous Arabic stories of apparitions existing in lonely places, specific jinn, and it is of interest how often these manifest as women, young or old, or spirits who make the transition of age before the startled eyes of the traveler, as in the *Saragossa Manuscript.* It is interesting that women are often hidden in public in Islamic countries, but in hallucinations they are unveiled, which, of course, indicates they are jinn.

If we examine lucid dreaming and the state of consciousness induced by peyote or LSD, we find numerous similarities. However, one element is of central interest and that is the ability of the individual to engage the experience, that is, to control or act within the dream or hallucination and make choices. In general hallucinations are considered events that impinge on the individual and cannot be altered; they can be projected outside the individual as a miracle, or only present in the inner eye of the person experiencing them (Sacks 2012). But there are variations to this paradigm, and some people do interact in dreams and hallucinations. The idea of miracles is a wide subject that varies by religion and culture. Saint Augustine argued that the conversion of a sinner or evil person was a miracle. The Catholic Church holds that miracles are preternatural or supernatural because total "Reality" is not visible to the human eye (Catholicism.org 2020). To some people, like the Jivaro (Harner 1972) access to true or total reality can only be attained by using psychedelics. Elements of culture may precondition such perceptions as when Harner (1972) uses ayshuasca and meets bird-headed people during his experience who assure him they are the true gods. Miracles in this dogma can be "above the laws of nature," that is, raising the dead or contrary to the laws of nature, as in parting the Red Sea. They are expressions of power and knowledge by the godhead. In the ancient world miraculous cures would be included, the action of magic and manifestations of power in nature as volcanoes and massive storms are clear examples. The variety is so great and the number so stupefying in the "supernatural" make up that classifying has a quality of absurdity, as Ashe (1978) has shown. But this depends on interpretation, as in some ancient societies gods walked the earth, in others spirits are expected to meet people and interact with them. Verifying such events today, however, is near-impossible and requires belief for their survival (talking animals, signs or images of gods in omelets, etc.).

Most historically recorded miracles relate active interaction between the individual and the miraculous entities or events, as in the partridges that landed on Sidi Slima's body to pick off the lice (Vansina 1985) or apparitions of a malevolent nature. Freud (1966, 498) attributed some of these to the power of belief, or individual skill, as in the séances of his time or conjuring tricks when more than one person claims to have seen a supernatural event. The confusion of crowds (or mass hypnosis) leads to claims of miracles, as in the bread and fish of Matt. 4.17. In some groups ritual and belief are prime members for the experience of miracles, as in the Mahikari of Japan (Bowen 2002). The cult of Mary among some Catholics, has produced a number of interactive miracles, especially where children are participants, as at Fatima in 1917 (Bowen 2002). Many hallucinations are static while in others, like those of Huxley (1954), we find pictures or settings like flowers seem to become "alive" only in the sense that they visually "vibrate" or show pulsations and mimic movement of elements in them, as in the perceptions of Krippner (1970) in paintings. But other people have more active hallucinations where people move, paintings come alive, and objects appear and disappear.

There are also aberrations of normal perception as when one sees only half a face; this can be the result of a chance combination of reception and called a "misperception." There are also conditions where one person present will see only one feature in a scene, while another sees five or more after the feature is moved. This is a "polyopia." If the person sees multiple images while the one is still present, this is called "palinopsia." Sometimes this is also referred to as "visual perseveration," and is reported in CBS. The sensation of movement of the image can also revert to its original position or repeat the change. These are both examples of preservation of image and are usually considered to be distinct conditions, though they have been reported to appear together in the same person in a case of occipital lobe epilepsy, which is interpreted to mean that they are related in some way (Kataoka and Ueno 2009). Some epileptics also report multiple images and repeated images or words in the air or on walls that can be read, as opposed to CBS (Sacks 2012). In some cases these images can be superimposed over actual objects and, if they possess writing, can still be read. More frequent or typical are bright spots or blue spots, which often rotate. So, to a certain extent, these two pathologies share some forms of expression in hallucinations, though some epileptics experience "dream-like fantasies" and "reminiscences." And there appears to be a link in some epileptics where they dream vivid scenes and some of the images of dreams appear in the epileptic visions—these appear as false flashbacks of places once visited (Sacks 2012). Then we might say that the scene is familiar but the qualia, the essential aspects that make up the reality of a memory to a particular person, is strange.

What is curious is not that drugs can limit or reduce seizure in epileptics, but that surgery can result in either better drug control or their silence. This is remarkable given that some one third of epilepsy patients' seizures cannot be controlled by drugs. Those with "lesional epilepsy" respond poorly to antiepileptic drugs, but vagus nerve stimulation can provide relief for some patients (Miller and Hakimian 2013). Removal of "focal areas" of the temporal or other lobes of the brain or surgeries usually involving tumors or vascular malformations (abnormal blood vessel groups) often are undertaken in some epileptic conditions. Why such surgery can be effective is curious. In one case a patient had a seizure-related vision of Christ telling him to kill his wife and then himself, of which he did only the first part. But after surgery he no longer had seizures (Sacks 2012). This kind of "command hallucination" is much like those in psychosis and are often related to delusions, yet distinguishing them from "intrusive thoughts" is difficult (Hersh and Borum 1998). But some epileptics have hallucinations that are only "feelings," some of a spiritual nature (though in one case the person "converted" to atheism after it) or in combination with auditory or visual sensations, as in the case of a conductor who felt he was in heaven (Sacks 2012). Sacks ponders this result, wondering if interpretations of the "sacred disease" of epilepsy imply some universal basis for spirituality or, as Durkheim would have it, a feeling of social unity. One neurologist made a specific examination of this idea (Nelson 2010).

Mesial temporal sclerosis (MTS) is a common finding in patients with temporal lobe epilepsy. It appears that this abnormality is both the cause and the result of seizures, especially prolonged ones. The main theory regarding MTS is that it is due to excessive excitability after release of excitatory amino acids, primarily glutamate. Agents that produce MTS in adult animals when applied experimentally do not do so in immature ones (Liu et al. 1995), while injury to the head can induce epilepsy and so can electrical stimulation of the brain. Penfield and Jasper (1954) developed a method of stimulating the exposed brain with an electrical probe that could locate areas that produced seizure. Removal of these often resulted in improvement for the patient. Certain chemicals can also induce epileptic conditions in animals. One of these, pilocarpine, causes local injury to the brain, leading to hippocampal sclerosis and reorganization of neuronal networks (Curia et al. 2008). Pilocarpine induces an increase in glutamate levels in the hippocampus following the appearance of seizures. Penfield and Jasper's probing often produced images of past events; he called them "flashbacks," and such remembered images have been reported from traumatic events as in PTSD and in drug use, especially LSD. Dostoevsky experienced epileptic seizures that were ecstatic or of transcendent joy and mystical (Sacks 2012).

Recent studies have found that about half of all people questioned have experienced some form of lucid dreaming. But only 11% have had two or more lucid dreams. So this brings up the issue of initiation of a lucid dream (Vallat and Ruby 2019). Since many people express an interest in engaging in a lucid dream, why are so few able to initiate one or to have one at all? Even rarer are people who report lucid dreaming but also controlling behavior—that is, they can make choices in the dream that can change events or act on the dream or dream entities. It is of interest that attempts to induce lucid dreaming are largely unsuccessful; these mostly rely on interrupting sleep and especially deep sleep. Some experience multiple appearances of objects, first one and then the repeated image over and over again, called polyopia.

Oster (1970) gives a general explanation and Cervetto et al. (2007) a more technical one. Usually people perceive patterns with their eyes closed that are similar to swirls or rotating streams. William James, like others, had a "feeling illness" and later headache, but does not describe his visions, but notes them (Kluver 1928/1966, 25). We will discuss other physiological examples in due course (Fig. 2.3).

Types of Psychedelic Experience

These are mainly visual a great many people have auditory hallucinations. These are discussed in the text and can largely be divided between musical and voices.

	Mescaline	LSD	MDA	Shaman/religious
1. Brilliant colors	x	x	x	
2. unstable conditions	x	x	x	
3. seeing self as dead	x	x	x	x/
4. seeing spiritual beings	x	x	x	x/x
5. speaking w/ spirits	x	x	x	x/x
6. geometric designs	x	x	x	
7. seeing the future				x/x
8. seeing gems/gem palaces	x	x	x	x/x

Frequency and Source

1. Mescaline 1, 2, 3, 4,5 Osmond, 1970
2. LSD
3. MDA
4. Religious (via pain, self-abuse, starvation, meditation, etc)
5. Psilocybin
6. Peyote

(Mescaline–the active ingredient of psilocybin and peyote-is listed separately simply to identify the source)

7. Ayahuasca
8. Anadenenanthera peregina, A. colubrine (Mimosa hostilis)

Examples

A Visions (NDV)

1. in Ezra
2. Abram of Yahweh: Gen. 15:1
3. Daniel 2:12
4. Handsome Lake
5. Milarepa

Hallucinations

1. Glass of water becomes a vortex of time (m) Osmond, 1970

Fig. 2.3 Types of psychedelic experience

2. Zelda sees walls becoming pink lattice
   a. flowers, shapes of animals, blue dots (p) Sacks, 2012
   b. nose grows in size on person's face
   c. she sees one person become many copies of self= polyopia

6. Handsome Lake (Seneca Prophet)
   a. Sees 4 messengers pleading for him to come
   b. See a pathway covered with grass
   c. Sees a woman speaking
   d. Sees an overgrown pathway

7. Thomas Hennell (p) Hennell, 1938
   a. Orchestra tuning up (discordant sounds)
   b. Fields of plantings boiling
   c. "Van Gogh" like sky

8. Robert Sinnett (M) Sinnett, 1970
   a. geometric grid with vivid color

8. Stanley Krippner (Ps) Krippner, 1970
   a. intense taste, colors
   b. images of oriental palace, space travel, music
   c. complex hallucination with movement and action
   d. prediction of Kennedy murder
   e. interactive he is in boat on violent sea
   f. meets god

9. Jonathan Clark (Ps) Clark, 1970
   a. while listening to music, notes float and skate across a floor

10. Bernard Aaronson (LSD) Aaronson, 1970
   a. color changes, flashing lightning, man turns to clown. Euphoria. Saw Hebrew letters,
   b. sees friend transformed into devil
   c. see self in strange city with brown skin but is familiar with scene
   d. perceived person as tree
   e. Cave appears with shaft of light
   f. ground bubbles
   g. goblins and red devils, comical
   h. floating yellowish squares
   i. human changes into elf, wolf & leprechaun

Fig. 2.3 (continued)

11. Richard Bucke (NVD) Bucke, 1901
    a. vision of being wrapped in a flame – colored cloud & euphoria
12. Hebb's student experiments (SD) Bexton, et al. 1954
    a. dots and llines, geometric patterns, little yellow men with hats
13. Santhouse, et al., CBS patients (p) Santhouse, et al. 2000
    a. facial distortion, grids or latticed networks
    b. small figures wearing hats in biological motion
    c. multiple copies of objects in rows
    d. armies, ancient ones
    e. small children standing by bed
    f. road maps with tiny cities 6 feet away
    g. musical notes
    h. multiple particles like rain drops over everything
    i. car approach, then turn off abruptly

14. Aldous Huxley (M) Stevens, 1988
    a. field of little squares, then blue spheres
    b. Creation and eternity in his pants, flowers, etc.
15. Experiments by Pascual-Leone (SD) Merabet, et al., 2004
    a. flashing lights, phosphenes
    b. geometrical patterns
    c. figures, faces, hands, animals, buildings, landscapes
    d. peacock feathers, sunsets
    e. transformations: butterfly to sunset to otter to flower
16. Anderson (NVD) Anderson, 2005)
    a. ancestors, angels, Alien beings
17. Michael Shermer (F) Shermer, 2011)
    a. UFOs
    b. horses, trains, phantom people, voices, strange animals
18. Jerry Richardson (LSD) Richardson, 1970
    a. faces in mirror change to animal, aged to grotesque to ethnic
    b. an endless stream of human forms moving toward him, sad, suffering, but perhaps related to music playing in the setting.
19. Gerald Heard (LSD) Stevens, 1988)
    a. Great Void, darkness, world boundless, pointless
20. Marie Persaud (LSD) ZoeHelene.com
    a. self in colorful God's eye nebula
21. Marie Persaud (NDV) ZoeHelene.com
    a. celebration float lighted up on road
    b. communication with grasshopper

Fig. 2.3 (continued)

22. Marie Persaud (SA) ZoeHelene.com
    a. on Hoffman's bicycle on yellow brick road with flowers
23. Jeffrey Linzer (Y) Linzer, 1970
    a. becomes snake, frog and sea lion
    b. experiences a jungle
24. Laura Bridgman (NDV) Tylor, 1889
    b. her breath taken by god to heaven
25. Janiger's sujects (LSD) Stevens, 1987
    a. Became bird
    b. Images beyond images to infinity (Anais Nin diary)
26. Milarepa (NDV) Milarepa, 11th century
    a. demons
27. Sacks subjects (L) Sacks, 2012
    a. faces on tv screens
    b. pictures come alive
    c. cars attacking female subject (L, P and A Sacks, 2012)
    d. fierce chimerical animal elephant –like (L and P Sacks, 2012)
    e. human brain from noodles (L and P Sacks, 2012
    f. missing cat appears repeatedly (L and P Sacks, 2012)
    g. strangers invade room, take notes, photos of subject, have sex. (L and P Sacks, 2012)
    h. tattoos appear on peoples faces (L and P Sacks, 2012)
    i. image of Taj Mahal with chanting (L and P Sacks, 2012)
    j. old photos appear on ceiling lamp (L and P Sacks, 2012)
    K. women trying on fur coats (L and P Sacks, 2012)
    L. furry black animal jumps at (L and P Sacks, 2012)
    m. urine stream becomes video of recent past (LSD Sacks, 2012)
    n. sees cells of self functioning (LSD Sacks, 2012)
    o. levitates, travels through tunnel to beautiful light, total love, voices, relives life (LSD Sacks, 2012)
    p. stars, tunnel, flame, colors, kaleidoscope of Images (eyes closed) eyes open: room changes size, face covered with
    q. lice, geometric patterns, laughter
    r. see non-existing people & conversation& Helicopter (Ar, Sacks 2012)

Fig. 2.3 (continued)

s. philosophical conversation with spider
t. face turns to gorilla (P, Sacks. 2012 & Ebin, 1965)
u. friend turns into fake (LSA, Sacks, 2012)
v. Medieval battle scene on sleeve (O, Sacks, 2012)
w. coffee turns green, then blue; person has head like elephant seals, people on bus have huge white heads like eggs, with glittering eyes designed like compound eyes of insects. (O, Sacks, 2012)
x. "Amy" sees aliens as in Hollywood movies (P) Sacks, 2012
y. towers, gems tiny lights, colors, geometric images by Weir Mitchell (Pe)

28. Paul Radin (P. Radin, 1920)
a. sees eagle before him, then lion and then a small man in blue military suit, then flags, beautiful ones in house, sees Earthmaker spirit becomes spirit, feels all are linked
,b. sees self tied up, flowers, road, city
29. Ralph Metzner (from Spanish sources on Aztecs)(T, Metzner, 1970)
a. individuals attacked by worns, snakes
b. seeing future, own death, adultery, drowning, riches
30. Myerhoff (Pe, Myerhoff, 1974)
a. impaled on the tree of life
b. sees magic bird
31. Barbara (K, Barbara, 2021)
a. sees evil clowns, Jair Bolsonaro
32. Woman hospitalized other reasons (O, Kiyokawa and Haning, 2021)
a. sees bugs in hair and clothes
33. multiple images, same repeated one (P=Sacks, 2012)
a. sees man coming from manhole in street wearing white hat with flag on it
b. figure clad in white back only showing in large room with large windows
34. Tim Leary sees palaces, temples & bejeweled vistas like Huxley (Pe. Stevens, 1987)
35. Visions of memory, working walking down streets (P, Noda, 1993)
36. World of color, beauty and god (Adelle Davis, 1961)

Fig. 2.3 (continued)

37. Visions of spirit world, flowers, birds, clashing rocks destroying souls, Thunderbird shooting lightning (Schultes, 1972)
38. Gods judging humans & destruction of world (Masters & Houston, 1966)
39. In desert, becomes one with light gardens (de Rios & Janiger, 2003)
40. sexual feeling, enchanted gardens (de Rios & Janiger, 2003)

Abbreviations

1. M= mescaline
2. LSD
3. MDA
4. p= pathology, cancer, lesions in brain, trauma
5. NDV=No drug Vision/ hallucination
6. Ps = psilocybin
7. Pe = peyote
8. SD = sensory deprivation techniques
9. F = fasting, exhaustion
10. SA = Salvia divinorum
11. K = ketamine
12. L= L-dopa
13. A= amantadine prevents dopamine uptake
14. T= teonanactl or psilocybin species (e.g., Psilocybe mexicana)
15. Ar= Artane Sacks' experience with this drug produces what appears to be an entirely auditory hallucination, the interesting point is the "conversation" with imaginary people. The drug is an antispasmodic used to treat stiffness in Parkinson's.
16. Y = Yage / harmine / reserpine / ayahuasca
17. O = opioids
18. LSA= Lysergic acid amide, Morning Glory seeds, also Ololiuhqui, Pomoea violacea, etc.
19. I= iboga
20. Ap/c = Anadenenanthera peregina, A. colubrine (Mimosa hostilis) see Schultes, 1972

Fig. 2.3 (continued)

There is a problem with the 4th and 5th categories. Some of the features noted by individuals in these categories may be related by the natural history of disease and not external stimuli in #5. Teeple et al. (2009) have produced a table in an attempt to classify the etiology of the visual hallucinations. The simple patterns, spots, shapes or lines they associate with migraine, seizure and tumors. Macropsia, micropsia and metamorphopsia are associated with seizure and Crutzfeldt-Jakob disease. While this relation cannot extend to all cases where disease was not known at the time of study, it might indicate that stages of disease or factors of (as in seizure) might be developing or present yet unknown.

Entries from Sacks (2012), r, s, u and v are Sacks' own experiences with drugs.

Siegel (1977) produced a series of categories derived mainly from Kluver (1966) but inspired by Moueau and de Boismont, which showed that all these images appear in a variety of conditions where the central nervous system is excited by a number of agencies including sleep, hashish, fevers, delirium, alcohol and other hallucinogens. To Kluver and Siegel there appeared to be "form constants" of images drawn by the nervous system from memories, excitation and lack of stimulation. This entirely physiological explanation of hallucinations, can be extended to visions, dreams and auditory forms as well, including sensory forms like "presences" (Fig. 2.4).

J. J. Mouear collected during his career as a psychologist in the early nineteenth century descriptions of hallucinations and visions by his patients as well as experiments on the use of hashish. In 1845 he published a 400 page book based on these descriptions. Some of these were simple sensations like pleasure or pain, others vivid mental caricatures of life or natural phenomenon, some very strange. This book was republished in 1973.

Dose Again and Variations in Experience

Grof (1976), in describing his methods involving 3800 "records" from LSD sessions where patients were administered LSD of pharmaceutical quality, notes the effective dose at 75 mg and a high dose of 500 mg, with

Location of Hallucination Type and Area of Damage
Not a Comprehensive List

Area of Brain	Type of Hallucination
Left Fusiform gyrus	Visual Word Form Area Word texts
Frontal, parietal and medial Temporal cortex	illusions of motion
Temporal lobe seizures in epilepsy Nearly always right-sided	ecstatic-religious
Superior temporal sulcus	deformed, dismembered faces (neurological faces, Sacks, 2012)
Brain stem, Pons	Peduncular hallucination*
Frontal and caudate nucleus	PD patients with chronic visual Hallucinations*
Amygdala and parahippocampus	visual hallucination in Lewy Body pathology*
Frontal and Visual association area	degeneration in PD & visual Hallucinations*
Thalamic limbic nuclei	Lewy Body hallucinations*
Right intralaminar nuclei with Right dosomedial nucleus	auditory and visual**
Left intralaminar nuclei	
Occipital lobe Posterior Cortical Atrophy	Anton's Syndrome Hallucinations*
Degeneration of visual system (CBS)	Wide variety of hallucinations*
Brain stem	REM Behavior Disorder

*Lewis, Simon J.G. , James M. Shine, Daniel Brooks, and Glenda M. Halliday, 'Hallucinogenic mechanism: pathological and pharmacological insights," In *The Neuroscience of Visual Hallucinations*, (ed.) Daniel Collerton, New York, John Wiley & Sons, pp. 121-150.

** Noda, S. , M. Mizoguchi and A. Yamamoto (1993) "Thalamic experiential hallucinosis," *J. Neurosurg. Psychiatry,* Nov. v. 56, n. 11, 1224-1228.

Fig. 2.4 Location of hallucination in the brain

doses up to 1500 mg in certain unresponsive cases. He argues that the physiological response to the drug ends at 500 mg. Higher doses are of no use. One assumes 500 mg is what he is referring to as the "higher dose" that accelerates achievement of his Basic Perinatal sequences (Grof 1976, 150), which he reports can also be reached using eyeshades and stereophonic music. The 75 mg dose has been shown effective in eliciting psychological perimeters of the reported drug response, as verified by neuroimaging (Carhart-Harris et al. 2016). Holze et al. (2020), however, found a 100 mg dose to be effective. Some therapists in the 1950s and 1960s varied the dosage depending on the response of the patient, with beginning doses running from 25 mg up to 100 mg and then using higher doses (of 150 mg) at times but found 75 mg to be the most useful (Chandler et al. 1960). There have been reports of tremendous-sized doses, as in the case of a woman who took a dose 550 times the size of typical doses and experienced a reduction in foot pain that had dogged her for over 26 years and a 15-year-old girl who took a dose ten times the usual size and reported a substantial improvement of her mental health (Hunt 2020; Haden and Woods 2020). But these are difficult to document, as they occurred outside laboratory or clinical conditions.

While the issue of perinatal memories is uncertain, there is some basis in the ontogeny of the brain; specifically we see myelination of neurons in the hippocampus and prefrontal cortex prior to birth and these are the two main areas of memory storage and retrieval (Abraham et al. 2010; Nickel and Gu 2018). I should mention a curious report in Blum et al. (1964) that some of their subjects reported habituation to the drug, with a reduced response. They concede that this was difficult to measure, as they could not rigorously define the nature of this reduced effect. In another place in this book I mention subjects reporting such tolerance to LSD, but it was impossible to document or verify.

The fact that Grof reports patients who had no response at all to LSD and that there was no invariant physiological response ("drug effects") or uniform psychological responses, but produced a variety of responses highlights the range of variation. The individual patient's experience and outcome seemed based on the pre-existing status of the individual's mental state and history of experiences. Yet Grof reports a general series of transitions to be expected, as in the regression to childhood and an "oceanic," "peaceful," " intrauterine," and "cosmic unity" feeling. Some individuals, however, experienced pain, pain of birth, of past operations or injuries, emotional crises, and so on. It is interesting that the results of the Mogar Lab differed from those of Grof, but they were very similar to those reported by Janiger, with almost 1000 subjects who were screened as normal individuals without detectable psychological disease. The general experience and positive nature of the subjects' paralleled the Mogar Lab results. Janiger was associated with the University of California, Irvine at the time of this work (Dobkin de Reios and Janiger 2003). He was basically a psychiatrist in private practice who had rather loose methods for choosing subjects (Stevens 1988). These results were often reproduced in other laboratory settings and in the recently renewed research, for example, by Griffiths and Grob (2010), though much of this new work utilizes other chemical agents like psilocybin (also called "magic mushrooms") and mescaline. They report on a number of studies, but also on the use of before and after questionnaires to measure the effects of the drug experience (Bogenschutz et al. 2015; Carhart-Harris et al. 2016; Griffiths et al. 2006, 2016; Ross et al. 2016). A recent review is available by Nichols (2016) of this work. His results and of many others are indications of psychological improvement in subjects' state of being by a number of factors (Carbonaro et al. 2016). "Well-being" is one and, though subjective, later retesting seems to indicate a fair degree of stability. The use of hallucinogens in the Carbonaro et al. (2016) report has a number of positive results, including reduction of depression, breaking addictions, and reducing some symptoms of illness, as in obsessive-compulsive disorder. This is comparable to the findings of many anthropologists (Fabrega 1997, 144–150), where shamans and individuals seek out hallucinations as a means of entering the spirit world and communicating with ancestors to find answers, solace, or aid.

Documentation of the adaptive nature of these experiences for individuals and societies has been suggested (Johns 1990; Davis 2001; Winkelman 2015).

Just as with the purity of street LSD, often there is confusion about what mushroom has been consumed. In some cases people use *Amanita muscaria*, noted among some indigenous people of Siberia, or *A. pantheria* (Nyberg 1992). Siberian peoples like the Korjaks and the Chukchee people report the spirits speaking to them in ways similar to how indigenous people of Mexico have experienced its use (Wasson and Wasson 1957). These are mushrooms, different from peyote, which is from the spineless cactus *Lophophora williamsii* and its derivative is called mescaline. Another aspect of the variety of human response to psychedelics is La Barre's (1975) report that in many cases people do not experience visual hallucinations with psilocybin, but only gustatory or tactile, olfactory, or kinesthetic. One might consider the uniformity of the drug described in the specific case or, perhaps, variations in the product of the plant. Given that psilocybin is produced by more than 200 species of fungi of the genus *Psilocybe*, and about a dozen other genera (Passie et al. 2002), one might expect variations, as well as given the illicit use in many cases where specific quantities might be contaminated with a variety of other substances.

Sometimes the word mescal is used for mescaline, but this is an error, as the drink "mescal" is made from the agave plant and is indigenous to Mexico.

In our experiments these feelings were also present in subjects as well as in individual cases I observed outside of the scientific institutional setting, which took place in private homes, often with groups of people, with as many as eight or ten people present. I was present only once when a group attempted to follow Timothy Leary, Richard Alpert (Ram Dass) and Ralph Metzner's protocol of chanting from the *Tibetan Book of the Dead* (Leary et al. 1964; Greenfield 2006). In this case some individuals became agitated and left the room, a response that was not uncommon where such chanting did occur, without prior specific group agreement. I knew of several group houses (where people lived together, some couples of males and females and some single males). In a few of these, residents took LSD together, but seldom as a ritual, and when this was a practice, relations did not descend into the kind of "cult-like" behavior reported for Leary and Alpert's International Federation of Internal Freedom (IFIF) houses (Stevens 1988) or anything like the Manson group (O'Neill and Piepenbring 2019; Garber-Paul (2022) examines this work with some skepticism, and this brings up the issue of fake crash pads set up by various agencies, e.g., by West 1956). The same problem applies to stories Stevens (1988), among others, reports of the development of a "group mind" among IFIF followers. I think there is a confusion here, produced by outsiders unfamiliar with the specific context. A generalization is applied to one of any subculture or religious group that produces boundaries in shared experiences. The idea of a group mind, as in Star Trek's Borg or a field of slime mold is imagined, as are healing efforts, as when a scorpion bite produced a rash from head to toe in one person and in the retelling of the event it is assumed all present had only one interpretation. The entire IFIF group then dropped acid and the person was cured of the rash. While one might imagine a psychosomatic cure of some kind, a group hallucination is more likely. Descriptions of Leary's various locations, like Millbrook and its organizational products, including Castalia and IFIF, are usually described as quite male-oriented and focused affairs (Stevens 1988). This is also true of much of the San Francisco scene as expressed by Ken Kesey and the Merry Pranksters. The contrast Stevens describes between the Eastern philosophy/religious aroma of Leary's organization at Millbrook and that of the freewheeling Merry Pranksters, while a stark vehicle for the writer, does a disservice to the West Coast to make Kesey's traveling show representative of California or even those people I found in New Mexico and Arizona in the early 1970s. The description of the Merry Pranksters as anti-guide and anti-rules seems to contradict the "group entity" or gestalt they reported experiencing. How is one so freely disconnected and libertarian and yet part of a group mind? I do recall that group meetings in many of the communes and collective houses I visited in the 1960s and 1970s could be interpreted as a kind of "group think," as I describe in my study of the Goodman Building (Caldararo 2019), though that also could describe a town council meeting following Robert's Rules of Order (I was a town councilman for four years and experienced the constraints and cooperation of citizen meetings). The opposite of this kind of organized chaos would be the uniform tyranny of a People's Temple or a Trump rally. But I have to admit that Kesey's and the Pranksters' anti-authoritarianism and humor were effective means of dealing with the dogma of morality at the time.

Most of the people I knew at the time were experiencing some psychological connection with nature, taking LSD in the wild or forest. But this was also part of a general ethos that permeated the scene. From what I could see there were women involved in the scene in San Francisco like Lenore Kandel and some of those I met in the Diggers, but they were not prominent in the decision-making as far as I saw. Kandel is a bridge character, like some others in the Beat Generation (Burns 1994); Kandel was a poetess and a very articulate speaker, and her performance at the various trials was often more than entertaining (Bess 1967a, b). Her poetry brought about a series of arrests for its sexual nature in the 1960s and her lectures at San Francisco State were a regular event, where other poets and artists, young intellectuals of the general faculty, and students listened to her marvelously sensual and clever imagery.

In another case, I was at a gathering of friends and relatives in a house in San Francisco's Mission District in the 1970s. A high school friend of mine was visiting where I lived with another former high school friend. My brother came into the party and some time later I entered the kitchen, where one friend (Michael Canright, whom I describe taking LSD in an event during the Summer of Love elsewhere in this book) had been drinking some punch from the punch bowl. He was talking to my brother, who was smiling broadly and chuckling uncontrollably. All of a sudden Michael said to my brother, "You dosed me, didn't you. You put it in the punch!" My brother started laughing hysterically and said, "Took you a while to notice." I then realized that both were out of control and said to my brother, "That was not a fair or responsible thing to do." My brother, at that time a motorcycle mechanic who often rode with the Hell's Angels, replied, "Michael is an old hand at acid, he was bragging about it and I just wanted to see how he looked on acid." Needless to say, this was an ethical problem, but it did provide an interesting amount of information about how people can recognize they are experiencing a drug-induced event versus a natural insight or pathology. However, since Michael had been also drinking alcohol and smoking marijuana and perhaps other drugs, it cannot be used specifically to inform us of LSD. The fact that Michael was able to discern that he had been "dosed" with LSD reflects on his learning how the drug affected his consciousness.

I was present when a similar event took place at a party a few years later in San Francisco. Most of those present were actors, artists, and writers. It took place in someone's home and there was a large fruit bowl sitting on a table in the kitchen and next to it were several smaller bowls with white powders in them and a larger bowl with what looked like marijuana. Each small bowl was labeled, "PCP," "cocaine," and a smallish wooden box labeled "mystery pills, take a chance." Later I was told these were mainly "downners." The PCP was phencyclidine, also known as "angel dust." I had been at the party for about an hour when I noticed that a number of people were on the floor, crawling about and some howling. A few were sitting alone, looking vacant and some couples were engaged in amorous behavior. Shortly, it became obvious that someone had put something in the punch. I looked over at the table and saw that the bowl labeled "PCP" was empty. I then picked up the punch bowl that was still about half full and dumped it in the sink. The person who had invited me to the party was on the floor howling, but her girlfriend came over to me and said, "Ever the Boy Scout, aren't you?" I said, "People should have a choice about what experiences to have." She said, "It is a performance piece, they were invited to one of our parties. People do not expect a "Leave it to Beaver" evening."

PCP is a dopamine receptor agonist and an antagonist of the NMDA receptor subtype of glutamate receptors. It is well known to produce hallucinations as well as panic and a variety of other symptoms (Aronson 2016). Most of those engaged in the effects of the drug at the party seemed to be having mainly sensory enhancements and not describable visual images. Reported experiences include euphoria, omnipotence, superhuman strength, and sexual prowess (Bey and Patel 2007). It was clear to me that euphoria and sexual effects were present. Those affected seemed to take no notice of other people and acted in an immediate sphere of contact, if one could make that assumption. Audiovisual hallucinations were reported, but in this case, it was difficult to assess what experiences were taking place. Aggressive behavior was also reported but nothing of that type was seen as long as I was there, about two hours. While I had no idea what was to happen at this party, it is in my opinion dangerous for people to take drugs in a group setting and here I mean more than five people. In the "early Haight," as people often referred to the period 1965–1967, people I knew, and this included the Psychedelic Rangers, urged people to always have one or more persons "sober," that is, not on the hallucinogen, at any time. This name, "Psychedelic Rangers," was used by several people in the late 1960s, one was a band (formed by former Doors drummer, John Densmore) and another a group promoting social work, led by John Sinclair in Ann Arbor. I have no idea if any of these were connected in any way or who influenced whom.

In another setting, a woman was giving birth who had been a member of the theater group Angels of Light. Members had moved north of San Francisco in the early 1980s and formed a group-living situation. The birth was taking place as a party and there were about 30 or 40 people there. I had arrived in the later afternoon, visiting friends, and was invited to attend, as I knew some of the elders from the 1960s Haight scene. A group of women surrounded that pregnant woman and some sang, others administered to her needs. Men helped and there was a general busy nature about the place, where I had noted before a more relaxed milieu.

Most people were engaged cooking food, some were eating, and others smoking drugs were high on LSD or peyote or other drugs. As night unfolded, singing and dancing become more group oriented, though many danced to their own drum, so to speak. The woman giving birth was surrounded by friends, mainly females, and the female nature of the group had always been a keystone of its culture. After her water broke, they began to chant, and this brought the entire group to participate in "helping the birth." She gave birth about midnight or 1 am and festivities continued till dawn, when a celebration of birth and naming and the morning took place. Breakfast then was made with a variety of colors of pancakes, juices, and bread. I slept.

Some Interpretations, Expectations, and Origins

In this book I will often contrast the experiences either I had with psychedelics or others in scientific settings with those in private settings, though I will note when "structure," that is, a planned environment, was expected or created by either scientists or practitioners. For the scientists, the environments in the experimental settings I was present for were characterized as those of sensory deprivation conditions, designed to avoid influencing the subjects. In most private settings the opposite occurred, where practitioners, or "aids," "leaders," or "gurus," attempted to create conditions to produce a maximum of influence on the subjects. The outcomes of these two diametrically opposed conditions were often as different as the settings.

Two aspects of Grof's work bothered me. One was the idea that LSD had dramatically created a new model of human consciousness. Much of his 1976 book is taken up with arguing this point. The other problem was that of dose. It was taken for granted by most of the MDs and PhDs who came to the Mogar Lab that there was little evidence for microdosing and that the optimum dose required for a full human response was 300 mg. There were a number of discussions about this and reference to work done by other teams and published, but when I read Grof's book I was skeptical due to this atmosphere. In a later publication Grof and Halifax (1978) reported that 100 mg could produce a reduction of pain in patients as well as result in improved sleep.

One case at the Mogar Lab that I heard staff report on was of a young woman who was unaffected by any dose of LSD or any other hallucinogen. Later it was noted that Grof (1976, 217) had a patient who had been treated with an anti-depressive drug, Niamid, a monoaminooxidase inhibitor, which he found made a person almost immune to the effects of LSD. This was unknown in 1966–1967 and thus that young woman was considered unique, though I do not recall if her history had included any such drugs at the time. We do not have a big enough sample to determine the extent of population variation to LSD. I have noted a number of cases here of people who seemed to be unaffected. This is unclear and needs further research.

The new model Grof referred to was "a multidimensional and multilevel continuum of mutually overlapping and interacting phenomenon." This sounded to me like the pronouncement of Constantin von Monakow (1911), who argued that the idea of localization of function in the brain had to be more complex than that proposed by earlier anatomists in attempting to identify specific areas of histological significance and function, like Broca, for example. Rather, it seemed that as the evolution of the brain took place, primitive areas of function were extended into new areas like the neocortex, and so when certain areas of identified function were destroyed by trauma or disease, function could often be regained in other areas. There is some support for this idea in the work of people like Striedter (2005), though I hasten to mention that I am not attributing this idea to him. His book is a compendium of studies, very useful and well organized.

With Grof a form of archetype or ancestral core is the first level. The second level were encompassed by psychodynamic experiences, the third were perinatal experiences which seemed like Freud's model, and the fourth, transpersonal experiences, or out of body (associated with near-death experiences, DMT, and ketamine), and these seemed like those of shamans (Eliade 1964). Here we find the great visions of prophets like Ezckiel (Patai 1990) and religious formulators (Radin 1937). This includes Mohammed, who according to many reports in tradition deported himself as a prophet and was called a *Kahin* or seer based on ecstatic inspiration. Pre-Islamic *Kahins* interpreted dreams, acted as judges, and otherwise resolved conflicts (Wolf 1951). Though Mohammed denied being a *Kahin*, like Christ, whose behavior was similar and has been described as a shamanic healer in some views (Craffert 1999; La Barre 1975, 16, in Jesus' use of magic verbal formulas to cast evil spirits out of a man into swine), the vision or dream is a medium of action in the waking world that has great power in some cultures. Some characteristics of both of these men would place them in the category of charismatic leader as described by Fabian (1966), for example.

While some prophet's visions can be a reflection of threatening conditions of change, as in the Seneca Native American Handsome Lake (Parker 1912), and result in adaptations to resist or adapt, in other cases the prophet and his or her message can be mythological and be a justification for existing conditions, as in the people of Kano prior to the Arab invasion and arrival of Islam. The prophet Barbushe is a voice from the past telling the people they will be conquered and subjugated by another people and that resistance is futile, that they should resign themselves to defeat (Palmer 1908).

The expression and intensity of the experience was of great importance to Grof; he distinguished between the experience people had based on physiology, for example, whether their eyes were open or closed when the drug came to full force and the difference in later experiences from the first. Those who took LSD under Grof's care apparently often took the role of prophet, or attempted to situate their experience as someone who could predict events (Grof 1976, 177). Prophecy is often related to time travel in my experience, though Grof does not link them, except as the reliving of past life experiences, as in birth trauma, reincarnation, and so on. The idea proposed by Hofmann (Grob 2002) that the drug could function as an "entheogen" or a means to see the world anew in all respects (Ruck et al. 1979) comes to mind in reading many descriptions of use of the drug. Aside from the neurophysiological effects of the drug due to is modulation of serotonin (Liester 2014), it is clear from the variety of reports that come from illegal use that the drug has been adulterated with other chemicals, substituted and mistaken, or used in concert with alcohol and other agents. Dos Santos et al. (2016) review the potential mechanisms of LSD.

We often hear that serotonin is a neurotransmitter, which does not tell us much. We know it is conserved across all vertebrate groups as well as invertebrates (Striedter 2005). It is found in mast cells and causes constriction of small blood vessels and influences blood pressure and also increases the vascular permeability of capillaries and somewhat larger vessels called venules (Bloom and Fawcett 1975). In fact, only less than 5% of the serotonin in the body is found in the brain, most about 95% is found in the blood platelets and gut or gastrointestinal tract and retina (Fouquet et al. 2019; Barrett et al. 2010). This relates also to some other drugs like components of ayahuasca, where taking the drug orally would not be active without the monoamine oxidase inhibitor (Schultes 1972). Davis (2001), among others, argues that the combination could not have come about by accident by indigenous people. But this seems to demean the curiosity and creativity of people. Releasing serotonin, as with the drug reserpine, in treating high blood pressure, increases the permeability of blood vessels like capillaries and decreases blood pressure. If LSD blocks receptor sites for serotonin we might expect it to have effects on the immune system, digestion, and, most importantly, the brain. Increasing tryptophan in the diet can also increase brain serotonin content, but it is "recaptured" by a reuptake mechanism and inactivated by monoamine oxidase (Barrett et al. 2010).

This relates also to some other drugs like components of ayahuasca were taking the drug orally wouldnot be active without the monoamine oxidase inhibitor (Schultes, 1972). Davis (2001) among others, argues that the combination could not have come about by accident by indigenous people. But this seems to demean the curiosity and creativity of people.

Drug interaction with LSD or impurities and drug combinations may explain "bad trips" as well as exposure to unstable or threatening environmental conditions under which the drug experience took place and may include reported "flashbacks." The nature of this phenomenon has been disputed and lacks definition (Wesson and Smith 1976; Matefy et al. 1978); it was earlier argued that flashbacks wore off and became less frequent over time. Some researchers found that there seemed to be a relationship between the number of doses of LSD taken and the incidence of "flashbacks" (Batzer et al. 1999). In recent years the phenomenon has been divided into a benign temporary and mild occurrence, and a more persistent and pathological one, termed Hallocinogen Persisting Perception Disorder (HPPD) (Hermie et al. 2015). Some chemical treatments were found of use in ameliorating the symptoms of HPPD (Lerner et al. 2002). A comprehensive and retrospective study found that most reported experiences of "flashback" were pleasurable and that the few reports of HPPD and "flashback" as well as the variable description make the syndrome difficult to classify and categorize. I myself never experienced this or saw it in others. I do think that often people talked of "contact highs" involving meth, hash, peyote, and other drugs. Most reports I have heard of indicated that the experience was due to an evoked memory (smell, place, etc.). Also, again, street drugs made this difficult to quantify.

Mogar did an in-depth study of the so-called acid freak, a person who it is claimed took too many trips. Mogar concluded that most of these cases were difficult to attribute to LSD, as there was no or little documentation of their drug or psychological history. He was unable to find actual cases among clinicians he knew, but from the media reports at the time there should have been many. In an interview with Dave Brice he suggested from his inquiry that many had taken trips alone and without guidance and that too much use of the drug could estrange people from friends and family, causing isolation (Brice 1966). Mogar was critical of both the research being done on psychedelics and the promotion of their use by people who were not trained in psychology or medicine. He concluded from his work, "Turning to the psychedelics, it has become apparent that adverse psychological or behavioral effects are not drug-specific. More generally, the nature, intensity, and content of the experience are the result of past history and personality, the set and experiences of both subject and administrator, and the physical and psychological setting in which the experience takes place" (Mogar 1965). A ten-year follow-up study of LSD use in a medical experimental setting by McGlothlin (1971) of 247 individuals found 23% had additional LSD use after the initial experiment, but there was little change in personality and immediate indications of more contemplative feelings were not permanent.

The lack of controlled scientific conditions is typical of most reports of use of the drug. De Rios (1984) describes the variety of settings in which the indigenous context of various people shapes psychedelic experiences, including the very rigid to the unstructured, as in the New Guinea highlanders' non-ritual use and desired "amok" behavior. She also notes that changes in the role of psychedelics have taken place, often due to contact, as in the Fang in Africa, who used *Tabernanthe iboga* as a part of hunting preparation, but after European colonialism it came to play a part of a revitalization movement. Again, documentation and interpretation are a problem as in many of the studies and reports of "bad trips" or suicide are anecdotal or subjective regarding psychedelic use in urban settings. There is a preponderance of reports of unquestioned association of LSD with a variety of outcomes. Usually only on aspect of a subject's "trip" is reported, though one of Grof's (1976, 113) subjects reports an initial troubling experience that changes repeatedly into an oceanic pleasure, then cosmic understanding and then womb-like serenity and nipple-feeding security. This jumping back and forth from one experience "theme" to another, pleasure to pain or threat, is also common and was reported by Hoffman in his first use of the drug in 1943. He experienced pleasure and happy thoughts though also disorientation, but later saw devils and experienced anxiety (Hoffman 1980/2009). He also followed a course of discovery many see compelling; his perceptions come to discover that all life has perceptions or consciousness. He then compares this idea with his scientific and philosophical background to find it has some relevance. Here, in a similar mode, Grof's subject (1976, 114) interprets even his experiencing the phylogenetic history of life (similar to Shepard's 1978 idea in ontogeny of a human child and language or Deacon's system of developmental abstractions). At the end of his session, he expresses the overall result one of self-acceptance and unity with the world, a not uncommon result.

As Mogar (1965, 403) has said, however, subjects interpret their experience in terms of their past learning and exposure to knowledge and people. Researchers often have difficulty teasing out background from subjective impressions of subjects, especially where drug use was not confined to a laboratory setting. Often they found that several other stimulants were used and often depressants as well have been used; this influences the experience of the subjects. But past experience can be the source of the "bad trip" then, as Mogar argues, though in Grof's terms this is due to the reliving or latent effects of the birth experience, both pain felt by mother and/

or child. Though it is also interesting that many of Grof's female subjects experience trauma during the LSD sessions, these are tied to past sexual assault or experiences of a negative nature. It is known that childhood sexual abuse has specific association with hallucinations, which Bentall and Varese (2013) relate to the theory of internalization of social speech of Vygotsky, the development of "inner speech" as a process of "thinking in pure meanings." This is due to the fact that the voices of authority heard by psychotic patients are often chastising or directing behavior. Grof does note that some women who were LSD subjects and had had children were able to reinterpret the experience during the LSD influence.

Referring to the 1967 data Allan Rinker collected and I aided, it did seem that those persons who reacted strongly on LSD were those making the most significant personality changes, and/or are dealing with problems which related to themselves in some vital or important way. In my initial notes from reviewing Rinker's data, it seemed to me that those individuals who had problems on LSD resulted from a lack of context, and in Mogar's terms, they lacked a means of dealing with the massive change from language-oriented knowledge. However, we come to the issue of interpretation, of whether the subject is experiencing "poorly" or the analyst is poorly interpreting and this relates to the conclusions of Ungerleider and Fisher (1967) mentioned earlier. Given at least in the context of the Mogar Lab, subjects were screened using mainly the MMPI, as I have stated. However, Rinker did not always screen his subjects, at least from what my notes indicated. Yet the MMPI was not perfect, as I mentioned with regard to the student incident at Humboldt State. We know now that the test as designed and available in the 1960s failed to identify potential suicidal tendencies and redesigns, as in the MMPI-2-RF are effective (Gottfried et al. 2014).

Problems in source monitoring (knowing what is the origin of a sound or event) and "misattributed thoughts," especially of children and trauma, where the event was so overwhelming its origin is blocked, are associated with hallucinations. Bentall and Varese (2013) also found that people who score high on the mindfulness spectrum (ability to be in the present moment) also were prone to hallucinations but not intrusive thoughts. This differs from the quality of "attentive presence," where people have an overall perspective of themselves within the context of their social organization and culture that allows them to create specific opportunities that are unique and act on them. As Roy Wagner (1975) argued there is a constant invention of culture going on among people in a society, and to understand one's place and the intent of others requires more than language, but context and background. This constant innovation is also a process of discovery, as Paul Radin (1937) noted, where certain individuals, religious innovators, reconstruct the ideological and cosmological setting of human life to revalue why people do things. One must "see through" the cultural context of values and statuses to be able to innovate new routes for change and adaptation. This is the basis of attentive presence. It seems similar to Leary's idea of "breaking set" or "seeing through the cultural veil," a reference to the insight to a problem or the "Aha" experience described by Kohler (1925) and Kaplan and Simon (1990), where the "mental set" of life's conditioning is overcome in a moment's unique perception. The difference in my concept of "attentive presence" is a state of mind where one has stepped outside the framework of this cultural conditioning and makes several, if not continuous observations that change life relations. The most significant instance of this, in a non-human case, is that of the Japanese monkey on Kashima Island who made several "inventions" related to her situation (Kawai 1965).

Misreporting of studies is also found, as in the case of the Krebs and Johansen (2012) analysis that reviewed reports and studies from 1943 to 2010 and found significant short-term benefits in use of LSD. Also evaluated were six trials with a total of 536 patients, with benefits at three and six months. So the overall outcomes of the use of LSD and its benefits have probably been underestimated, and I would argue that the media concentration on supposed or real "bad trips" has been a factor.

Reports of overdoses of LSD have also been made as well as the idea that the drug can "build up in the body," though no analysis or mechanism for this has been identified or described (Das et al. 2016). From Hofmann's original work (2009) he determined that 250 mg were necessary to induce an effect—that is, the LSD experience seems dependent on at least this amount, which is why in the Mogar Lab the 300 mg was recognized as necessary. Recently LSD has been applied to other syndromes and illnesses, and Family et al. (2020) reported using doses as low as 5, 10, and 20 mg with effect. Carhart-Harris et al. (2016) administered 75 mg of LSD by i.v.

in 10 mL saline. They used fMRI to scan for changes in brain activity and found that this level of LSD had measurable effect and also subjects reported significant distortions in visual perception and dream-like visions characteristic of other psychedelics they had tested. This provides some degree of reference for dose and experience in brain activity.

What is also of interest is the setting of the experience. In earlier studies from the 1950s and 1960s the Mogar Lab had compared reports in clinical settings to results in their lab. The general experience seemed to be similar and this held true for those who were patients with conditions like alcoholism or healthy student volunteers. However, reports from outside laboratory and clinical settings had descriptions of experiences that were reported as similar with some differences. Different experiments and therapists reported a variety of outcomes in treatment with LSD in the 1950s and 1960s (Abramson 1967). Van Dusen et al. (1967) found in a survey of reports that trials without controls reported over 80% positive results, but those with controls only 25%. Their study was the only one reported I could find that had only women and controls, though their control protocol changed during the trial. They had an 18-month follow-up for their subjects and found no significant benefit from the use of LSD in producing a longer "cure" of alcohol use than in their controls. However, they did report that LSD aided therapy. It should be noted that the control group was given scopolamine, a drug that can cause dizziness and hallucinations (see MedlinePlus: https://medlineplus.gov/druginfo/meds/a682509.html). However, Van Dusen et al. (1967) reported that control members and those receiving LSD quickly discerned the difference and identified the scopolamine group.

While Mogar was critical of many of the experiments, he was also concerned about how people were mixing therapies and LSD treatment and how the therapy was organized and applied. The problem of outcome and measurement was also inconsistent. Goals for improvement seemed vague in many cases. In the hospital studies Mogar undertook, the focus was on how the patient felt, what find of change took place that gave the individual a greater sense of satisfaction and a more integrated personality. In one group, made up largely of women, he found a change where the women had been dissatisfied in their relationships due to clear incongruities with their husband's personalities. After LSD treatment, he found the change in the wives was a greater amount of self-control, and a more relaxed personal view of the world. Their husbands had generally a reverse change, becoming more emotional and expressive. One might speculate that this reflected a breaking of the conditioning of submission and resign which many women suffer from, and the husbands experiencing a loss of control. This would fit in information discussed later in the last chapter, from work by Manon Garcia (2021), though in a separate group of women there was only a short-term change that was positive, and a relapse within a few months. This might have been due to the fact that their relationships did not change (Mogar and Savage 1964).

After the reports in the press of the public use and "experiments" of Leary and Alpert research assessments changed and the experiences of people came to be reported as dramatically different. I have described some of these situations above, especially where experienced "helpers" had to be called in to "bring people down safely." There was a general feeling expressed by some people, both clinically trained doctors like Dr. David Smith (1969) and practically experienced community members of the broader Haight-Ashbury (I describe this community in my 2019 book), that the drug caused people to go on what might be described as inner journeys. Others argued, like Grof, that they were to be carried into the past of their ontogeny in ways that they could re-experience their past. When people got into "trouble" it was interpreted that they were reliving emotionally damaging experiences from their past and could fall into loops of repeating terror and pain, actually reliving their lives. "Reliving" is also the term used by Grof (1976). From this danger the "helpers" like the Psychedelic Rangers could extract people without harm. I witnessed several of these "extractions" once or twice with medical students present from nearby University of California, San Francisco (UCSF).

Some ten years later a very good friend of mine related that she often awoken in the middle of the night screaming and warned me of its likely recurrence when it happened one night and I was bolted into a waking state by her screaming. At first she seemed still asleep, and since she had been asleep beside me, I was startled to find her sitting upright, screaming and her eyes open. As someone who had once in his teens been a sleepwalker, I could understand how she could still be unconscious. She told me later when she woke that she never could recall why or if she had been in a dream and awakened by events depicted in the dream. Talking with her and her sister we were not able to find an event in her past that might have been traumatic enough to cause such a returning feature of her sleep. It seemed to me at the time that it was one of those violations of the control of Freud's so similar mechanisms of consciousness ordered to retard coming to consciousness but sometimes active during dreaming. Here, some event it seemed was breaking into sleep with the most terrifying strength.

Sometime later we were at a dinner where the host produced some LSD and all imbibed except myself. Not that I was opposed to its use, but rather I had come to the conclusion that I had nothing more to learn from such experiences, also, now it was illegal. Some two or three hours later with people continuing to eat, drink, consume ice cream and other pleasures, I found myself sitting next to her and thinking of her night terrors. I was unsure if I should mention them, so I instead began to ask her about her past and especially her childhood. I listened as she related early experiences at school, as a teenager, family events, and travel. I wondered if some typically tense problems of childhood might be a trigger, especially as I knew her parents had divorced, though I was ignorant if that was early or late in her life.

As I questioned her trying to push back her stories in time she came to a period when her family was in a rural area and all of a sudden she began to retell an experience where, as a little girl of some five or six years, she had heard a crash and a scream. Then, while inside the house they were staying in, she heard the screams and wailing of her farther who had cut down a tree that had fallen back on him with such violence that it smashed his face and broke his nose. The father was so injured that he could not walk but crawled to the door of the house and banged on it, calling her name. She opened it to find her father's voice coming from a battered and bleeding face.

Months went by after this event and, as I was her boyfriend, I slept with her night after night and did not experience the periodic awaking and screaming that had been a common event. After about six months I asked her about the story and the LSD experience. She remarked that she had not thought about it, but it (the repressed memory) seemed to be gone. While this story seems too pat to be true, it does indicate, and is typical of the kinds of stories people told me at the time of reliving their past and this was the typical experience of the patients discussed at the grand rounds of the Mogar Lab and their clinical associates. Yet such lingering problems and their immediate solution has been reported many times by individuals and therapists, as in Rivers' (1920) case of a shell-shocked soldier. Similar cases are often related to childhood trauma in schizophrenic patients (Blom and Mangoenkarso 2018). An interesting fact in Grof's reports was the form which subjects' bodies took when they went through the "reliving" process. They reported that their bodies returned to the age and size when the disturbing events took place. This could involve numerous changes in body size and age.

Grof (1976; 91) argues, however, that if a person had a "flashback" related to the core systems of condensed experience (COEX) system and it was not resolved during the session, it could put the person under its influence for an indeterminate time. Grof found that this could intensify symptoms or change one's perceptions of the physical environment as well as "exteriorize the general theme of the system." This change can take on an "approximate replica of the traumatic event" that had been repressed, was recalled by the session, not resolved, and instead comes to "life." This relates to my earlier comments on some peoples' belief (and apparently the military) in the 1960s that LSD was a "truth drug" (see Weinberger 2019; Ignatieff 2001 and below). Some saw the ability of the drug to change perceptions and attitudes as a means of manipulating political power or, in the case of some like Leary, Ram Dass, and Aldous Huxley, to arrive at world peace (Stevens 1988). However, I never saw this happen, and it was never mentioned at the Mogar Lab and I am unsure what exactly Grof meant by it. His later publications are no clearer on the subject in terms of case studies.

Recent research on PTSD (Przybyslawski et al. 1999) and repressed memories indicates a certain plasticity in the process of recall, especially regarding Reconsolidation Theory, where memories become fragile and subject to "disruption." In this view the initial memory of the core event if recalled and repressed might become so transformed (distorted?) that the means to resolve it might be lost (McKenzie and Eichenbaum 2011), though Li et al. (2020) demonstrate in experiments with Fragile X Syndrome mice that the efficacy of hippocampal engram reactivation might be enhanced by enriched environment prior to reactivation, improving memory recall. Therefore, Grof's idea that such flashbacks are unresolved might mean that they were no longer so coherent that the COEX system had become fragmentary and not amenable to correction. Li et al.'s (2020) findings might also indicate Grof's suggestion that positive COEX conditions can improve the "unfolding" of negative COEX systems and resolution. "Positive" here he defined as pleasant conditions.

Grof (1976, 129–130) generalizes to all people's experience that they have a fixation with sexuality and with bodily fluids and substances that can be disgusting or pleasurable. In my experiences with people and my own, this is variable, some do and some do not. There were some early reports (e.g., Klee 1963) that discussed memory impairment after LSD use; thus, LSD involvement in the hippocampus could be related, though these experiments were made with few subjects. Grof was not unique in using LSD in therapy, or in seeing stages of effects of the drug related to past experience, but some, like Stolaroff and his colleagues in Menlo Park, regarded the hallucinations or visions during the LSD experience as a "smokescreen" to cure, yet did spend considerable time evaluating them in light of the background of the patient (Harman et al. 1966; Sherwood et al. 1968). There was an element of Christian mysticism that bothered some of those who came into contact with their work (Stevens 1988).

The idea that "flashbacks" are unresolved parts of a pathological complex as Grof has defined, the COEX system, seems incomplete at best. These he describes as psychological events after the drug session has ended and the drug has worn off. These are largely daytime events, but not so limited. I have reviewed some of the disagreement over how long the drug lasts and problems of purity and dose elsewhere. In my experience, many people had after-"trip" flashbacks, which seemed to be continued experiences from the LSD. This is hard to prove or categorize. Reports of LSD "flashbacks" are diffuse and vague. Goldman et al. (2007) report a man who used what he called LSD in high school (of unknown purity or dose) and later when on a long period of alcohol abuse. Years later diagnosed with bipolar disorder he was put on an SSRI and experienced "flashbacks." He later took an unspecified dose of buspirone (presumably street version and not prescribed by a physician). One is concerned here if the effects of the SSRIs, paroxetine (can also cause music hallucinations) and buspirone, were the cause and not LSD. There is some complication concerning buspirone (Pantelis and Barnes 1993)

Once relived, the COEX system never reappears but Grof states many such systems may coexist in one patient. And, while these systems vary from patient to patient, once resolved the patient may arrive at the more normal "perinatal and transpersonal phenomena" (Grof 1976, 94). This reflects something of the experience I had (but no "rebirth"), and most of the private users and many of Mogar's subjects reflected on, though the idea of "rebirth" I think is subjective. The reliving of life, time, and origin is common. What is also interesting in Grof's description of his therapy cases is the remarkable variety of pathology. I do not deny these experiences of his patients, but do question some of his interpretations. On the other hand, some patient's views seem intuitive, as when he describes the categories of intrauterine experience, one being the calm stasis as a Buddha-like consciousness (Grof 1976, 110) related in Indian cultural terms. This could be interpreted as if the womb, as a normal environment, is the meditative world, real in all its supportive elements, yet threatened by the world beyond the womb. Interpretation, of course, has many problems, as we have discussed, yet Luria (1968) argued that the turn in medicine of his time was away from considering the abnormalities of patients with brain and nervous disorders as entirely pathological, to where the responses of the affected individuals expanded the nature of human consciousness and demanded our attention for study. Therefore, looking at such resulting perceptions in abnormal or pathological conditions as aberrations of reality, we might consider them as part of a distribution of potential perceptions, as in the turn of a kaleidoscope.

The question of "mind" brings up a number of questions, especially regarding its use by philosophers and in religious contexts. The forms of meditation historically associated with Indian religions, especially Buddhism, argue that the use of this method can reduce "mind" and allow one to have "pure thoughts" or achieve various states not encumbered with human ideas or social contexts. The separation of mind from nature was discussed also in Confucianism, especial the Neo-Confucianism of Chu Hsi. He argued that though the mind has nature within it (*li* in Chinese) it is also composed of substance or *ch'i*. It means in his view that by practice the reduction of mind produces a condition where the substance remains, but is opaque. The great Japanese teacher, Ishida Baigan, produced a systhesis of Buddhist, Confucian, and Shinto thought. He considered the interplay of principle (nature) and substance (mind) one of motion and function (see *Toimondo* in Bellah 1957).

Discussing consciousness brings up ideas of "mind" and the nature of human thought ideas fraught with circular definitions and a lack of clarity (as it is often confused with philosophical ideas like "soul," though fascinating), as Crick (1994) allowed. Some philosophers have argued, like Colin McGinn (2006), that the human mind is not equipped to solve the problem of consciousness—which is the kind of circularity that comes at the end of many of the discussions of "mind" and "human consciousness." But then, he also argues that an individual finds nothing surprising in their own imagery, which would surprise most people given the confounding nature of our dreams and hallucinations. William James (1892) began his discussion of consciousness with the idea of "simple forms of sensation" and then turns to thoughts and personalities. This leap from instinct to awareness of the environment (consciousness) to self-consciousness is one usually broached in terms of evolution. Here consciousness and self-consciousness can be reduced to conditioning, as was done by the Behaviorists (Skinner 1953, but also see Fletcher 1966).

Some scientists have considered that mind and consciousness are epiphenomenon, the result of the combination of brain structure and functions, or a feedback mechanism of them (Bunge 2019). Some have called this an emergent property often using analogies, for instance, that of water being the combination of hydrogen and oxygen but neither of these elements has the properties of wetness of water. See C. Lloyd Morgan's version of this idea in his 1923 book.

The question of the "rich inner life" of individuals and intense personal experiences seemed to contradict the ideas of Behaviorists and their strict conditioning model of consciousness. Philosophers of the mind and consciousness, like David Chalmers (1996, 2012, 2020), try to escape the mind/body dualism and the mechanistic model of Behaviorism by constructing special cases for human language and consciousness. Chalmers has constructed a paradigm called "panpsychism" much like, in part, the work of sixteenth-century philosopher Francesco Patrizi (1591), who argued that all things in the universe have "mind" (Skrbina n.d.). One might align this with the idea of "being" in chemistry, where all atoms have electrons and give off energy signals under a variety of physical conditions (see a complex description of this in Linus Pauling's 1988 master work). Interactions of all forms of life and inorganic material is communication. As an anthropologist this sounds a lot like animism, the religion of many traditional people that holds a form of life and communication is inherent in all things, or more generally, all things are animated by energy (animatism) (Herskovits 1966). But for the panpsychist like Chalmers, the human mind is a more refined form, seen as a unique entity, different from other organisms' minds.

However, on examination we find this verges on metaphysics only in the view that communication and understanding between two people with the same language is due to complex conditioning set on context. This is essentially Behaviorism. The idea of communication from other worlds or universes seems undermined by the fact that other worlds have existed on the earth before 1492 without affecting or communicating. That the Aztec or Maya had no idea of the existence of France or Rome seems clear. Or the opposite that the English or Spanish "seers" or paranormals of the last 1000 years knew of Native Americans. In reviewing the Native American literature and that of European fantasies, one finds little to build on, though one must reflect on the fact that almost all of the Native American literature was destroyed shortly after the conquest (Caldararo 1994). While there were science fiction stories of great imagination written as early as the ancient Greeks (space travel to the Moon by Lucian of Samosata), it was mainly after the discovery of the Americas that fantastic worlds began to be proposed (e.g., Thomas More's *Utopia* 1516). Though a thousand years before More and about 300 years after Lucian, Chinese poet Tao Yuanming published a story of a utopia in *The Peach Blossom Spring*. Golden Ages like Eden or Hesiod's *Theogoy* are different, as they are linked to this world, as was Plato's *Republic*.

But Chalmers (2012) is attempting to go beyond this linkage of minds; he is after an understanding of how minds come into being and thus how information is transmuted into knowledge on which minds are constructed. He begins his 2012 book with a quote from the French Chemist Pierre-Simon Lapace and then boils it down to his purpose: "Laplace suggests that given the right basic information, and sufficient powerful reasoning, all truths about the universe can be determined." He then produced exceptions to this idea from a fundamental question of "is the world scrutable," then to problems in quantum theory, his "scrutability thesis." Why his discussion appears so circular to an anthropologist is that it occurs in one context of reality at one time. One is reminded of the effort to produce a comprehensive system of meaning in the 1920s by scholars organized for the purpose by Ogden and Richards (1923). Yet Chalmers falls into the dilemma that Umberto Eco argues for the participants in the creation of the book *The Meaning of Meaning* (Ogden and Richards 1923) that he terms the "therapeutic fallacy," the idea that more precise language can reduce misunderstanding and mistake. This applies to Chalmers' endeavor concerning reality, especially his 2012 book, where reality becomes simply a special case, an individual experience, thus an accident in exercises in phenomenology. Yet this goes back to meaning and learning. Rottier et al. (2011) found that some languages, like English, are structured with significant ambiguity compared to others, like Dutch. We learn to respond to ambiguity by reference to context and memory, which is why some psychedelics alter meaning so intensely; special relations, time, and memory often are altered. The idea of LSD's effect on the inner world structure and meaning of conditioning to cope with the external world, the Freudian paradigm, evaporates, leaving one entirely rootless, and then as Richard Alpert relates, quoted in Stevens (1988) and described in detail by the panelists at the 1961 Napa State Hospital Symposium in "LSD and Therapeutic Uses, there is theorized a transformation." The space where the self dissolves is followed by a broad and comprehensive examination of reality and the reconstruction of the self in the process, one that is individual by "an interaction by the person with themselves." Obviously in cases of therapist intervention, as in Grof's cases, the process is not individual, but in Grof's analysis it is made authentic by the trained and experienced therapist who attempts to avoid conflict with that process of healing. This is the "quiet therapist" described by Dr. Sidney Cohen (see audio recording by Skene 1961). We might say then that the only authentic world, cosmos, or mind is that produced by the individual in such a process.

In another attempt, Anil Seth (2021) fashions a mechanism for consciousness in humans by fabrication of the experience of hallucination into a system of reality as "shared hallucinations." However, if momentary hallucinations contain information, how are they shared and tagged for social significance? How much variation is tolerated, or does Vygotsky's zone of proximal development that provides a map of translation of individual experience or Chomsky's ideas might also be of use here? Kandel (2007) argues that we must consider the "complex memory" animals lodge in the hippocampus for a means of organized information useful for survival and this gives us an evolutionary context for consciousness, shared experience, and language. So in a way we have returned to both Behaviorism and a form of reductionism. Recently, discussions of consciousness have been resolved into a systems feature of complex feedback between different parts of the brain, especially from studies of visual awareness, visual attention, and vision-guided behavior (Li and Geng 2009).

The idea of consciousness being simply an evolutionary development related to both organic evolution and perfected by human civilization failed to provide a paradigm for the problems of psychological injuries that resulted from the American Civil War and then the First World War. While the trauma of railway accidents and other kinds of violent crash could be seen as a physical explanation for a general collapse of consciousness, it did not suffice to address the torrent of psychopathologies that came with modern warfare. W.H.R. Rivers (1920) especially, as a wartime physician, was faced with what we would call today PTSD in all its variety of expression. He came to suggest that consciousness was an adaptation, learned in a context of social interaction that helped the individual both to organize behavior characteristic of his or her culture and to provide a means of checking the onslaught of stimuli, positive and negative, from the environment. A theory of self-preservation, or instinct of survival, came to be associated with these pathologies. For Rivers (1920), Freud's theories of repression and the unconscious provided a logical means of protection and survival of soldiers in war. As an organizational complex it produced an interface of the individual's self that is often called "personality" (Kelly 1963). However, this complex could become damaged and disoriented into forms of catatonia (e.g., "shell shock") or other sustained pathology. While there is some evidence that soldiers in the American Civil War did suffer forms of PTSD, reports are few and it was not recognized (Horwitz 2015).

Where Crick (1994) begins his study of consciousness in functions of the brain, as in depth perception or overcoming optical illusions, Rivers (1920) argues these are just late adaptions in ontogeny, as in reflexes or the suppression of some routine stimuli that led Head to more substantial questions of brain integration of perception. While it is well known that the hippocampus, being part of the basal brain, is involved in many reflex actions in mammals, for example, the startle response (Gambarian et al. 1979; Lee and Davis 1997) and that these can be affected by LSD (Radulovacki and Adey 1965), what Rivers (1920) proposed was that the unconscious was made up of millions of parts of memories of reflect action, as well as both internal and external stimulation responses as well as repressed memories. He called the last, along with forgotten information, "unwittingly" lost memories. Therefore, consciousness is the result of constant testing of sorts of all these memories of self. The ability of the brain to "fill in" missing or lost information in perception, a process of abstracting from similar experiences, is also well known, as in the so-called blind spot of the eye (Ramachandran and Gregory 1991). A similar process may underlie what takes place not only in hallucinations and visions, but also in dreams. We have already looked at the hippocampus in earlier pages and will revisit its role in what is often called "mind," "subconscious," and "unconscious" in later sections.

Here then we could say that the "world-denying" nature of Buddhism is reflected in biology. The question of where does consciousness go when one develops coma or amnesia (even temporary) or under sedation or meditation is central. Yet this may misinterpret the idea from Weber's original account. He used the German word "Liebesakosmismus" which has been translated in English as "the acosmism of love" or a "cosmos without love," but given the more popular phrase by Bellah (1999), as "world-denying love." In some of Weber's work the idea of "religious rejections of the world" is clearly stated, and for Bellah (1999) this seems apt. Achieving the denial of the value of consciousness is a goal of Buddhism, as is separation from the mirage of life as defined by its philosophers. Thus, one might say a rejection of the world and of the body is an effort in the rejection of consciousness.

Bellah tries to join Weber's idea of "the prophetic age" of ancient Greece with Jasper's Axial Age. They produce time periods that are about

400 or 500 years apart, and established to try and explain Western "rationality" which seems an artificial distinction from all other complex societies (e.g., ancient Egypt or Sumer) as a desire to found Western society on rationality as a means to "modernity." This modernity, to me, is no more than a form of complex society with enhanced conditioning schedules and population control and has existed in each past civilization. See my criticism of the concept of modernity (Caldararo 2014) and also Goody's revision of the idea (Goody 2004).

On the one hand, some religions, especially the classical polytheist ones and those animistic, seem to have a message of living in the world and enjoying it as a mortal without reference to an afterlife, or a specifically individual reference. I say this in regard to animistic ideas of reincarnation as a positive path, as opposed to, for example, reincarnation as a negative one in India, with exception of the "Twice-Born" Brahmins. The world-denying religions, like Hinduism, Buddhism, and the Judeo-Christian-Islamic tradition, define the world as the province of evil and the post-life period as one of unity and bliss with their god. Perhaps this is less true of Orthodox Judaism or its pre-Hellenistic form. Bellah (1999, 278) quotes Hegel on Spinoza regarding the understanding of the context of mortal and cosmos. Hegel argues that Spinoza was not an atheist, one who denies God, but rather an acosmist, one who denies the world, because God is all things. This is a Deist approach, and if people do not experience love, it is not due to a god, but due to the context of their experience in the cosmos. Intention is lost here and love becomes either an accident or an achievement.

The Revolution That Was and Is

I will return to this idea later, but now I should continue with rebirth. What greater revolution could there be than the transformation of the self, either in personality, sensual outlook, from illness, or in belief? This was one of the claims of Leary and the Pranksters. But it also reflects on the common actions that can take place and produce a joy of being together in some action. This is ritual in many cases, and I note this in regard to Turner's (1967) idea of communitas in indigenous communities. One did experience this feeling of joy in the company of small groups, dozens, hundreds at the beginning of the Haight. The Diggers argue it was a part of the drugs, the music, and the sense of excitement of begin alive and aware. It was a revolution of the self, joined with others in a place and period of time. Then it was over. The temporary nature of that "revolution" had consequences that I think transformed how people think and act. The assessment of that transformation will be made in perhaps a hundred years.

Digger David Simpson put the Digger's part this way, "We were trying to promulgate a spirit—a way of being. And we really succeeded. We gave it away. When you give it away, you don't know where it's gonna go. Human social accomplishment is a strange deal, isn't it? If you hold on to it too tightly, you strangle it; if you let it go, freely, it morphs into something that to you might not be in the spirit."

I should mention that Grof (1976, 131) associates birth trauma with rebirth violence, where his subjects experience destruction of negative experiences as historic epic changes in war, revolution, and so on. He also uses the idea of birth as a renewal and thus conceives of the subject on LSD coming to each experience of sensory information as new or as if just born (Grof 1976, 140). I never saw another person experience this nor did I, but the opposite positive view was common where people experienced being born and passing through light into the world. It seems to me this could have significance as an "archetype" for many forms of religious visions which are often bright, colorful, shiny, and indistinct and for the prevalence of gems and begemmed rooms and buildings (especially in dreams), as noted by Huxley (1954). Light at birth and in the immediate post-natal period is extremely important for the development of normal vision (Yates 2018); thus, the flood of light at birth must have a role in that process.

An additional characteristic of this form of recall and relearning was something I discovered in group sessions and in informal conditions. Often when a number of people took LSD together, they might intervene with each other's experience. In a clinical setting some researchers would question subjects now and then depending on their protocols, but in these informal settings one person expressing interactions with people not present in body, but only in mind, would evoke a comment by another person. This interaction could produce involvement of two or more people, but often it was ignored. If someone did "break in" to another's memory sequence, it could be troubling or informative. Sometimes it could end one sequence for a person, in others it could elicit a series of questions and answers, as often happened in a clinical setting. Yet often it could also change the tone to one of an absurd realization that involved all in laughter. A certain quality of some of these interactions seemed to me like trance and the shaman exchange with spirits (the difference between "trance," "daydream," "hallucination," and "vision" is vague in most definitions; more on this later).

There was some discussion of setting in the Mogar Lab and psychiatric treatment that was negative. Many of the people involved who were not doctors and not academics felt that the laboratory and treatment conditions were too limiting, that they constrained the free experience of individuals. They argued that in nature or in a person's room at home was the best setting. Also, some felt that the treatment reports were so varied, and especially the negative ones, that they reflected the attitudes of the psychiatrists and were polluting the best outcomes of the drug. I was not sure if this was a valid criticism, due to the fact that what I had seen of the Mogar team's work appeared consistent no matter who was the therapist and the results were generally positive.

Though Sacks (2012) emphatically states that dreams are nothing like hallucinations, we should keep this in mind that it is a matter of what people are personally experiencing and this is a phenomenological problem. Grof does criticize the opinion of other psychologists who believe that trance is pathological, and one might argue that, given the similarity of reports regarding trance, dreams, hallucinations, and visions, one might expect at least some beneficial aspects for mental health and society. Bourguignon (1972) distinguishes between dream and hallucination on the one hand, and possession trance on the other by the apparent motor arrest of the former. In possession trance, movement is typical and often exaggerated. Simple trance she classed with dream and hallucination and produced a chart with these all set in a continuum. You can see "hallucination" at the center of this chart. Sacks (2012) would remove it, considering from a psychopathological standpoint that hallucinations are highly varied and due to very many different underlying conditions, only some being the result of trauma to the brain, including lesions.

The difference would then hold that from dreams, visions, and trance, some aspect of meaning is associated with symbols and images, whereas in hallucinations, the link to meaning is lost and only a jumbled junction remains as a shade of the whole that was meaning and memory. I am not sure I agree with this interpretation, but will consider it as we move forward. Likewise, Bourguignon (1972) does find in her survey of ethnographic examples of possession trance that there are cases where the trancer must convince his audience that his or her hallucination has cultural meaning; otherwise, it is only a deviant chaos of one person segmented from social context. One missing element in the chart as well, this is the "negative hallucination" described by B.F. Skinner (1953), where someone is shown an object, or confronts a stimulus, whether visual or auditory, and has normal physiology, but does not "see" or experience the stimulus. This can result from conditioning, a child "paying no attention to a parent" and develop into a "functional deafness," though momentary mistaken recognition can be called an illusion (la Barre 1975). In general, however, Skinner makes the distinction noted already concerning illusion as a temporary false mental appearance capable of correction, and delusion, which he argues, as a fixed false concept occasioned by external stimuli that remains largely "insusceptible to correction." However, this can also be seen as a less clear definition in phenomenological terms, as when a cultural cosmological context identifies a spirit emanation, as in the case of the Punan Dyaks, whose behavior is a sign language spoken via a bird from the forest god. We then have neither an illusion nor a delusion, but instead a hallucination in daylight (Blair and Blair 1988). ffytche (2013) produced a chart I reproduce here as Fig. 2.6, using instrumentation and subject responses to specific questions as to the nature of their experience and logical classifications resulting.

There is another caveat here, one La Barre (1975) seems unsure of, the suffering of many women until the latter part of the twentieth century as hysterics. Their conditions of pain were discounted by physicians as psychological or psychosomatic. La Barre (1975), following Freud, discerns these are "somatized" erotic repression or need for attention that becomes expressed as a "hallucination of pain." La Barre also considers the social milieu and roles for psychological variation described by Benedict (1934a, b) and detailed by Oesterreich (1922) for Europe in the pre-modern period. Here social expectations of a variety of expression of behavior considered today abnormal were quite common and accepted. The constraints of modern society, in this view, have reduced the tendency of human performance of feelings of repression to a minimum, contained in alcohol, drugs, and distractions like TV.

Such a state goes both ways in La Barre's interpretation of the ethnographic record, for in the relation to the divine, revelation, the act of the supernatural world to introduce humans to facts unknown until the moment of exposure, can be seen at the foundation of many religious ideas of hallucination, illusion, and prophesy. This provides another opportunity for a series—the shaman, seer, priest, and prophet are vessels of the divine revealing to man facts about nature and man's place in it. The magician, sorcerer, and scientist study the natural world with the facts they possess, either handed down as part of cultural dogma or discovered method, and reveal to man the nature of the function of the natural world. Divination can be placed halfway, between the seer, who is a passive transmitter of divine signs, and the magician, who can use the knowledge of the cosmos to bend the forces of nature to his or her use. A relation as that below is, perhaps, a clearer spectrum. The priest is, in most cases, the most passive of all. While most discussions of psychedelics in terms of their evolutionary role point to the origin of human consciousness and healing (e.g., McKenna 1992) it is clear that they are also associated with shamanic acts of murder, manipulation and acquisition of power and status (Harner 1972).

Priest—shaman—seer—diviner—magician—sorcerer—scientist

Sacks (2012) would have us consider hallucinations as "a special category of consciousness and mental life." He also argues that the hallucinations of schizophrenics are separate from other kinds. In this way we must demand an examination of whether there can be a classification called "hallucination." In so demanding, we should ask if there are characteristics that allow grouping, and I do think we have a general trait that Sacks (2012) provides himself, "a special category of consciousness and mental life." There is much agreement that the mental life of those suffering from neurological trauma and disease differs from that causing the mental life of schizophrenics or people on drugs or otherwise normal but hallucinate at times. This difference then, can be seen as a type to be distinguished by the character of both expression of that mental life and the location in the brain where it originates. Yet this argument seems vague and confusing given the variation seen in all mentioned groups. Some examples of these locations are given in the chart on Types of Psychedelic Experience.

Wakefulness is a quality usually assigned to the multiple interacting neurotransmitter systems in the brain stem, hypothalamus, and basal forebrain that converge into effector systems in the thalamus and cortex (Brown et al. 2012). A variety of states, both exogenous and endogenous, can interrupt or disorganize the coordination of these systems, disrupting sleep or blocking it. Sleep results in the inhibition of wake-promoting systems by sleep factors such as adenosine, nitric oxide, and GABAergic neurons in the preoptic area of the hypothalamus. Congenital narcolepsy results from a lack of a wake factor, orexin, as in sleep deprivation, these people also experience hallucinations (Sacks 2012). Non-REM sleep results in conservation of brain energy and facilitates memory consolidation via modulation of synaptic weights (Brown et al. 2012).

In the cases I have mentioned above, especially in a group setting, people did influence one another. Some individuals on LSD would act out events of their lives. One person is involved in a very complex interaction in memory and they could recite an entire exchange that happened two, ten, or more years before the present. Sometimes, the scene appeared to me derived from a novel or movie I was familiar with and the subject was living in the movie or book action. Other times, the scenario was too strange or foreign and confused to such an extent that no interaction or sense could be extracted from it. Bourguignon (1972) argues from her research and that of others that possession trance can be induced by contagion, a "contact high," as some people refer to that of drug experiences with LSD. But in these cases the cultural foundations of how one learns what a trance is, what possession means, and how others respond to it create a powerful context for learning. The film *Holy Ghost People* (1967), about a religious group in Scrabble Creek, West Virginia, has very effective examples of this, where adults engage in individual and group trance and possession in the company of children, who then mimic what the adults do. But induction of such states has a variety of means, including hypnosis, hysteria, and mass psychogenic disease. Hypnosis, or the loss of conscious control, must be a vehicle for the study of the unconscious, as it seems to be a force of distraction in a particular area of the brain, lingual gyrus, involved in higher order processing (Landry et al. 2017). However, research has also shown the involvement of anterior cingulate and prefrontal cortices in hypnotic responding and that high hypnotic suggestibility is associated with atypical brain connectivity profiles (Jensen et al. 2017). This indicates a role for connectivity in consciousness. Hoffman (1980/2009), among a host of others, associates the mass behavior reported in the Middle Ages as "poisonings" with ergot, called "ergotism" or St. Anthony's fire. This, and other examples of people acting in stereotyped ways, as automatons, or as under anesthetic without or with pain but aware of some aspects of the environment, brings up the question of what "happens" to the unity of consciousness under these conditions (Fig. 2.5).

Grof, like Freud, places a great deal of emphasis on the birth experience and fears of death. This seems to me to contaminate his findings, and like the concentration of ideas by Leary and Ram Dass, influences his subjects and his interpretation considerably. In my experience, few people had such concerns, but then my data comes from the West Coast and before Leary and Ram Dass' fetish with the *Tibetan Book of the Dead* took hold or the publication of Grof's book. During the 1961 Napa Hospital Symposium there was a discussion that some LSD experiments were so rigidly designed that they prevented a number of experiences seen in other contexts, as, for example, the oceanic, cosmic unity feeling.

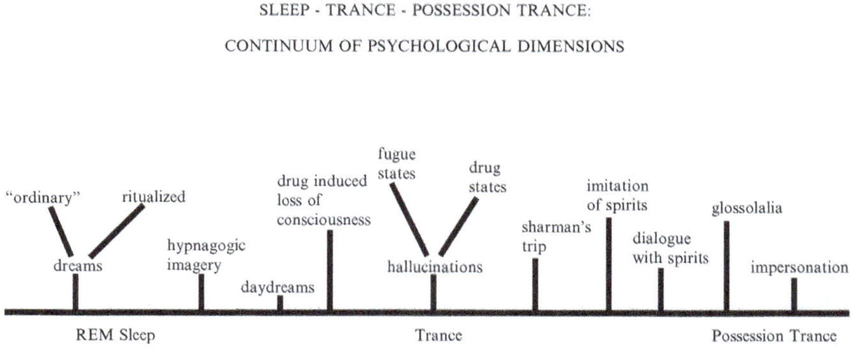

Fig. 2.5 Chart on relation of trance, dreams, and other forms . From Bourguignon, 1972, reprinted with permission by Schenkman Publishing Company, Inc.

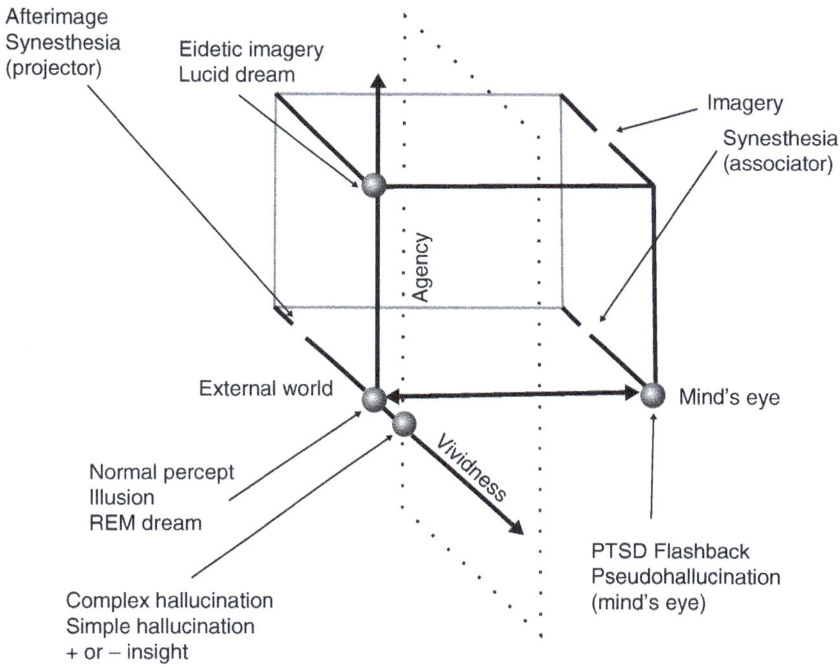

Fig. 2.6 From ffytche (2013), showing a number of intricate relationships between types of experience from hallucinations to visions as they are reported or tested. Reproduced with permission by MIT Press

References

Abramson, H.A. (1967) (ed.) *The Use of LSD in Psychotherapy and Alcoholism*, Indianapolis, Bobbs-Merrill.

Abraham, Hajnalka, Andras Vincze, Ilja Jewgenow, Bela Veszpremi, Andras Kravjak, et al., (2010) "Myelination in the human hippocampal formation from midgestation to adulthood," *Int. J. Dev. Neurosci.* Aug, 28 (5), 401–410.

Adair, Peter, (1967) *Holy Ghost People*, Film, distributed by Thistle Films and available on YouTube.

Adler, Shelley (2010) *Sleep Paralysis: Night-mares, Nocebos, and the Mind-Body Connection*, Piscataway, NJ, Rutgers University Press.

Aiken, John W., (1970) "The church of the Awakening," In Aaronson, Bernard and Humphry Osmond, (eds) (1970) *Psychedelics, The Uses and Implications of Hallucinogenic Drugs,* Garden City, Anchor Books: 165–182.

Anderson, Robert (1996), *Magic, Science and Health*, Orlando, Harcourt Brace & Co.

Anderson, Robert (2005) *The Ghosts of Iceland*, Independence, KY, Cengage Learning.

Anderson, T., R. Petranker, D. Rosenbaum, C.R. Weissman, L.A. Dinh-Williams, et al., (2019) "Microdosing psychedelics: personality, mental health, and creativity differences in microdosers," *Psychopharmacology*, v. 236, 731–740.

Andrade, Chittaranjan and Rajiv Radhakrishnan, (2009) "Prayer and healing: a medical and scientific perspective on randomized controlled trials," *Indian Journal of Psychiatry*, v. 51, n. 4, 247–253.

Aquinas, Thomas St. (1922) *Summa Theologica,* Part II, Question 95, 6, Benziger Brothers, New York.

Aronson, J.K. (2016) "Phencyclidine" in *Meyler's Side Effects of Drugs*, (ed.) J.K. Aronson, Elsevier, pp. 670–2.

Ashe, Geoffrey (1978) *Miracles,* London, Routledge and Kegan Paul.

Bachofen, J.J. (1861) *Das Mutterecht,* Stuttgart: Verlag von Krais und Hoffmann.

Bachofen, J.J. (1926) *Der Mythus von Orient und Okzident,* edited by Manfred Schroeder, Munich, Becksche Buchhandlung.

Baird, Benjamin, Anna Castelnovo, Olivia Gosseries and Giulio Tononi, (2018) Frequent lucid dreaming associated with increased functional connectivity between frontopolar cortex and temporoparietal association areas," *Scientific Reports*, v. 8, n. 17798, https://doi.org/10.1038/s41598-018-36190-w

Balasubramaniam, B. and G.R. Park (2003) "Sexual hallucinations during and after sedation and anaesthesia," *Anaesthesia*, v. 58, n. 6, 549–553. https://doi.org/10.1046/j.1365-2044.2003.03147.x

Barrett, Kim, Heddwen Brooks, Scott Boitano, Susan Barman, (2010) *Ganong's Review of Medical Physiology,* 23rd edition, New York, McGraw Hill.

Basso, Ellen (1987) "The implications of a progressive theory of dreaming," in Barbara Tadlock (ed.) Dreaming: Anthropological and Psychological Interpretations, Cambridge, Cambridge University Press, 86–104.

Batzer, W., T. Ditzler and C. Brown, (1999) "LSD use and flashbacks in alcoholic patients," *J. Addict Dis.*, v. 18, (2): 57–63.

Bellah, Robert N. (1999) "Max Weber and world-denying love: a look at the historical sociology of religion," *Journal of the American Academy of Religion*, v. 67, n. 2, Jun. 277–307.

Bellah, Robert N. (1957) *Tokugawa Religion*, Boston, Beacon Press.

Benedict, R. (1934a) *Patterns of Culture*, Boston: Houghton Mifflin.

Benedict, R. (1934b) "Anthropology and the abnormal," *Journal of General Psychology*, 10, 5-82. (b).

Benson, Herbert, et. al., (2006) "Study of the therapeutic effects of intercessory prayer (STEP) in cardiac bypass patients, a multicenter randomized trial of uncertainty and certainty of receiving intercessory prayer, " *Amer. Heart J.*, Apr. v. 151 n. 4, 934–942.

Bentall, R.P. and F. Varese, (2013) "Psychotic hallucinations," in *Hallucination: Philosophy and Psychology*, (eds.) Fiona Macpherson and Dimitris Platchias, Cambridge, MA, MIT Press, pp. 65–86.

Bergson, Henri (1914) *Dreams,* Trans. By Edwin E. Slosson, New York, B.W. Huebsch.

Beringer, K., (1927) Der Meshalinrausch, Berlin.

Berrios, G.E. and Ivana S. Markova, (2015) "Visual hallucinations: history and context of current research," in *The Neuroscience of Visual Hallucinations*, (ed.) Daniel Collerton, New York, John Wiley & Sons: 3–22.

Berwick, R.C., A. D. Frederici, N. Chomsky and J.J. Bolhuis, (2013) Evolution, Brain and the nature of language," *Trends in Cognitive Sci.*, https://doi.org/10.1016/j.tic.2012.12.002.

Bess, Donovan, (1967a) "Lenore defends the Love Book," *San Francisco Chronicle*, 9 May, page 3.

Bess, Donovan, (1967b) "Love Book Poet keeps her cool," *San Francisco Chroncile*, 9 May, page 3.

Bey, Tareg and Anar Patel, (2007) "Phencyclidine intoxication and adverse effects: a clinical and pharmacological review of an illicit drug," *Cal. J. Emergy Med.*, v. 8, n 1, 9–14.

Black, Carmen (1975) *The Catalpa Bow*, London, George Allen & Unwin.

Black Elk (1932) *Black Elk Speaks, Being the Story of a Holy Man of the Oglala Sioux*, As told to John G. Neihardi, Lincoln, University of Nebraska Press.

Blair, Lawrence and Lorne Blair (1988) *The Dream Wanderers of Borneo*, PBS/C.

Blom, Jan Dirk and Esmeralda Mangoenkarso, (2018) "Sexual hallucinations in schizophrenia spectrum disorders and their relation with childhood trauma," *Frontiers in Psychiatry*, v. 9:193: https://doi.org/10.3389/fpsyt.2018.00193.

Bloom, William and Don W. Fawcett (1975) *A Textbook of Histology*, Philadelphia, W.B. Saunders.

Blum, Richard, Nevitt Sanford, Eva Blum, Mary Lou Funkhouser, Joseph J. Downing, et al., (1964) *Utopiates: The Use and Users of LSD-25, A Publication of the Institute for the Study of Human Problems*, Stanford University, Atherton Press.

Blumer, Dietrich and A Earl Walker, (1969) "Memory in temporal lobe epileptics," in George A. Talland and Nancy C. Waugh (Eds.) *The Pathology of Memory*, New York, Academic Press, pages 65–74.

Bogenschutz MP, Forcehimes AA, Pommy JA, Wilcox CE, Barbosa PC, Strassman RJ. (2015) Psilocybin-assisted treatment for alcohol dependence: a proof-of-concept study. *J Psychopharmacol.*;29(3):289–299.

Bourguignon, E. (1972) "Dreams and altered states of consciousness in Anthropological research," in *Psychological Anthropology*, Francis L.R. Hsu (ed.) Cambridge, MA., Schenkman Publishing Co.,: 401–434.

Bourguignon, E., (1954) "Dreams and dream interpretation in Haiti," *American Anthropologist*, 56, 262–268.

Bowen, John R. (2002) *Religions in Practice*, Boston, Allyn and Bacon.

Brice, Dave (1966) "Acid freaks," Golden Gater, Insert Section, May, 31–35.

Briggs, Chantalle, Sherri C. Bowes, Kazue Semba and Michiru Hirasawa, (2019) " Sleep deprivation-induced pre and postsynaptic modulation of orexin neurons," *Neuropharmacology*, August, v. 154, 50–60.

Brown, Emery, Ralph Lydic and Nicholas D. Schiff, (2011) "General anesthesia, sleep and coma," *New England J. of Medicine*, Dec. 30, v. 368 (27), 2638–2650.

Brown, Ritchie E., Radhika Basheer, James T. McKenna, Robert E. Strecker and Robert W. MaCarley, (2012) "Control of Sleep and Wakefulness," *Physiol. Rev.* July, 92(3) 1087–1187.

Buchborn, T., G. Grecksch, D.C. Dieterich, V. Hollt (2016) "Tolerance to Lysergic Acid Diethylamide: overview, correlates and clinical implications," Chapter 79, In *Neuropathology of Drug Addictions and Substance Misuse*, Volume 2, Stimulants, Club and Dissociative Drugs, Hallucinogens, Steroids, Inhalants and International Aspects, (Ed.) Victor R. Preedy, Amsterdam, Academic Press 846–858.

Bucke, Richard M. (1905) *Cosmic Consciousness: A Study in the Evolution of the Human Mind*, Philadelphia, Innes & Sons Edition facsimile. Originally published in 1901.

Bunge, Mario (2019)" Is Consciousness an epiphenomenon?" in N,R, Matthews (eds), *Mario Bunge: A Centenary Festschrift*, Cham., Springer, 377–385.

Burgy, de Martin (2008) "The concept of psychosis: historical and phenomenological aspects," *Schizophr Bull.* Nov 34(6) 1200–1210.

Burns, Jeffrey M. (1994) "Lenore Kandel," *The Argonaut*, v. 5, n. 1,

Burridge, Ken (1960) *Mambu, A Melanesian Millennium*, London.

Burridge, Ken (1969) *New Heaven, New Earth*, London, Blackwell.

Caldararo, Niccolo (2014) *The Psychic Unity of Mankind*, Saarbrucken, Scholars' Press.

Caldararo N. (1994) Lost libraries of the Americas, *Library History*, 10, 9–18.

Caldararo, Niccolo (2019) *An Ethnography of the Goodman Building, The Longest Rent Strike*, New York, Palgrave/Macmillan.

Caldararo, N. (2020) "Social Complexity, Pathogen Adaptation and Covid-19: History of Disease Avoidance, Social Spacing and Work/Home Matrix," in, *City Life and Beyond in Times of Pandemic*, Special Issue—Edited by G. B. Prato, Urbanities, Vol. 10 · Supplement 4 · September 2020.

Cameron, Lindsay P. (2021) "Citizen science: asking questions of psychedelic microdosing," *eLife*, March 2, https://elifesciences.org/articles/66920?utm_source=content_alert&utm_medium=email&utm_content=fulltext&utm_campaign=3-March-21-elife-alert.

Carbonaro TM, Bradstreet MP, Barrett FS, MacLean KA, Jesse R, Johnson MW, Griffiths RR (2016) "Survey study of challenging experiences after ingesting psilocybin mushrooms: acute and enduring positive and negative consequences," *J Psychopharmacol* 30(12): 1268–1278. https://doi.org/10.1177/0269881116662634.

Carbonell, Xavier, Ursula Oberst and Marta Bernuy (2013) "The cell phone in the Twenty-First century: a risk for addiction of a necessary tool?," Chapter 91, in *Principles of Addiction*, Peter M. Miller, (ed.) Volume 1, 901–909.

Carhart-Harris, Robin L., Suresh Muthukumaraswamy, Leor Roseman, Mendel Kaelen, Wouter Droog, et al., (2016) "Neural correlates of the LSD experience revealed by multimodal neuroimaging," *PNAS*, April 26, v. 113, n. 17:4853–4858.

Cawte, J.E. (1964) "Australian ethnopsychiatry in the field: a sampling in N. Kimberley," *Medical Journal of Australia*, v. 1, 467–472.

Cerf, Moran, Nikhil Thiruvengadam, Florian Mormann, Alexander Kraskov, Rodrigo Quian Quiroga, et al., (2010) "On-line, voluntary control of human temporal lobe neurons," *Nature*, Oct, v. 467, n. 7319: 1104–8.

Cervetto, L., G.C. Demontis, and C. Gargini (2007) "Cellular mechanisms underlying the pharmacological induction of phosphenes" *Brit. J. Pharmacol.* Feb, 150 (4) 383–390.

Chalmers, David J. (1996) *The Conscious Mind*, New York, Oxford, Oxford University Press.

Chalmers, David J. (2012) *Constructing the World*, Oxford, Oxford University Press.

Chalmers, David J. (2020) *Reality +: Virtual Worlds and the Problems of Philosophy*, New York, W.W. Norton.

Chandler, Arthur L. and Mortimer A. Hartman, (1960) "Lysergic Acid Diethylamide (LSD-25) as a facilitating agent in Psychotherapy," *Amer. Medical Association Archives of General Psychiatry*, March, v. 2, 286–299.
Charles T. (1972) *Altered States of Consciousness,* Garden City, Doubleday.
Charles T. (1975) *States of Consciousness,* New York, Dutton.
Christoff, K., K. C. R. Fox, J. M. Windt, and U. Voss. 2018. Spontaneous Thought, Insight, and Control in *Lucid Dreams,* (Eds) Kalina Christoff and Kieran C.R. Fox, Oxford, Oxford University Press, 385–410.
Codrington, R.H. (1891) *The Melanesians,* New York, Dover Publications, 1972 edition.
Colten, H.R. and Altevogt, V.M. (2006) "Sleep disorders and sleep deprivation: an unmet public health problem," Chapter 2 in Committee on Sleep Medicine and Research, Institute of Medicine, Washington, D.C.
Cook, Christopher, C. H, (2015) "Religious psychopathology: the prevalence of religious content of delusions and hallucinations in mental disorder," Int. J. Psychiatry, 61(4) 404–425.
Craffert, Pieter F., John R. Baker and Michael J. Winkelman, (eds) (2019) *The Supernatural After the Neuro-turn,* New York, Routledge.
Craffert, Pieter F. (1999) "Jesus and the shamanic complex: first steps in utilizing a social type model," *Neotestamentica,* v. 33, n. 2:321–342.
Crick, Francis, (1994) *The Astonishing Hypothesis, The Scientific Search for the Soul,* New York, Simon and Schuster.
Cumming, Paul, Milan Scheidegger, Darlo Dornblerer, Mikael Painer, Boris B. Quednow, et al., (2021), "Molecular and functional imaging studies of psychedelic drug action in animals and humans," *Molecules,* v. 26, n. 9: https://doi.org/10.3390/molecules26092451.
Curia, Giulia, Daniela Longo, Giuseppe Biagini, Roland S.G. Jones and Massimo Avoli, (2008) "The pilocarpine model of temporal lobe epilepsy," *J. Neurosci Methods.*, Jul 30, v. 172, n. 2–4, 143–157.
Das, Saibal, Preeti Barnwal, Anand Ramasamy, Sumalya Sen and Somnath Mondal, (2016) "Lysergic acid diethylamide: a drug of 'use,'" *Ther. Adv. Psychopharmacol.* June v. 6, n. 3:214–228.
Davis, Wade (2001) *Light at the Edge of the World,* Vancouver, Douglas & McIntyre.
Dean, Sanford J and Luise Hiesinger, (1964) "Operant level, awareness, and the Greenspoon Effect," *Psychological Reports,* v. 15, n. 3, 931–938.

De la Herran-Arita, Alberto K., Magdalena Guerra-Crespo and Rene Drucker-Colin, (2011) "Narcolepsy and orexins: an example of progress in sleep research," *Front. Neurol.* V. 2, https://doi.org/10.3389/fneur.2011.00026.

de Rios, Marlene and Oscar Janiger (2003) *LSD Spirituality and the Creative Process,* Rochester Vt., Park Street Press.

de Rios, Marlene Dobkin (1984) *Hallucinogens: Cross-Cultural Perspectives,* Albuquerque, University of New Mexico Press.

Dhossche D, Ferdinand R, Van der Ende J, et al. (2002) Diagnostic outcome of self-reported hallucinations in a community sample of adolescents. *Psychol Med*; 32:619–27.

Dos Santos RG, Osório FL, Crippa JAS et al (2016) "Antidepressive, anxiolytic, and antiaddictive effects of ayahuasca, psilocybin and lysergic acid diethylamide (LSD): a systematic review of clinical trials published in the last 25 years," *Ther Adv Psychopharmacol* 6(3):193–213. https://doi.org/10.1177/2045125316638008.

Du Bois, Cora, (1945) "The Alorese," in *The Psyhological Frontiers of Society,* eds., Kardiner, Abram, Ralph Linton, Cora Du Bois and James West, New York, Columbia University Press, 101–145.

Dyck, Erika (2008) *Psychedelic Psychiatry: LSD from Clinic to Campus,* Baltimore, Johns Hopkins University Press.

Eisner, Betty Grover and Sidney Cohen (1958) "Psychotherapy with lysergic acid diethylamide," *Journal of Nervous and Mental Disease,* v. 127, n. 6, 528–539.

Ekman, Paul and Wallace V. Friesen (2003) *Unmasking the Face: A Guide to Recognizing Emotions From Facial Clues,* Los Altos, Malor Press.

Eliade, Mircea (1964) *Shamanism*, Bolligen Foundation, Princeton, Princeton University Press.

Emerson, Ralph Waldo (1883) *Lectures and Biographical Sketches,* "Demonology," The Riverside Press, Cambridge, Houghton Mifflin, Co., Boston and New York, p 7 & 8.

Ermentrout, B. and J.D. Cowan, (1979) "A mathematical theory of visual hallucination patterns," *Biological Cybernetics*, v. 34, 137–150.

Etzioni, Amitai (1961) *A Comparative Analysis of Complex Organizations,* New York, Free Press.

Evans-Pritchard, E.E. (1956) *Nuer Religion,* London, Oxford University Press.

Fabian, Johannes (1966) "Dream and charisma, 'theories of dreams' in the Jamaa Movement (Congo)," *Anthropos*, 61, 544–560.

Fabrega, Horacio Jr., (1997) *Evolution of Sickness and Healing*, 172–181.

Fadiman, James (2011) *The Psychedelic Explorer's Guide, Safe, Therapeutic, and Sacred Journeys*, Park Street Press.
Family, Neiloufar, Emiline L. Maillet, Luke T.J. Williams Erwin Krediet, Robin L. Carhart-Harris, et al., (2020) "Safety, tolerability, pharmacokinetics, and pharmacodynamics of low dose lysergic acid diethylamide (LSD) in healthy older volunteers," *Psychopharmacology*, v. 237:841–853.
Feen, Richar Harrow (1984) "The historical dimensions of infanticide and abortion: the experience of classical Greece," *The Linacre Quarterly*, v. 51, August:248–254.
Ffytche, Dominic H. (2013) "The hallucinating brain: neurobiological insights into the nature of hallucinations," Chapter 3, in *Hallucination: Philosophy and Psychology*, (eds.) Fiona Macpherson and Dimitris Platchias, Cambridge, MA, MIT Press, pp. 45–64.
Firth, Raymond, (1936) *We, The Tikopia,* London, George Allen and Unwin.
Fletcher, Ronald (1966) *Instinct in Man,* New York, Schocken Books.
Fouquet, G., T. Coman, O. Hermine and F. Cote (2019) "Serotonin, hematopoiesis and stem cells," *Pharmacol. Res.*, v. 140:67–74.
Freud, Sigmund (1966) *The Complete Introductory Lectures on Psychoanalysis,* trans. James Strachey (ed.) New York, W.W. Norton.
Freud, Sigmund (1901) *The Psychopathology of Everyday Life*, New York, W.W. Norton, 1990 edition.
Fromm, Erick (1951) *The Forgotten Language: An Introduction to the Understanding of Dreams, Fairy Tales and Myths,* New York, Grove Press.
Furst, Peter T. (1972) *Flesh of the Gods, the Ritual Use of Hallucinogens,* New York, Praeger.
Gambarian, I.S., K. Gekht, G.T. Sarkisov, I.N. Koval and G. M. Kazarian, (1979) "[Role of the hippocampus in conditioned reflex activity," in Russian, *Zh Vyssh Nerv Deiat Im I P Pavlova.* 1979;29: 56–63.
Garber-Paul, Elisabeth (2022) "RS Recommends: Choas: Charles Manson, the CIA and the Secret History of the 60's," *Rolling Stone*, July 9.
Garcia, Manon (2021) *We Are Not Born Submissive*, Princeton, Princeton University Press.
Gearing, Robin Edward, Dana Alonzo, Alex Smolak, Katie McHugh, Sherelle Harmon, et al., (2011) "Association of religion with delusions and hallucinations in the context of schizophrenia: implications for engagement and adherence," *Schizophrenia Research*, v. 126, n.1–3, 150–163.
Goethe, Johann Wolfgang, (1836) *Conversation with Eckermann*, (edition of 1898) Trans, John Osenfort, George Bell & Sons, 315.

Goldman, Sarah, David Galameau and Richard Friedman, (2007) "New onset LSD flashback syndrome triggered by the initiation of SSRIs." *The Ochsner Journal,* Spr, 7(1), 37–39.

Goody, Jack (2004) *Capitalism and Modernity: The Great Debate,* New York, Polity.

Gottfried, Emily, Lindsay Bodell, Joyce Carbonell and Thomas Joiner (2014) "The clinical utility of the MMPI-2-RF suicidal/death ideation scale," *Psychol. Assess.,* Dec. v. 26, n 4, 1205–1211.

Graf, Stanislav, (1976) *Realms of the Human Unconscious Observations from LSD Research,* New York, Dutton.

Graham, Laura R. (2003) *Performing Dreams: Discoveries of Immortality Among the Xavante of Central Brazil,* Fenestra Books.

Granberg-Axèll, A., I. Berghom-Engbery, D. Lundberg, (2001) "Clinical signs of ICU syndrome/delirium: an observational study," *Intensive Crit Care Nurs.,* v 17, 72–93, https://doi.org/10.1054/iccn.2000.1539.

Grant, Frederick C., (1953) *Hellenistic Religions,* New York, The Liberal Arts Press.

Greenfield, Robert, (2006) *Timothy Leary, A Biography,* New York, Harcourt.

Gregor, Thomas (1981) "A dream content analysis of Mehinaku Dreams," Ethos, v. 9:353–390.

Griffiths, Roland R. and Charles S. Grob (2010) "Hallucinogens as Medicine," *Scientific American,* Dec., v. 303, n6:76–79.

Griffiths RR, Richards WA, McCann U, Jesse R. (2006) Psilocybin can occasion mystical-type experiences having substantial and sustained personal meaning and spiritual significance. *Psychopharmacology (Berl)*; 187(3):268–283.

Griffiths RR, Johnson MW, Carducci MA, et al. (2016) Psilocybin produces substantial and sustained decreases in depression and anxiety in patients with life-threatening cancer: a randomized double-blind trial. *J Psychopharmacol.*;30(12):1181–1197

Grinspoon, L. and J.B. Bakalar, (1979) *Psychedelic Drugs Reconsidered,* Basic Books, New York.

Grob C. (2002) Conversation with Albert Hofmann. In: Grob C. (ed.), *Hallucinogens: A Reader.* New York: Tarcher/Putnam, pp. 15–22.

Grof, Stanislav (1976) *Realms of the Human Unconscious: Observation from LSD Research,* New York, E.P. Dutton.

Grof, Stanislav and Joan Halifax, (1978) *The Human Encounter with Death,* New York, Dutton.

Gudjonsson, Thorsteinn (1976) *Astrobiology: The Science of the Universe,* Reykjavik, Bioradii.

Gumilla, Padre (1741) *El Orinoco Illustrado*, Madrid.
Guthrie, Stewart E. (2004) "Review of *Shamanism, The Neural Ecology of Consciousness and Healing*," *Journal of Ritual Studies*, v. 18, n. 1, 97–100.
Haeckel, Ernst (1866) *Generelle Morphologie der Organismen (General Morphology of the Organisms)* Berlin, G. Reimer.
Haden, Mark, and Birgitta Woods, (2020) "LSD over doses: three case reports," *J. of Studies on Alcohol and Drugs*, v. 81, 1.
Hallowell, A.I. (1942) "The role of conjuring in Salteaux society," *Publications of the Philadelphia Anthropological Society*, volume II, Philadelphia, University of Pennsylvania Press.
Harman, WW, McKim, RH, Mogar, RE, Fadiman, J., Stolaroff, MJ. (1966) Psychedelic Agents in Creative Problem-solving: A Pilot Study. *Psychol Rep.* 1:211–27.
Harner, Michael (1972) *Hallucinogens and Shamanism*, Oxford, Oxford University Press.
Harner, Michael (1973) *The Jivaro: People of the Sacred Waterfalls*, New York, Doubleday.
Harner, Michael (1968) "The sound of rushing water," *Natural History*, v. 77, n. 6, 28–33.
Hermie, L., M. Ruchsow and K.L. Taschner, (2015) "Hallucinogen persisting perception disorder (HPPD) and flashback phenomena- differential diagnosis and explanation models," (in German) *Fortschr Neurol Psychiatr.* Sept, v. 83, (9) 506–515.
Hersh, Keith and Randy Borum, (1998) "Command Hallucinations, Compliance, and Risk Assessment," *J. Am. Acad. Psychiatry Law*, v. 26, n. 3, 353–359.
Herskovits, Melville (1966) *Cultural Anthropology*, An abridged revision of *Man and His Works*, New York, Alfred A. Knopf.
Hobson, Allan (1999) *Dreaming as Delirium: How the Brain Goes Out of its Mind*, Cambridge, MA, MIT Press.
Hoffmann A. (2009) *LSD my problem child.* Santa Cruz: Multidisciplinary Association for Psychedelic Studies, originally published in 1980 by McGraw-Hill, Boston.
Hollan, Douglas (2003) "The cultural and intersubjective context of dream remembrance and reporting," Chapter 9 in *Dream Travelers: Sleep Experiences and Culture in the Western Pacific*, (ed) Roger Ivar Lohmann, New York, Palgrave Macmillan,169–188.
Holze, Friederike, Patrick Vizeli, Laura Ley, Felix Muller, Patrick Dolder, et al., (2020) "Acute dose-dependent effects of lysergic acid diethylamide in a

double-blind placebo-controlled study in healthy subjects," Neuropsychopharmacology, 15 Oct. 46, 537–544.

Horiguchi, Jun, Tsuyoshi Miyaoka and Hideto Shinno (2009) "Pathogenesis and symptomatology of hallucinations (delusions) or organic brain disorder and schizophrenia," *Psychogeriatrics,* Jun, 9(2), 73–76.

Horwitz, Tony (2015) "Did Civil War soldiers have PTSS?" Smithsonian Magazine, January, https://www.smithsonianmag.com/history/ptsd-civil-wars-hidden-legacy-180953652/.

Howard, R., A. David, P. Woodruff, J. Mellers, M. Brammer, E. Bullmore, and S. Williams (1997) "Seeing visual hallucinations with functional magnetic resonance imaging," *Dement Geriatr Cogn Disord, Brain Imaging,* 8(2), 73–77, https://doi.org/10.1159/000106610.

Hunt, Katie (2020) "A woman took 550 times the usual dose of LSD with surprisingly positive consequences," *CNN Health,*https://www.cnn.com/2020/02/27/health/lsd-overdoses-case-studies-wellness/index.html accessed Jan 2 2021.

Huxley, Aldous (1954) *The Doors of Perception, and Heaven and Hell,* New York, Harper Colophon Books.

Ignatieff, Michael (2001) "What did the C.I.A. do to his father?" *The New York Times Magazine,* April 1, 56–61.

Inserra, Antonio, Danilo De Gregorio, Tamim Rezai, Martha Graciela Lopez-Canul, Stafano Comai and Gabriella Gobbi, (2021) "Lysergic acid diethylamide differentially modulates the reticular thalamus, mediodorsal thalamus, and infralimbic prefrontal cortex: an in vivo electrophysiological study in male mice," *Journal of Psychopharmacology,* v. 35, n. 4, 469–482.

Jackendoff, Ray (1987) *Consciousness and the Computational Mind,* Cambridge, MA, Bradford Books, MIT Press.

James, William (1892) *Psychology, New York,* Henry Holt & Co. reprinted 1907.

Jaspers, K. (1959) *Allgemeine Psychopathologie.* 7th ed. Berlin, Germany: Springer.

Jaynes, Julian (1976) "The origin of consciousness in the breakdown of the bicameral mind," *Philosophy and Rhetoric,* v. 14, n. 2:127–129.

Jaynes, Julian (1986) "Consciousness and the voices of the mind," *Canadian Psychology,* v. 27, n. 2.:1–20 From Bauer Lectures, 1983.

Jensen, Mark P., Graham A. Jamieson, Antoine Lutz, Giuliana Mazzoni, William J. McGeown, et al., (2017) "New directions in hypnosis research: strategies for advancing the cognitive and clinical neuroscience of hypnosis," *Neurosci. Conscious,* Apr 12. https://doi.org/10.1093/nc/nix004.

Jiang, Qiaolei, Xiugin Huang and Ran Tao (2013) "Internet addiction: cybersex," in *Principles of Addiction,* (ed.) Peter Miller, London, Elsevier, 809–818.

Johns, T. (1990) *With Bitter Herbs They Shall Eat It,* Tucson, University of Arizona Press.

Johnstad P (2018) "Powerful substances in tiny amounts: An interview study of psychedelic microdosing, "Nordic Studies on Alcohol and Drugs **35**:39–51.

Kaberry, Phyllis M. (1939*) Aboriginal Woman, Sacred and Profane,* London, Routledge.

Kandel, Eric R. (2007) *In Search of Memory: The Emergence of a New Science of Mind,* New York, W.W. Norton.

Kant, Immanuel (1900) *Dreams of a Spirit Seer,* Trans. E.F. Goerwitz, New York, Macmillan.

Kaplan, C.A., & H.A. Simon (1990) "In search of insight," *Cog Psychol* 22:374–419

Karig, David, K. Michael Martini, Ting Lu, Nichola A. DeLateur, Nigel Goldenfeld, et al., (2018) "Stochastic Turing patterns in a synthetic bacterial population," *PNAS,* June 25, v. 115, (26) 6572–6577.

Kataoka, Hiroshi and Satoshi Ueno, (2009) "Cerebral polyopia and palinopsia in a patient with occipital lobe epilepsy," *Epilepsy Behav*. Apr, v. 14, (4):684–6.

Kawai, M., (1965) "Newly-acquired, pre-cultural behavior of the natural troop of Japanese monkeys on Kashima Islet," *Primates*, v. 6, 1–30.

Kehoe, A. B. (2000) *Shamans and Religion: An Anthropological Exploration in Critical Thinking,* Prospect Heights, Waveland Press.

Kellener, Ian, Helen Keeley, Paul Corcoran, Fionnuala Lynch, Carl Fitzpatrick, et al., (2012) "Clinicopathological significance of psychotic experiences in non-psychotic young people evidence from population-based studies," *Brit. J. Psychiatry*, July, v. 201, n. 1, 26–32.

Kelly, George A. (1963) *A Theory of Personality*, New York, The Norton Library.

Kempf, Wolfgang and Elfriede Hermann (2003) "Dreamscapes: Transcending the Local in Initiation Rites among the Ngaing of Papua New Guinea, " in *Dream Travelers: Sleep Experiences and Culture in the Western Pacific*, (ed) Roger Ivar Lohmann, New York, Palgrave Macmillan: 61–86.

Kent, John (2010) *Psychedelic Information Theory*, Seattle, PIT Press.

Kitto, H.D.F (1966). *Poiesis*. University of California Press. pp. 236–242.

Klee, G.D. (1963) "Lysergic acid diethylamide (LSD-25) and ego functions," *Archives of General Psychiatry,* VIII, 461–473.

Klein, Richard, (1989) *The Human Career*, Chicago, University of Chicago Press.

Kluver, Heinrich (1942) "Mechanisms of Hallucinations," in Q. McNemar & M.A. Merrill, *Studies in Personality*, McGraw-Hill: 175–207.

Kluver, Heinrich (1966) *Mescal: The Divine Plant and Its Psychological Effects*, Kegan Paul (originally published in 1928).

Kohler, W. (1925) *The Mentality of Apes*. London, Routledge and Kegan Paul.
Kracke, Waud, (1987) "Myths in dreams, thought in images: an Amazonian contribution to the psychoanalytic theory of primary process," in Barbara Tadlock (ed.) *Dreaming: Anthropological and Psychological Interpretations*, Cambridge, Cambridge University Press: 55–85.
Krebs T., Johansen P. (2012) "Lysergic acid diethylamide (LSD) for alcoholism: meta-analysis of randomized controlled trials." *J Psychopharmacol* 26: 994–1002.
Krippner, Stanley, (1970) "An adventure in psilocybin, " in Aaronson, Bernard and Humphry Osmond, (eds) (1970) *Psychedelics, The Uses and Implications of Hallucinogenic Drugs*, Garden City, Anchor Books: 35–39.
La Barre, Weston (1975) "Anthropological perspectives on hallucination and hallucinogens," in *Hallucinations: Behavior, Experience and Theory*, (eds.) R. K. Siegel and L.J. West, New York, John Wiley, & Sons, 9–52.
Laing, R.D. (1959) *The Divided Self*, Harmondsworth, Pelican Books.
Landry, Mathieu, Michael Lifshitz and Amir Raz, (2017) Brain correlates of hypnosis: a systematic review and meta-analytic exploration," *Neuroscience and Biobehavioral Reviews*, v. 81, 75–98.
Latham, Larry M. (1972) "Hallucinations induced by sensory deprivation: fact or fiction?" *Scholarly Commons @ Ouachita Baptist University*, Honors Thesis, https://scholarlycommons.obu.edu/cgi/viewcontent.cgi?article=1278&context=honors_theses
Laughlin, Robert M. (1976) *Of Wonders Wild and New: Dreams from Zinacantan*, Smithsonian Contributions to Anthropology, n. 22, Washington, D.C., Smithsonian Institution.
Lazzari, Carlo, Ahmed Shoka, Basavaraja Papanna and Georgios Mousailidis, (2017) "Oneirophrenia in dementia: when the difference between dream and reality becomes clouded," *Sleep Medicine and Disorders*, v. 1, n. 5, 110–111.
Leary, Timothy, Metzner, Ralph, Alpert, Richard, *The Psychedelic Experience*, New York, 1964.
Lee, Younglim and Michael Davis (1997) "Role of the hippocampus, the Bed Nucleus of the Stria Terminalis, and the Amygdala in the Excitatory Effect of Corticotropin-Releasing Hormone on the Acoustic Startle Reflex," *J. Neurosci.*, Aug. 15, v. 17, n. 16, 6434–6446.
Lerner, Arturo G., Marc Gelkopf, Irena Skladman, Igor Oyffe, Boris Finkel, et al, (2002),"Flashback and hallucinogen persisting perception disorder: clinical aspects and pharmacological treatment approach," *Isr. J. Psychiatry Relat. Sci*, v. 39 (2): 92–99.

Levy-Bruhl, Lucien (1966) *Primitive Mentality*, (originally published in 1923) Boston, Beacon Press.
Lewis-Williams, J.D. (2009) "Cognitive and optical illusions in San Rock art research," " In Warms, Richard, James Garber and R. Jon McGee, (2009) *Sacred Realms: Readings in the Anthropology of Religion,* Oxford, Oxford University Press, 217–226.
Li, Jie, Rena Y. Jiang, Kristin L. Arendt, Yu-Tien Hsu, Sophia R. Zhai and Lu Chen, (2020) "Defective memory engram reactivation underlies improved memory recall in Fragile X Syndrome," eLife, Nov. 20th; 9:e61882 https://doi.org/10.7554/eLife.61882
Li, Qi and Haiyan Geng (2009) "Progress in cognitive neuroscientific studies of visual awareness," *Progress in Natural Science,* v. 19, n. 2, 10 Feb, 145–152.
Liester M. (2014) "A review of lysergic acid diethylamide (LSD) in the treatment of addictions: historical perspectives and future prospects." *Curr Drug Abuse Rev* 7: 146–156.
Lincoln, J. S. (1935) *The Dream in Primitive Cultures,* London, Cressett Press.
Liu, Z., M. Mikati and G.L. Holmes, (1995) "Mesial temporal sclerosis: pathogenesis and significance," *Pediatr Neurol.,* Jan, v. 12 n. 1, 5–16.
Luria, A.R. (1968 *The Mind of a Mnemonist,* New York, Basic Books.
Lutz, C and G. M. White (1986) "The Anthropology of Emotions," Ann. Rev. Anth., 15(1) 405–436.
Macpherson, Fiona (2013) "The philosophy and psychology of hallucination: an introduction," in *Hallucination: Philosophy and Psychology,* (eds.) Fiona Macpherson and Dimitris Platchias, Cambridge, MA, MIT Press, pp. 1–38.
Malone, Noreen (2016) "Why power women are microdosing at work," *Marie Claire,* Nov. 17, https://www.marieclaire.com/culture/news/a23669/power-women-microdosing-lsd/
Matefy, R.E., C. Hayes and J. Hirsch, (1978) "Psychedelic drug flashbacks: subjective reports and biographical data," *Addict. Behav.* V. 3 (3–4, 165–178.
McBrearty, Sally and Allison S. Brooks, (2000) "The revolution that wasn't: a new interpretation of the origin of modern human behavior," *Journal of Human Evolution,* v. 39, 453–563.
McGinn, Colin (2006) *Mindsight, Image, Dream, Meaning,* Cambridge, MA, Harvard University Press.
McGlothlin, William H. (1971) "LSD revisited: a ten-year follow-up of medical LSD use," *Arch Gen Psychiatry,* v. 24, n. 1, 35–49.
McKenzie, Sam and Howard Eichenbaum (2011) "Consolidation and reconsolidation: two lives of memories?" *Neuron,* Jul 71(2), 224–233.

Metzner, Jeffrey L. and Jamie Fellner, (2010) "Solitary confinement and mental illness in U.S. prisons: A challenge for medical ethnics," *Journal of the American Academy of Psychiatry and the Law,* v. 38, n 1, 104–108.

Miller, John and Shahin Hakimian, (2013) "Surgical treatment of epilepsy," *Continuum (Minneap Minn.)* June, v. 19, n. 3, 730–7e42.

Mogar, Robert E., (1965) "Current status and future trends in psychedelic (LSD) research," *Journal of Humanistic Psychology,* Oct. 1, v. 5, n. 2, 147–166.

Mogar, Robert E., and Charles Savage, (1964) "Personality change associated with psychedelic (LSD) therapy: a preliminary report," *Psychotherapy: Theory, Research & Practice, 1*(4), 154–162.

Monakow, Von Constantin (1911) "Lokalization der Hirnfunktionen (localization of brain functions)" *Journal fur Psychologie und Neurologie,* v. 17:185–200.

Moore, James W. (2021) "'They were noble automatons who knew not what they did:' volition in Jaynes' *The Origin of Consciousness in the Breakdown of the Bicameral Mind,*" Front. Psychol. 20 Dec. https://doi.org/10.3389/fpsyg.2021.811295

Morewedge, Carey K. and Michael I. Norton, (2009) "When dreaming is believing: the (motivated) interpretation of dreams," *Journal of Personality and Social Psychology,* Vol. 96, No. 2, 249–264.

Morokuma, Yoko, Kaori Endo, Alushi Nishida, Syudo Yamasaki, Shuntaro, Ando, et al., (2017) "Sex differences in auditory verbal hallucinations in early, middle and late adolescence: results from a survey of 17, 451 Japanese students, aged 12–18," BMJ Open, v. 7(5) https://doi.org/10.1136/bmjopen-2016-015239.

Moueau, J.J. (1973) *Hashish and Mental Illness,* New York, Raven Press.

Munn, Norman L., (1961) *Psychology: The Fundamentals of Human Adjustment,* Boston, Houghton Mifflin Co.

Myerhoff, Barbara G. (1974) *Peyote Hunt: The Sacred Journey of the Huichol Indians,* Ithaca, Cornell University Press.

Nagel, T. (1974) What is it like to be a bat?" *Philosophical Review,* v. 83, n. 4, 435–450.

Napier, A. David, (1986) *Masks, Transformation, and Paradox,* Berkeley, UC Press.

Naranjo, Claudio (1972) Psychological aspects of the yage experience in an experimental setting," in Michael Harner, (ed.), *Hallucinogens and Shamanism,* Oxford, Oxford University Press:177–190.

Nelson, Kevin (2010) *The Spiritual Doorway in the Brain: A Neurologist's Search for the God Experience,* New York, Fenguin/Plume.

Nichols DE. (2016) Psychedelics. *Pharmacol Rev.*;68(2):264–355.

Nickel, Mara and Chen Gu, (2018) "Regulation of central nervous system myelination in higher brain functions," Neural Plast, March 5, https://doi.org/10.1155/2018/6436453

Nyberg, H. (1992). "Religious use of hallucinogenic fungi: A comparison between Siberian and Mesoamerican Cultures". *Karstenia.* **32** (71–80): 71–80.

Oesterreich, T. K. (1922) *Die Bessessenheit.* Halle: Wendt und Klauwell, (Translated as Possession, demoniacal and other, among primitive races, in antiquity, the middle ages, and modern times. New York: Richard R. Smith, 1930; University Books, 1966

Ogden, Charles K. and I.A. Richards, (1923) *The Meaning of Meaning: A Study of the Influence of Language Upon Thought and of the Science of Symbolism,* London, Routledge.

O'Neill, Tom and Dan Piepenbring, (2019) *Chaos, Charles Manson, the CIA, and the Secret History of the Sixties,* Boston, Little Brown.

Osmond, Humphry and John R. Smythies, (1953) "The present state of psychological medicine," *Hibbert Journal,* 133–142.

Oster, Gerald (1970) "Phosphenes," *Scientific American,* Feb, v. 222, (2), 82–87.

Ouellette, Jennifer (2018) "A math theory for why people hallucinate," *Quanta Magazine,* July 30, https://www.quantamagazine.org/a-math-theory-for-why-people-hallucinate-20180730/.

Pahnke, Walter (1963) *Drugs and Mysticism: An Analysis of the Relationship Between Psychedelic Drugs and the Mystical Consciousness,* Thesis, Harvard University, https://maps.org/images/pdf/books/pahnke/walter_pahnke_drugs_and_mysticism.pdf.

Palhano-Fontes, Fernanda, Katia C. Andrade, Luis F. Tofoli, Antonio C. Santos, Jose Alexandre S. Crippa, et al., (2015) "The psychedelic state induced by ayshuasca modulates the activity and connectivity of the default mode network," PLoS One, Feb. 18, v. 10, n. 2, https://doi.org/10.1371/journal.pone.0118143

Palmer, H.R. (1908) *The Kano Chronicle,* Translated with an introduction by Palmer, H.R., The Journal of the Royal Anthropological Institute of Great Britain and Ireland, v. 38, Jan.-June:58–98.

Pantelis, Christos and Thomas R.E. Barnes, (1993) "Acute exacerbation of psychosis with buspirone?" *Journal of Psychopharmacology,* May 1, 7(3), 295–300.

Parker, Arthur C. (1912) The Code of Handsom Lake, The Seneca Prophet, Education Department Bulletin, n. 163, University of the State of New York, Nov 1.

Parsons, Neil (2010) *Clicko: The Wild Dancing Bushman,* Chicago, University of Chicago Press.

Passie T, Seifert J, Schneider U, Emrich HM (2002). "The pharmacology of psilocybin". *Addiction Biology*. 7(4): 357–364

Patai, Raphael (1990) *The Hebrew Goddess*, Detroit, Wayne State University Press, third edition.

Patrizi, Francesco (1591) *Nova de universis philosophia*, Ferrara.

Pauling, Linus (1988) *General Chemistry*, New York, Dover Publications, altered and corrected from the 1970 edition.

Penfield, Wilder and Herbert Jasper (1954) *Epilepsy and the Functional Anatomy of the Human Brain*, Boston, Little Brown and Co.

Petre-Quadens, O., H. Hussain and C. Balaratnam, (1975) Paradoxical sleep characteristics and cultural environment," *Acta Neurological Belgique*, 74, 85–92.

Przybyslawski, P. Roullet and S. J. Sara, (1999) "Attenuation of emotional and non-emotional memories after their reactivation: role of beta-adrenergic receptors," J. *Neurosci.*, 19, 6623–6628.

Radin, Paul (1937) *Primitive Religion*, New York, Viking Press.

Radulovacki, M. and W.R. Adey (1965) "The hippocampus and the orienting reflex," *Experimental Neurology*, v. 12, n. 1, 68–83.

Ramachandran, V.S. and R.L. Gregory, (1991) "Perceptual filling in of artificially induced scotomas in human vision," *Nature*, 350, 699–702.

Ratsch, Angela, Kathryn J. Steadman and Fiona Bogossian (2010) "The pituri story: a review of the historical literature surrounding traditional Australian Aboriginal use of nicotine in Central Australia," *Journal of Ethnobiology and Ethnomedicine*, v. 6, n. 26, 12 Sept.: https://ethnobiomed.biomedcentral.com/articles/10.1186/1746-4269-6-26.

Rechtschaffen, Allen (1983) "Physiological correlates of prolonged sleep deprivation in rats," *Science*, v. 221, n 4606, 182–184.

Rechtschaffen, Allen and J.M. Siegel (2000) "Sleep and Dreaming," in *Principles of Neuroscieince*, (eds.) E.R. Kandel, J.H. Schwartz and T.M. Jessel, New York, McGraw-Hill, 4th edition.

Rector, N.A. and M.V. Seeman (1992) "Auditory hallucinations in women and men," *Schizophr Res.*, Sept. v. 7(3) 233–236.

Reiter, Keramet, Joseph Ventura, David Lovell, Dallas Augustine, Melissa Barragan, et al., (2020) *Am. J. Public Health*, January, v. 110, Suppl 1, S56–S62.

Ritchie, Elspeth Cameron, Jerald Block and Remington Lee Nevin, (2013) "Psychiatric side effects of mefloquine: applications to forensic psychiatry," *Journal of the American Academy of Psychiatry and the Law*, June, v. 41m n.2, 224–235.

Rivers, W.H.R. (1920) *Instinct and the Unconscious*, Cambridge, Cambridge University Press.

Ross S, Bossis A, Guss J, et al. (2016) Rapid and sustained symptom reduction following psilocybin treatment for anxiety and depression in patients with life-threatening cancer: a randomized controlled trial. *J Psychopharmacol*, 30(12): 1165–1180.

Rottier, Bart, Nannette Ripmeester and Andrew Bush (2011) "Separated by a common translation? How the British and the Dutch communicate," *Pediatric Pulmonology*, v. 46, n 4, 409–411.

Ruck C., Bigwood J., Staples D., Ott J., Wasson R. (1979) Entheogens. J Psychedelic Drugs 11: 145–146.

Russell, James A. and Jose Miguel Fernandez-Dols, (1997) *The Psychology of Facial Expression,* Cambridge, Cambridge University Press.

Sacks, Oliver (2012) *Hallucinations*, New York, Vintage Books.

Santhouse, A.M., R.J. Howard and D.H. Ffytche, (2000) "Visual hallucinatory syndromes and the anatomy of the visual brain," *Brain*, v. 123, 2055–2064.

Schultes, Richard Evans (1972) "An overview of hallucinogens in the Western Hemisphere, in *Flesh of the Gods, The Ritual Use of Hallucinogens*, Peter T. Furst (ed.) New York, Praeger Publishers: 3–54.

Serko, A., (1913) "Im mescalinrausch," *Jahrb. F. Psychiat.*, 34, 355.

Seth, Anil (2021) *Being You: A New Science of Consciousness,* Faber.

Shepard, Paul (1978) *Thinking Animals*, New York, The Viking Press.

Sherwood, J.N., M.J. Stolaroff and W.W. Harman (1968) "The Psychedelic Experience—a new concept in psychotherapy," *Journal of Neuropsychiatr.* Nov.–Dec, v. 4: 69–80.

Shevlin, M., J. Murphy, M.J. Dorahy, et al., (2007) "The distribution of positive psychosis-like symptoms in the population: a latent class analysis of the National Comorbidity Survey, " *Schizophr Res*, 89, 101–109.

Siegel, Jerome M. (2001) "The REM sleep-memory consolidation hypothesis," *Science*, v. 294, 1058–1063.

Siegel, Ronald K. (1977) "Religious behavior in animals and man: drug-induced effects," *Journal of Drug Issues,* v. 7, (3) 219–236.

Sinnett, E. Robert, (1970) "Mescaline: Experience and reflections," in Aaronson, Bernard and Humphry Osmond, (eds) (1970) *Psychedelics, The Uses and Implications of Hallucinogenic Drugs,* Garden City, Anchor Books, 29–34.

Skene, Gordon (1961) LSD: Clinical and Therapeutic Uses—Napa State Hospital Symposium, November 7th 1961, Gordon Skene Sound Collection, https://pastdaily.com/2020/03/28/clinical-and-therapeutic-uses-of-lsd-the-napa-symposium-1961-past-daily-pop-chronicles/.

Smith, David E. (1969) "LSD and the psychedelic syndrome," v. 2, n. 1, 69–73.
Skinner, B.F. (1953) *Science and Human Behavior*, New York, The Free Press.
Smith, Scharff Peter (2006) "The effects of solitary confinement on prison inmates: a brief history and review of the literature," *Crime and Justice*, v. 34, n 1, 441–528.
Spaulding, John (1981) "The dream in other cultures: anthropological studies of dreams and dreaming," Dreamworks, v. 1, n. 4, Summer, 330–342.
Spielberger, Charles D. and L. Douglas De Nike, (1962) "Operant conditioning of plural nouns: a failure to replicate the Greenspoon Effect," *Psychological Reports*, v. 11, n. 2, 355–366.
Stevens, Jay (1988) *Storming Heaven: LSD and the American Dream*, New York, Harper and Row.
Stewart, Pamela and Andrew J. Strathern (2003) "Dreaming and ghosts among the Hagen and Duna of the Southern Highlands, Papua New Guinea," in *Dream Travelers, Sleep Experiences and Culture in the Western Pacific*, (ed) R. Lohmann, New York, Palgrave Macmillan, 43–60.
Skrbina, David (n.d.) "Panpsychism," in *The Internet Encyclopedia of Philosophy*, (eds) James Fieser and Bradley Dowden, ISSN 2161-0002, https://iep.utm.edu/
Skrzypinska, Dagna, Malgorzata, Holda, Barbara Szmigielska, and Monika Slodka, (2018) "The phenomenology of dream-reality confusion: a quantitative study," *Dreaming*, v. 28, n. 3, 245–260.
Striedter, Georg F. (2005) *Principles of Brain Evolution*, Sunderland, Mass., Sinauer Associates.
Sundkler, B. (1961) *Bantu Prophets in South Africa*, London.
Szasz, Thomas S. (1960) The myth of mental illness," *Amer. Psychol.* 15:113–118.
Szigeti, Balazs, Laura Kartner, Allan Blemings, Fernando Rosas, Amanda Feilding, et al., (2021) "Self-blinding citizen science to explore psychedelic microdosing," *eLife*, Mar 2, https://elifesciences.org/articles/62878.
Tedlock, Barbara (1987) "Dreaming and dream research," in *Dreaming: Anthropological and Psychological Interpretations*, (ed.) Barbara Tedlock, Cambridge, Cambridge University Press, 1–30.
Teeple, Ryan C., Jason P. Caplan and Theodore A. Stern (2009) "Visual hallucinations: differential diagnosis and treatment," *Prim Care Companion J. Clin Psychiatry*, v. 11(1) 26–32.
Tien AY. (1991) Distributions of hallucinations in the population. *Soc Psychiatry Psychiatr Epidemiol*; 26:287–92.

Tobin, Joseph J. and Joan Friedman (2009) "Spirits, Shaman and nightmare death: survivor stress in a Hmong refugee, " In Warms, Richard, James Garber and R. Jon McGee, (2009) *Sacred Realms: Readings in the Anthropology of Religion,* Oxford, Oxford University Press, 327–332.

Todorov, Tzvetan (1984) *The Conquest of America*, New York, Harper and Row.

Tonkinson, Robert (2003) "Ambrymese dreams and the Mardu dreaming," in *Dream Travelers: Sleep Experiences and Culture in the Western Pacific*, (ed) Roger Ivar Lohmann, New York, Palgrave Macmillan: 87–106.

Trigoni, Thalia (2019) "Thomas De Quincey and the fluid movement between literary and scientific writings on dream-inducing drugs," in *Histories of Dreams and Dreaming: An Interdisciplinary Perspective,* (Eds.) Giorgia Morgese, Giovanni Pietro Lombardo and Hendrika Kemp, Cham, Palgrave Macmillan, 63–90.

Trulson, M, and T. Crisp, (1983) "Tolerance develops to LSD while the drug is exerting its maximal behavioral effects: implications for the neural bases of tolerance," *Eur J. Pharmacol,* Dec. 23, v. 96, n. 3–4: 317–320.

Turner, Victor (1967) *The Ritual Process, Structure and anti-structure,* Chicago, Aldine.

Ungerleider, J. T. and D.D. Fisher, (1967) "The problems of L.S.D. 25 and emotional disorder," *California Medicine*, v. 106, 49–55.

Vallat, Raphael and Perrine Marie Ruby (2019) "Is it a good idea to cultivate lucid dreaming?" *Frontiers in Psychology,* 15 Nov, https://www.frontiersin.org/articles/10.3389/fpsyg.2019.02585/full.

Van Dusen, Wilson, Wayne Wilson, William Miners and Harry Hook, (1967) "Treatment of alcoholism with Lysergide," *Quarterly Journal of Studies on Alcoholism*, v. 28,: 295–303.

Vansina, Jan (1985) *Oral Tradition as History,* Madison, University of Wisconsin Press.

Voltaire, Francois-Marie Arouet, (1764) *A Philosophical Dictionary,* section on Somnambulists and Dreamers, Trans. F. Fleming, E.R. Dumont, v. VII, pp 2, 9.

Voss, U., R. Holzmann, I. Tuin, A. Hobson, (2009) "Lucid dreaming: a state of consciousness with features of both waking and non-lucid dreaming," *SLEEP*, 32, 9, 1191–1200.

Vygotsky, L. S., (1978*) Mind in society: The development of higher psychological processes.* Cambridge, MA: Harvard University Press.

Wagner, Roy (1975) *The Invention of Culture,* 2nd edition with a forward by Tim Ingold, Chicago, University of Chicago Press.

Wallace, Lord Alfred Russel (1905) *My Life: A Record of Events and Opinions*, Vol. 1, London, Chapman & Hall.

Wamsley, E.J. (2014) "Delusional confusion of dreaming and reality in narcolepsy," *Sleep*, v. 37, n. 2, 419–422.

Wamsley, E.J. (2020) "Memory: how the brain constructs dreams," *eLife*, June 8, 2020;9:e58874. https://doi.org/10.7554/eLife.58874.

Wasson, R. Gordon and V.P. Wasson (1957) *Mushrooms, Russia and History*, New York, Pantheon Books.

Weinberger, Sharon (2019) "When the C.I.A. was into mind control," *The New York Times*, Sept 10., https://www.nytimes.com/2019/09/10/books/review/poisoner-in-chief-stephen-kinzer.html.

Wesson, D.R. and D.E. Smith (1976) " *Am. J. Drug Alcohol Abuse*, v. 3, (3): 425–438.

West, M.L. (1971) *Early Greek Philosophy and the Orient*, Oxford, Oxford University Press.

Wilson, Monica (1963) *Good Company: A Study of Nyakyusa Age Villages*, Boston, Beacon Press.

Winkelman, Michael J. (1992) *Shamans, Priests and Witches*, Tempe, School of Human Evolution and Social Change.

Winkelman, Michael J. (2000) *Shamanism, The Neural Ecology of Consciousness and Healing*, Westport Ct, Bergin and Garvey.

Winkelman, Michael J. (2015) "Shamanism as a biogenetic structural paradigm for human's evolved social psychology," *Psychology of Religion and Spirituality*, v. 7, n. 4, 267–277.

Winkelman, Michael J. (2017) "The mechanisms of psychedelic visionary experiences: hypotheses from evolutionary psychology," *Frontiers in Neuroscience*, v. 11, 539: 10.3389/fnins.2017.00539

Winson, Jonathan (1990) "The Meaning of Dreams," *Scientific American*, v. 263, n. 5, 86–97.

Wittmann, Marc, (2018) *Altered States of Consciousness: Experiences Out of Time and Self*, Cambridge, MA, MIT Press.

Wolf, Eric R. (1951) "The social organization of Mecca and the origins of Islam," *Southwestern Journal of Anthropology*, v. 7, n, 4, 329–356.

Yates, Jacuqueline, (2018) "Perspective: The long-term effects of light exposure on establishment of newborn circadian rhythm," *J. Clin. Sleep Med.*, Oct 15, v. 14, n. 10, 1829–1830.

3

Pursuit of the Miraculous or Just Piling up Confusion

Historical ideas of the transport of souls or the place of original life of humans have been quite diverse. As human society has expanded across the globe and social life has become more complex, the place of paradise has receded or been lost. Eden is nowhere. The assumed location of the Biblical Eden in the land between the two rivers of the Tigris and Euphrates is now more of a desert than a paradise, due to man's over-population and the results of his technological use of land, overgrazing, pollution, and salt buildup. Even the word "paradise" is an interesting combination. "Para" usually means almost and "dise" could be associated with roots for "to say" or "dios". So, we might conjecture a meaning of "almost god." The general meaning in Indo-European languages can be heaven, abode of the gods. But in Latin it can mean park, garden, or orchard. In Old Indo-European roots it can refer to "making of clay," or as different as "place of happiness."

In search of an original experience of contact with the gods we often resort to scripture, Moses, and the old prophets of Israel or the Chaldeans. Shamanic experience is also called upon. The main problem of all religions, secular constructs as well, is that of ultimate cause. What gave birth to god, the cosmos, life? For the Hindus the cosmos is recreated after its

N. Caldararo, *A Mental Ethnography: Conclusions From Research in LSD*,
https://doi.org/10.1007/978-3-031-13745-7_3

destruction, and such scenarios are not rare in religions (Campbell 1949). For the scientific world, there is the Big Bang, which like the Hindu system either expands and contracts or is beyond our knowledge in its expansion. In science fiction we have novels like *Simulicron-3* (Galouye 1964), where people discover they are in a computer program that crashes, but are saved by the programmers. But who saves the programmers?

Anthropologists investigating problems of ultimate causes, as in identity with god or its absence in anomie (loss of association) or individual experiences as believing they are robots, find themselves with some psychologists considering these to be pathologies or these to be abnormal dysfunctions of the brain of neurotics or induced by drugs or deprivation (Opler 1959), but all this is more complex (Devereux 1961; Ackerknecht 1943). Baudrillard (1981) argued that in humans our consciousness lacks the ability to distinguish reality from a simulation, which appears to agree with most of the philosophical discussions concerning hallucinations and dreams (Pagondiotis 2013). Our increasingly artificial realities created by new media produce virtual experiences that seem like hallucinations though are fantasies (see Tiffin and Terashima 2005 for ideas on "hyperreality"). Google's Deep Dream project began by looking at where dreams occurred in the brain and has expanded to study the nature of how dreams unfold and can be manipulated in their algorithm: https://deepdreamgenerator.com/. In a reversal of the discussion of how to tell hallucinations from reality, Google's experiments with volunteers produced results that were similar to the effects of psilocybin. This work has been done in collaboration with Anil Seth and some of it has been published (Suzuki et al. 2017). This has resulted in a "Hallucination Machine" that they claim induces most of the experience of reported hallucinations, both visually and in terms of brain activity. This certainly makes difficult distinguishing "natural" and "machine" or describing a pathological hallucination. This all reminds me of the science fiction movie *Forbidden Planet*, the 1956 movie where humans arrive at a distant planet where intelligent beings had created a super-civilization based on technology much like the internet and Artificial Intelligence software. The screenplay by Irving Block and Allen Adler tells how the beings, the Krell, eventually created programs based on their nervous system, then pouring all their conscious thoughts and desires into the program they fell victim to the AI of their most base desires.

The history of modern medicine in separating abnormal behavior from ideas of the possession of spirits or the devil provides a unique picture of concepts of the boundaries of religion and science, as in the work of seventeenth-century English physician Richard Napier (Fabrega 1997). Unusual experiences often interpreted in the Middle Ages as possession or the work of devils came to be identified in many cases as physical maladies and the purview of medicine, even by some members of the Inquisition in Spain (Keitt 2005). Can they be distinguished from delusions or temporary perceptions such as hearing voices or sounds, or chronic conditions like ringing in the ears (tinnitus) and symptoms that become so, as with Covid-19 patients who smell fire or lose their sense of taste or smell? Other cases of this, called anosmia, occur after injuries, sinus infections, or operations and are often incomplete, all smells replaced with bad ones (called cacosmia) or come and go somewhat (Sacks 2012). Many schizophrenics hear voices from objects, but not all people who hear voices are diagnosed as schizophrenic.

Such indications of presence are also common in other cultures. Among the Pondo of South Africa (Hunter 1961) possession by a "familiar" or spirit called an izulu can be recognized if certain conditions develop, some physiological, some behavioral, and some psychological or revealed in dreams. For example, a woman may find that her child will not suckle—such an event is typically explained as the presence of a izulu spirit in her. A woman may dream of an izulu, which usually means she is possessed by one or is about to be. Such a familiar can become an integral part of a person, but if caught early, it can be removed by a ceremony and the full confession of dreams. Thus, dreams form part of a process to achieve action in the realms of waking and sleeping life.

Experiencing and "Seeing": Art and Spirituality

Grof made a distinction between differences in experience when the eyes were kept shut and when the eyes were held open. Reports of eyes closed found visual hallucinations are commonly reported (e.g., Carhart-Harris et al. 2016; Teeple et al. 2009). Grof (1976) also reported that subjects often noted marked afterimages that could be perceived for long periods. Other dramatic visual effects with eyes closed could be seen by subjects as geometrical designs.

He records typical responses of kaleidoscopic displays, arabesques, decorations of objects and fields of color, patterns like the paintings of the Fauvists, Klimt, and Matisse, and a variety of others. All this was noted in the subjects of the Mogar Lab as well as in my own experiences and those of people I knew and met. In discussions with people at the Haight-Asbury Free Medical Clinic and the Psychedelic Rangers, all these were common before the Leary/Alpert media circus. If anything was clear it was that the setting, background, and people involved were major factors in the type of experience people had. This idea of the number of people involved during an LSD session was discussed at the 1961 Napa State Hospital Symposium, with some arguing that more than two could be a problem and others that groups were effective if all were familiar.

Here it is necessary to address the issue of what is a hallucination. Is it different than a delusion, or some physical change in perception, as in the effects of atropine poison on the optic nerve? Chaudhury (2010) repeats the story of Christoph Friedrich Nicolai, who in 1799 saw a "specter or phantom" of a dead person one day in the presence of his wife. His wife saw nothing and yet the apparition haunted him the rest of the day. The number of such images increased in the following weeks. Nicolai was among a number of literary figures of the time that experienced such apparitions or hallucinations; others included Daniel Schreber (1842–1922), Victor Kandinsky (1849–1889), Vaslav Nijinsky (1889–1950), Guy de Maupassant (1850–1893), Fyodor Dostoevsky (1821–1881), and Ludwig Staudenmaier (1865–1933). While there is some overlap in the life periods of these individuals, what is interesting perhaps is that they are all French, German, or Russian. But this is not a comprehensive list and at any rate, the concept of hallucination, delusion, or apparition remains vague (Ferriar 1813; Nicolai 1803; Sacks 2010). Some references at the time led to Absinthe as a productive agent of hallucinations, but Padosch, et al., (2006) question this given repeated analysis of its likely components (e.g. wormwood). Since opium was very popular at the end of the 19th century and beginning of the 20th (often called the aspirin of the time) it is more likely mixtures of a number of agents, perhaps opium as well, could have given Absinthe its visions. One in five people in Great Britain and the United States have experienced a ghost or apparition of some kind, in some cases associated with religious experiences (Klemperer 1992). There is the opposite perception, one reported by Laing (1959, 166), of schizophrenics who believed they were invisible and many of whose symptoms related to attempts to "prove existence." A similar feature of the LSD experience is one where the world as experienced seems unreal, as in the case of Michael C., who runs into traffic believing he could not be killed. In some subjects this feeling comes to be associated with ideas of Buddhism where reality is a sham of sorts. Joseph Campbell argued that the LSD experience was like an induced schizophrenia, common among yogis and other religious practitioners who engaged in trance, but difficult for the uninitiated (Campbell 1972). In some cases, "trance" is distinguished from visions or hallucinations by the ability of people to converse with the person in trance. But the term "possession" or "possession state" often appears in similar contexts. Bourguignon (1972) refers to Batson and Mead's (1942) and Belo's (1960) use of these terms in this regard. She argues that trance reflects a more demonstrative state that can be seen by others in the actions of the person in trance, either by running from demons, chasing, or speaking in tongues (Bourguignon 1972, 417). Trance is usually temporary, but can last a lifetime if of a certain kind of possession, as in the case of the Shilluk (Lienhardt 1954), where a king goes into a trance during the installation ceremony, but the resulting possession continues after the dissociative state ends. Trance can be contagious and even lead to large groups engaged in devotional acts, especially of self-mortification, as in the Shia flagellates or those of Christian sects in the Middle Ages and today as well as other events mentioned earlier as mass psychogenic events in some locates (Schneider 1986; Bartholomew and Wessely 2002).

Bourguignon (1972) notes that in many cases of trance as explained in cultural context, the idea of possession is a frequent one. The "entranced" one has allowed another spirit to join in his or her body, or a spirit (or agent, often a shaman or witch) has removed the person's spirit from the body, replacing it with their own. Or the person has gone on a spiritual journey or dream or been sick and their soul lost and left their body vulnerable. This idea of the separation of the body and the soul is one common in descriptions of Voodoo (or Vodoun) in Haiti by people like Wade Davis (Press 1987). The skill or power of the sorcerer, or Bokor, "captures the soul" of the victim. The loss of volition creates the zombie. The process is apparently aided by a drug, or a combination of drugs (Booth 1988). Grof reports a similar condition in some people, who in LSD sessions he administered found themselves in such identification with another person at the end of the session that separation was difficult and seemed to reflect some aspects of possession after trance (Grof 1976, 208).

The importance of the relation of dream to trance is that the two experiences are seen often as windows, almost confirmatory in information that can be extracted from spirit worlds. Bourguignon (1972) created a table of people where dream and trance are interpreted as either inseparable in effect or as part of the same process. I have reproduced it in (Fig. 3.1). The Diegueno dream doctor experiences the trance dream, the Toloache, as a kind of reference dream or one that opens a door to worlds that are then accessible and can be used to cure and interpret other dreams (Toffelmier and Luomala 1936, 201). Thus, in reference to the table, where trance exists, it is used as dreams are to influence the spirit world. Also, where trance exists we find the greatest variety of dreams reported. This feeling of an all-encompassing experience that opens the world to the shaman has some similarity to that reported by many people who experience LSD and peyote.

TABLE I Relation of Trance to Use of Dreams to Seek and Control Supernatural Powers

	Total		*Trance Present*		*Total*		*Trance Absent*		*Total*	
	No.	*%*	*Trance*	*Trance/Possession Trance*	*No.*	*%*	*Possession Trance*	*0*	*No.*	*%*
	54	100			37	100			17	100
	28	52	Paiute a,b,c,d	Semang a,b,c,d	23	62	Ifugao c	Cuna a,b,c	5	29
			Comanche a,b,c,d	Iroquois a,b,c,d			Wolof b			
Use			Crow a,b,c,d	Jivaro a,b,c,d			Nyakyusa b			
of			Ojibwa a,b,c,d	Pukapukans a,b,c			Bemba b			
Dreams			Omaha a,b,c,d	Copper Eskimo a,b,c						
Present			Papago a,b,c,d	Rwala b,d						
			Kaska a,c,d,	Yaruro b,d						
			Chukchee a,b	Kapauku a,b						
			Lapps a,b	Yakut d						
			Mundurucu a	Araucanians b						
			Trobriands c	Azande d						
			Fang a							
	26	48	Karen	Yoruba	14	38	Kurtatchi	Aymara	12	71
			Callinago	Mataco			Ganda	Min Chia		
Use			Riffians	Burmese			Tanala	Mossi (Yatenda)		
of			Iban	Lepcha			Bhil	Tallensi		
Dreams			Tupinambe	Thai			Samoans	Tiv		
Absent				Somali				Nama		
				Ifaluk				Siriono		
				Marquesas						
				Ashanti						

$X^2 = 4.97$ $P < .05$

Altered States of Consciousness 419

Fig. 3.1 Table 1 of trance use in seeking to control supernatural powers from Bourguignon. Reprinted with permission by Schenkman Publishing Company, Inc.

Bourguignon (1972) also notes associations in comparing her data with that of Textor (1967). Trance societies are more likely than those with possession trance to be: (1) found in North America, be migratory or semi-nomadic, smaller populations, and no jurisdictional hierarchy beyond the local level. They also tend to lack stratification and slaves, kinship cognatic, marriage unlikely to have any form of bride price, segregation of young boys absent, nuclear family typical, as in monogamy. (2) Societies with possession trance tend to be greater in scale and in social complexity. Those with both trance and possession trance are intermediate between these two in clusters of traits. In general, Bourguignon's sample represents ideological concepts of the utility of dreams and trance in effective communication with supernaturals. Since in possession trance (and to an extent trance in general), it takes on a public performance in an interaction of the individual and spirits or via an impersonation of spirits or other supernaturals that can be questioned or used as sources of action and power in this life. However, Bourguignon (1972) notes that in much of trance behavior, the ideology of religion argues that the performer does not recall the experience that others hear and see. We have to keep in mind that what is shared, especially with a stranger, scientist, or physician, may be edited and is a sample of what the individual desires to reveal or the culture allows. Tedlock (1987) describes this limitation for the Zuni and Hopi.

What the shaman or seer encounters, often in a personal language of his or her spirit guide, is recalled by the audience and is related back to the performer, who then interprets it—except in some cases where there are other specialists, as among the Pomo, who interpret the journey of the traveling shaman and concoct a cure from it. One can see that in the paradigm of Assagioli, where there are different kinds or levels of unconsciousness that is drawn on in dreams, the complications can be very complex. For Assagioli too, the other major complication to interpreting dreams and visions (hallucinations, etc.) is the "forgotten language of dreams" (Parfitt 2003). To some shamans, as in the Punan Dyaks, "the language of before being born and after dying" is partially available in travel of trance or in some cultures, through the spirit guide (Blair and Blair 1988).

The vehicle for the trance performance and supernatural journey can be deprivation; self-abuse, peyote, or any other drug that a people have found creates the necessary link to the spirit world. Whether the shaman takes the vehicle alone, with a guide, or the entire audience varies by group, task, and individual. For the Warao of Venezuela, the *baharnarotu* shamans used tobacco in hallucinogenic amounts (and the species of tobacco is significant here). By use of tobacco they were able to "travel in trance to the "banana-spirit realms in the eastern cosmic vault, and to feed with smoke the *kanabo* (ancestral spirits) and the *hoarotu* (spirits of the dead shamans), or to initiate new *hoarotu* into shamanhood" (La Barre 1975; Wilbert 1972). One wonders how the Warao developed the narrative and imagery of the "banana-spirit realms" from their experiences with tobacco. How did the physiological reaction with the drug produce the key to this journey? For someone who has only smoked tobacco a few times and was made sick from it (coughing fits, etc.) its seems strange, yet the effect of different species of tobacco and whether it is ingested or smoked and the amount can have varied effects, as can the experience of "sickness."

For the people of the Native American Gulf Coast, they brewed a stimulant and emetic, Black Drink, from *Ilex vomitoria* (*I. cassine* and *I. yaupon*) and some mixed it with tobacco for purification rites or initiation ceremonies. Caffeine is considered to be the main component (Hudson 1979). Such purification rites sometimes bring on vomiting, as does peyote. Visions then occur or hallucinations are expected of certain types.

The presence of a reality that is invisible to an audience is a central part of the communication of the shaman or priest in performing trance. Yet this reality often seems similar to aspects of pathological passages of individual patients, as Grof (1976, 217–8) describes for Otto. Otto experiences his hands becoming those of his father and this perception Grof turns into an interpretation, albeit suggested by Otto, of homosexuality or self-stimulation. But Grof also refers to the missing father and possessive mother and his hands become a surrogate for the father in contact with the mother. The background that the patient is living with, his father dying and his mother using him as a substitute in a rather sexual and incestuous manner, presents a number of scenarios. In Grof's description it seems simple and clear. However, in other cases, for example, one

I watched unfold in 1966 was unclear and confused on the surface, but clearly interpreted by authorities. A student in the men's dorm at the time at San Francisco State set his hands on fire one evening. He was heard shouting in his dorm room and then he came out of the room and broke into a run down the corridor. Most students were shocked at what they saw, but since individual students came out of their rooms at different moments of the event, they had different experiences, somewhat like a Rosamon Effect. What I saw, since I had just left the central bathroom at the time he was shouting and I had stopped to see what was happening, was a man coming out of a room with his hands on fire and running toward me. His face was distorted in terror, yet some who saw it thought he was laughing, and others, crying.

We later found out that his father had been a psychiatrist who had attempted to stop his son's masturbation. The student had told the police and a nurse that his father had told him as a child that if he masturbated worms would come to eat his penis and his hands. He apparently hallucinated such a thing happening and had splashed lighter fluid on his hands and set them on fire to kill the worms. The resident assistant later filled in a bit of information from the police, that it seemed he had done this several times at other schools before being suspended. This event struck me as very significant, as the student was experiencing an alternative reality that came and went depending upon his behavior. One might say he was possessed by an entity that caused him to initiate the burning sequence, but one wondered if his father appeared in it as well. What the students in the hall experienced was a performance of an alternative reality of someone else, but it impinged on theirs. I thought this was clearly similar to people having other kinds of visions and hallucinations that were not so personal, but instead, could be interpreted in a wider sense, like the Salem Witch Trials, or visions during plagues, as in the Black Plague, that cause people to kill someone or animals that appear in an affected individual's altered reality.

In some of these otherworldly adventures or journeys, we find similarities in the spirit guides (or animal familiars, see de Rios, 1984) of many cultures, where the individual meets with a familiar spirit, parent, lover, friend, and so on or a friendly demon who gives meaning to their life after a tremendously strange introduction of being lost. In some of these we find motifs similar to preserved literature, as in Dante's visit to the underworld led by Virgil, or that by Ulysses, or Gilgamesh. The recognition of the spirit guide has also its own literature among various peoples. The key is sometimes simply to search for a cure, or answer to life's crises, but in some we find the spirit passing from death to a vague landscape where a thread must be found to achieve a new life either among the happy souls, or return to their old life or some less valuable place. In a number where reincarnation is established, the soul, as among the Punan Dyaks, exists in a world after living and before being born, where a different language is present and the soul must arrive at some clarity or task to recognize rebirth. Though my description here is pieced together from several examples, I can cite none to be exact. John Lilly (1972) gives a description of guides of this type in his book *The Center of the Cyclone*. Other subjects report alien worlds of fantastic or incomprehensible nature. A few people related to me that they thought they "caught" waves of transmissions of such worlds as if watching TV; only in one case they had entered the "band" of transmission and interacted as if in a world millions of years old and billions of light years away. One wonders on hearing such reports if sensory variations do not produce the creativity of science fiction, or that dreams are refuse of embedded experience in the histones of our DNA mixed with a variety of complications in our hippocampus; similar to a theory proposed by McKenna (1993).

Grof describes the experience of some people on LSD, which parallels those of trance participants who leave reality and describe worlds of no known explanation. Usually there are some cultural contexts for the shaman in trance, patterned by the fact that shamans often are from families or learn their passage techniques from older shamans (Eliade 1964). Grof (1976, 194) argues that these experiences take the "form" of patterns reported by historians or anthropologists in different cultures. Grof (1976, 202–3, e.g., on Tantric practices) often describes subjects' responses using the term "naïve," with the implication that the person has no prior knowledge of the cultural pattern he or she describes, and Grof makes it appear as if the subject is reproducing the description for the first time from endogenous biochemical responses. Cross-cultural interpretations are of interest here, as I will describe later in this book, where a Yaqui Native American applies his cultural context to young Americans using a drug his people have long developed means of interpreting its effects is a substantial cross-cultural intervention.

When we come to discuss the variety of dreams and trance in a later section we must still consider the problem of desire and susceptibility. Some people are said to be susceptible to visual hallucinations and others to hypnosis (Naish 2013), but why—what are the factors that cause this susceptibility? Is it related to da Silva's (2013) continuum? Naish (2013) notes that there is a correlation between hypnotic susceptibility and schizophrenia, though some researchers argue that hypnosis is really a form of suggestibility and compliance that are so heavily conditioned in many people (Wagstaff 1981). I think the nature of hallucination, delusion, and vision is complicated by the individual experience and the difficulty of convincing someone that what they perceive is not real. My experience, and what I saw at the two hospitals as well as in the Mogar Lab, gives rise to the conviction that while drugs like LSD are operating in the individual, while the pathological conditions are functioning, and while belief is embedded in a person's character armor, there is little hope of a transformation back to normality (real experience), a point brought up at the Napa Symposium in 1961. This contention might seem contradictory to what I have said of the work of psychological practitioners and the ad hoc trained people like the Psychedelic Rangers. However, in my experience, these interventions functioned to calm a person and distract them long enough for the drugs to subside. One might compare this to Leary's findings in the Kaiser Clinic (Leary and Barron 1955) that people who waited compared to those treated turned out with the same statistical outcomes. But again, while LSD may not be a panacea for all human pathology, the experimental models have differed so much, and the street LSD is so uncertain in content that our knowledge of its effect is still superficial.

Both dreams and trance are utilized in different cultural contexts to achieve contact with the supernatural; thus, individuals develop, discover, or learn methods to accomplish this as usually a culturally defined process. They can prepare for the experience. In some cases a supernatural being may attack them and seize some aspect of their life or consciousness and generally establish some kind of relationship with the dreamer/trance traveler (Wallace 1958). To some extent this may not be desired and the chosen one may attempt to escape the relationship or task, which is why Henning (1951) considered arguments of Zoroaster and figures like Christ to be shamans, as they reflected typical healing exercises, interpretation of illness and dreams, and each attempted to escape his destiny, though in different ways. But the central question of both involuntary election and possession or nightmare is the lack of desire of the individual to be involved. The nature of nightmares may have psychopathological origins as Kleitman (1963) suggested, but the main fact is that they appear to be uninvited and generally indicate that the individual would not have them, if possible, though aspects of guilt and repression are certainly present in some cases.

But to many in the "oceanic" mode, a friendly, positive, and pleasurable world is all that exists; to Grof, this is due to the re-experience or a combination of drugs and fetal experience of the womb in the initial perinatal state. And Grof emphasizes the general perceptions of many of his volunteers and colleagues who were physicians, as quite parallel to those of schizophrenics, and he also equates the LSD experiences to those of shamans and mystics (Grof 1976, 110). In both cases, he argues the intrauterine experience makes for the foundation of both, negative schizophrenic-like and positive LSD-like. In some schizophrenics, like Julie in Laing's (1959, 199) discussion of the performance of selves in hallucinations, several "partial assemblies" of selves can interact with each other, one ordering the other to perform some task. One might suggest that this appearance and temporary persistence of a "self-hallucination" in such a schizophrenic can be related to the "ability" of some people to call up lucid dreaming states, control them, and have them persist for several episodes. This might be another reason why lucid dreaming might be dangerous either to cultivate or to provoke in the susceptible individual (Vallat and Ruby 2019).

This brings up an interesting phenomenological question on the relation of schizophrenia to lucid dreaming. Mota et al. (2016) found that psychosis enhances the experience of internal reality in detriment of external reality by use of lucid dreaming. They argue that lucid dreaming may further empower deliria and hallucinations, "giving internal reality the appearance of external reality." Other researchers, like Aviram and Soffer-Dudek (2018), found that the intensity of lucid dreaming and the techniques to induce it were associated with psychopathology, but not frequency. It seems that the main difference between schizophrenia and normal individuals who use lucid dreaming is exit access. Most schizophrenics, as reported by clinicians like Laing, are trapped in a version of internal reality similar to the lucid dream. One might relate this to Chalmers' ideas or even Seth's. A recent study of a large database of dreams and psychedelic drugs found a significant similarity with dreams in general in normal dreamers, and an association of LSD with the kind of dreaming intensity of lucid dreamers, and least similarity with the use of *datura* (Sanz et al. 2018).

While persona of the schizophrenic can order actions on other persona, being able to exit the reality at will seems lost to them. In a study of over 690 administrations of LSD, Chandler and Hartman (1960) noted that there was no evidence of impairment of the major ego functions, people were able to dive deeper into analysis or experiences and then extract themselves, either by consciously changing the scene or meaning or by focusing attention on some aspect that changes. What I noted in sessions was that the scene often "morphed" into something else. Here one could say that this was a conscious effort, but then the idea of the scene changing without "intention" would be the same outcome, but the question of volition remains. If, as Seth (2021) argues, our reality is a continuous stream of hallucinations, what happens when the stream stops? Nirvana? Or psychosis? But "no exit" as Grof (1976, 120) describes it emanating from experiences of dissatisfaction with life, depression, a failure to find meaning, are often associated with a creative phase. But for Huxley (1954) creativity can also be on the cusp of insanity.

Grof argues that the realization of the Buddha of the Four Passing Sights creates the releasing experience of meaning and understanding. Thus, one can conclude that from depression, anomie, or chaos comes an opening and end of the "no exit" lock. Some might call this a cure, as in the condition of the woman I describe who under LSD realizes that the figure of her nightmare is that of her injured father. She no longer has the dream, no longer wakes in the night screaming (good for the people she lives with) and feels relieved. However, often the realization is incomplete—the result not a cure for no exit, but immediately is followed by a new block. This was clear in a number of cases of people who married and were unhappy with their arrangement, ending the marriage via forms of therapy, which to the clinician seemed to be a solution, only resulting in a new relationship, a new infatuation, loss of familiarity, and depression. This seemed to be part of the initial response of a man I knew who one night jumped from the Golden Gate Bridge. He had been depressed, drunk, and supremely unhappy with who he was and life in general. Like Buddha he was intelligent, but could find no meaning in life, no feeling that could anchor him to relationships, pleasures, or goals. He had lived a very conservative life, and then moved to San Francisco, when his realizations of religion and ideologies failed to mask a hunger for truth. In San Francisco he tried drugs, alcohol, and sex (all kinds, including homosexual) but all left him empty. Finally, he jumped and survived. I spoke with him about his experience and why he now continued to live among people who had dissatisfied him and led him, as everything else in his life, to suicide. His answer was that the experience was so intense that it had taken his experience to a higher level of reality. In the moments before he hit the water, the feelings were the most uncommon and strange and he felt he had passed through worlds and beings that existed on planes that were hidden otherwise. Soon after he jumped again, and I never saw him after that. Did he jump into another world?

I have no idea if he really jumped twice; I was told by other people he had, one who had been at his first attempt and had called authorities. He apparently had gone to the hospital. Some have survived, like Kevin Hines, and say they regretted the jump the moment they left the bridge (Hines 2013). The fatality rate of people who jump from the Golden Gate Bridge is purported to be 98%, and there are an estimated 1700+ who are believed to have done it and a couple who are documented "double jumpers"; the statistics are shaky. No one knows how many have jumped. Cameras were installed in recent years but there is no way of knowing how many jumped before. In 2020 more than 30 people were known to have jumped and survived. In 1988 Sara R. Birnbaum at age 18 jumped a second time and is thought to have died. When pulled from the water the first time she was sobbing. Friends said she was disappointed at not being accepted to Stanford University and had had trouble as a student at UCLA. No matter what the motives of people, or the psychological condition that drives them to the act of suicide, it is an old means of release from the cares of the world.

In many cultures the choice of a person to end it is considered a personal decision, in America today it is largely seen as a sign of illness, though in some cases, as in cancer, a form of suicide is gaining acceptance, euthanasia. Rising rates of suicide are concerning to most people and efforts are spent to find means of understanding and reducing its frequency (Goldsmith et al. 2002). But Grof associates this theme also with the fear of engulfment and the birth experience. The appearance of monsters and entities to destroy a person seems similar to the idea Carl Sagan presents of a mammalian ancestral memory of dinosaurs (Sagan 1977, 151), and quotes a passage from Darwin suggesting a primeval origin for children's dreams. Such notions are interesting and grab attention when presented, but I think lack any rigorous scientific underpinning. These "monsters" have been interpreted by some people as omens or representations of conflict, as with the Mae Enga of New Guinea, where a child's dream represents the male child's struggle with the father for family estates with the help of the mother in the dream. The demon (father) is killed and the son and mother live happily ever after (Meggitt 1962).

Sagan (1977) also cites experimental research that seems to suggest that the left hemisphere of the neocortex is suppressed during sleep, allowing the right hemisphere to gain ascendance, whose insights Fromm (1951) called "the forgotten language." Sagan argues that in dreams people usually experience a kind of "watcher" or eye of normal consciousness, as Humphrey (1986) calls it, or perhaps a viewer of the self as if seeing the dream action from afar. But Darwin links dreams in most animals to the effect of daily impressions, and notes that this can be seen in their movements and sounds when asleep. He also thought that unclear impressions of experience could be the origin of superstitions in vague images remembered as dreams (Darwin 1871, 72–3).

Fromm's (1951, vi) approach, however, is a universalist one; he argues that there is one "forgotten" dream language or secret code. One might think that this could be equated with Freud's theory of ego, superego, and id via repression as a road to untangling the life history of an individual's adaptations. Fromm seems to allow for local adaptations, that there are dialects of this symbolic secret language due apparently to "differences in natural conditions" based on experience, as when fire can be beneficial (produces warmth) or destructive (forest fires). Fromm (1951) also contrasts the cultural influences, especially logic, from the contradictions in life. There is a pathway to understanding the illogic of dreams; they are attempts to create a bridge from the expected and culturally logical values and the real behavior of people, a bridge that reflects the confusion created by that contradiction. Yet Fromm asserts that the dream can be an expression of the lowest and most irrational as well as the highest and most "valuable functions of our minds."

One could also see Grof's system of the perinatal matrices I–IV or his COEX classification as a universal method. Yet in both of these, the "language" is individual in expression. A beginning assertion of Fromm's is that we are the author of our dreams and that they are our dreams, that is, of our invention. He argues for a universal set of symbols to his code and an accidental one that is unique to a person, place, experience prior to sleep. This makes his examination of dreams quite modern and a bit clinical, as he is immediately creating a distinction from the dreams of antiquity or ethnographic dreams, that dreams can be created in other worlds, and that they can be communications or journeys that we experience at the hands or bidding of other beings. However, Fromm's (1951) distinction between universal and accidental is parallel to other systems, especially some ethnographic examples, as in the Zinacantecans. However, there is also the possibility that people sometimes believe in the absolute veracity and originality of their ideas as if seeing them "written on the wall" by a god or spirit, specially this may be true of some pathological conditions, as in extreme cases of egoists, where they attribute their ideas to hallucinations, dreams, or visions, thus often giving them a form of sanction related to religion or ancestors.

I think that people do experience a lack of borders on LSD, and to some the idea that they have lost the self, but generally, and in my experience as I have noted, this is only a temporary sensation. I am unconvinced in the stages of gestation and their relation to the LSD experience that Grof has produced. He calls this "cosmic engulfment," and makes it into a typical feature of the LSD experience, which I think is forced, and that in many instances the issue of engulfment or borderlessness is more individual and situational, what is happening to this person, in this place given their history and the impresses they receive from the milieu. The description Allan Watts gives (Stevens 1988) is of being stripped of his attachments, job, status, and so on to a nakedness of humanity. This is also something other people have reported to me. In fact, a tense moment appears in the 1961 tape (Napa State Hospital Symposium) where Abramson objects to the rigid patterning of a spiritual nature described by some of the clinicians.

The idea of individual set nature and LSD experience was discovered by Mogar and Savage (1964). They found that "the nature, magnitude and stability of post-LSD changes were related to personality variables and modal defense patterns." This is why they came to have us administer MMPI tests to prospective subjects; the data indicated that subjects with "well-defined but flexible self-structure responded most favorably to the drug, while those with either underdeveloped or overtly rigid ego defenses responded least favorably." In Mogar's interpretation this finding was often found in the distinction between creative processes and psychotic states (Mogar 1965b, 404). There were other methods, for example, Huxley's friend Al Hubbard used Carbogen gas as a test procedure. The gas is a combination of oxygen (usually about 95–98%) and carbon dioxide. It has come to be used in cancer treatments to potentiate the production of oxygen radicals during radiation therapy. However, it achieves its effect by a drastic increase in blood acidity and the resulting changes in brain chemistry. While its inventor, L.J. Meduna (1950), claimed his patients had mainly positive experiences, many therapists using it have found it can produce "horrifying experiences beyond description" (Wellington et al. 2021). It is claimed to produce euphoria and Hubbard is cited as examining people intoxicated with the gas to ascertain if they would be stable subjects for psychedelics (Stevens 1988). I never heard of people using it at all in the 1960s or 1970s.

Many stories and dreams come to represent explanations for the status quo or revolutions. The Adam and Eve story in the Bible explains the subjugation of women in the Judeo-Christian-Islamic tradition. Dreams and visions of prophets and seers give legitimacy to changes in government or tradition or justify a war or starting a battle. From the dream world come communications of the ancestors or gods, which can bring healing skills or power (Elide 1964). To Luther the appearance of the Popes as the Anti-Christ in his dreams was a verification of his own analysis of the corruption of the Papacy and his visitations with angels, who drove him on, though his father asked him how to tell angels from devils.

To many who experienced it, evil and pain are foreign and non-existent (as Grof also described for his subjects, 1976, 107). It seems to me this is a confusion of the simple lack of regularity in perception they experienced and not a temporary mimic or "induced" state of schizophrenia. This led some to argue that the oceanic and friendly perception reflected the "Blank Slate" idea of human nature. In a recent book journalist Michael Pollan (2018) makes the same argument I often heard in Mogar's Lab and on the streets of the Haight-Ashbury in the 1960s, that LSD could erase the conditioning of civilization and open mankind to a new age of creativity and love. In a way this view holds that all evil and pain are external to human nature, all that is needed is some cleansing process. This is a very primitive concept, one that is typical in most religions. The dogma of Original Sin was a means of theologians to separate the responsibility for sin from god. Adam was pure, but Eve and Adam sinned and that sin is passed to every human born. Of course, what is missing in logic is that we learn that the prohibition to eat from the tree of knowledge is made before the creation of Eve, so it was Adam's prohibition not hers. The other problem is if humans were created pure, then how could they come to sin? What purpose could it have to make creatures you fashion so weak they violate laws? It appears only for the nature of the game between Yahweh and Lucifer. But these ideas of purity and danger, pollution, taboo, and sacrifice vary across cultures for a variety of social organizations to act as boundary markers and discipline measures, as Mary Douglas describes (1966).

Grof (1976) equates the oceanic experience with Walter Pahnke's mystical categories, mainly Category One: Unity (Pahnke 1963, 128). Pahnke had done his thesis work at Harvard in the late 1950s and early 1960s. He had studied the effects of psychedelics on different subjects. Pahnke found a continuum of mystical experiences, of which unity was the first often encountered. Others ranged from Unity as Category I, Category II: Transcendence of Time and Space, Category III: Deeply Felt Positive Mood, Category IV: Sense of Sacredness, Category V: Objectivity and Reality, Category VI: Paradoxically, Category VII: Alleged Ineffability, Category VIII: Transiency, and Category IX: Persisting Positive Changes in Attitude and Behavior. The lack of discrete limits was notable, and these categories, though I only became aware of them in 2020, are quite similar to the states or transitions of subjects I was familiar with and my own experiences. Pahnke's work included follow-up testing and interviews over a six-month period. Pahnke had received his MD from Harvard Medical School in 1956 and began study at the Harvard Divinity School, where his doctoral advisors were Timothy Leary and Ram Dass (Richard Alpert). He organized his research also to include the Good Friday Experiment (aka the Marsh Chapel Experiment). In this experiment students were divided into those receiving 10 mg of psilocybin and those receiving niacin as an active placebo. He reported that 90% of the psilocybin-receiving students had significant religious experiences, while only 10% of those receiving placebo did. A restudy undertaken by Rick Doblin in 1991 found no difference (Doblin 1991). Doblin has continued this research to the present, concentrating his work on mainly supplementing various routine therapies with the drug MDMA (Jacobs 2021). It is also known as "Ecstasy" and belongs in the group of entactogens (or empathogens, for the distinctive emotional and social effects they elicit) described by Ralph Metzner and David Nichols independently in 1982–1983 and includes other phenethylamine-related substances (Metzner et al. 2001; Nichols et al. 1993).

MDMA is called Ecstasy for its pleasurable effect, but it also induces a considerable sombulence or hypnotic effect and few if any visions or hallucinations (Olson 2021), though the phosphene threshold is reduced significantly more in users than in controls (Oliveri and Calvo 2003). Jacobs also is the founder and executive director of the Multidisciplinary Association for Psychedelic Studies (MAPS).

Pahnke (1963) administered LSD, psilocybin, and mescaline to subjects and studied the similarities and differences in their experiences with those of religious practitioners. He was both a physician and a priest. He claimed never to have taken any of the drugs before or during the study. The main finding of his study was in the significant difference of those who took psilocybin and experienced mystic consequences than those who did not. This was a difference in what Pahnke defined as "sacredness." However, those taking the other drugs did experience more instances of sacredness than did controls. This choice of word is unfortunate, as the experience is often related to "peak experience" and can be associated with everything from beauty to satisfaction in realization of non-spiritual existence, as noted by Maslow.

Grof also utilized Maslow's "Peak Experiences" as a reference (Maslow 1961, 1964). To Maslow such experiences are a paradox of development of the self and identity (Maslow 1962), as they tend to cause a transformation in the nature of the individual's identity. For Maslow, these experiences are not unique to religious dogma or orientation, but instead appear to be elicited by recognition of states of "perfection." A famous religious experience of this kind was that of Jacok Boehme, who in 1600 looked into a beam of light as it was reflected in a pewter dish and the nature of the universe and god's relation to man was revealed to him. He wrote of this in a book, *The Rising of Dawn*, later titled *Aurora.* But such experiences are rather common. This can be music, art, nature, or a general feeling of belonging and unity, what some have called, communitas. Maslow (1964) addresses the contradiction of such experiences, as in when one hears "inner voices" (see George Bernard Shaw's Saint Joan and our discussion of auditory hallucinations), sees visions, or experiences sensory events that others do not. These are upsetting to the homeostasis of the integrity of the individual's consciousness and yet they are also seen, not just in psychology, but also in primitive society and religious life in general, as necessary steps in achieving self-actualization and communion with the sacred. This is complicated by the fact that there is a great deal of variation in defining such experiences. But a related problem is the tendency, noted by Maslow (1964), for people to think in terms of black and white, either/or, and polarizing experience of a dichotomizing nature. I would call this the "Aristotlilization" of human thought. Aristotle described experience in this way and it has been one of the key elements in describing human cognition ever since (Bickerton 1990).

The main thesis of Maslow's 1964 book was to attempt to stanch the tendency of people to "bureaucratize" religious experience. This is perhaps what has happened with the LSD experience and other avenues to paranormal perception. Many have tried to so define the way people undergo the chemistry of the drug that the indescribable becomes so rigidly charted that the only authentic experience one can have is one that has been defined. To this point, Maslow states,

> Organized Religion, the churches, finally may become the major enemies of the religious experience and the religious experiencer. (Maslow 1964, Preface)

Maslow (1964) finds that there is a continuum of personal type and peak experience—one where the person comes to be completely absorbed in the event and focuses entirely on his or her own personal interpretation to the rejection of the world, to a "self-absorbed and inwardly searching" life, whether monastic, hermit, or ascetic. This can be turned outward, where the person attempts to explain, share, or even convert others to their own experience and its meaning. Here the division between insight, obsession, and pathology lies. Then, to Maslow, the failure of others to "see" what the seer has experienced as an all-powerful vision of reality or meaning of life can degenerate into rejection, separation, violence, and murder in the name of the "higher insight." The obverse of this is the possession of the vision, its protection from others, the embellishment of the secret against its dilution among others. But Maslow comes to a conclusion that these flights to the exotic, whether personal or secret, are escapes from the true sacred that is to be found in the ordinary, and he defines this as one's community, daily life, neighborhood. He thinks that in the search for the miraculous and miracles, people overlook the ancient feeling of social pleasure Robertson Smith (1894) talks about at the root of religion. Maslow also accepts Grof's negative "trips" as a wider case of human visions and hallucinations; he calls it the "nadir experience" as opposed to the "peak experience." And he recognizes a category that is mid-range between, the "plateau experience," that is less sacralized and more cognitive but still contains an element of the unitary, or oceanic. It can be seen as a "cognitive blissfulness" with a milieu of "casualness." He describes the two as often associated with age—younger people experiencing the peak type and having rebirth as an element, while older individuals feel pure enjoyment and happiness. I cannot agree with this distinction about age, as I have seen young people have both peak and plateau experiences as well as the nadir type. I have been around people in their 30s who were on LSD, and read and heard descriptions of older people, as in Tim Leary and Ram Doss' cases, as well as some older individuals in more recent reports. In general, though, I do think Maslow

(1964) is right in the case of older individuals. Ultimately, Maslow is motivated to undertake writing his book by the need he sees to counter both popular ideas on drug use and being "turned on" as both a hedonistic means and a shortcut to enlightenment, as well as how he sees both religion and philosophy (especially Existentialism) negating positive roles in human biology and "specieshood." Maslow posits a transcendent "project" for humanity, an empirical and "holistic" making of himself. He considered Freud "at his poorest with all the questions of transcendence."

Transcendence was a problem for Freud; he states that he felt that the mass of the people do not appreciate "what is of true value in life" (Freud 1962, 11) but he reflects on this in his book *The Future of An Illusion*, which was on religion, that he had overlooked "how variegated" human mental life was. He speaks of the feeling of eternity, of limitlessness and an "oceanic" perception as of value, but lacking the experience himself, it gives rise to analysis, which was his means of determining the world. Here the achievement of detachment from the mother and the world is interpreted by Freud as normal; any return to a loss of ego would then seem to be a regression. But instead he argues that this feeling would seem to be a preserved part of ego development, of a period of positive early life, and that since nothing can be lost in his view of mental ontogeny and aging, then the existence of the "oceanic" feeling is retained. Thus, reflections on this feeling in later life are a means of satisfying the ego, of consolation, and could develop into foundations of religious feeling. This would certainly be consistent with ideas of religion expressed by Durkheim (1915) and Robertson Smith as extensions of individuals as group feelings of, as Freud put it, "oneness with the universe" (Freud 1962, 19).

Thus. Freud is not dichotomizing transcendence from an objective scientific view; rather, he is using an ontological approach, saying perceptions differ as we develop or age, and this would be the same in looking at cultural differences in structuring reality. If people perceive of "supranormal" experience, of hidden worlds and spirits and ghosts, these perceptions have something to do with their ontogeny and enculturation. The descriptions Lohmann (2019) reproduces from Oceania, the "haunting" of people by "other-than-human-persons," are similar to those reported from the same area by Codrington (1891), or by Anderson (2005) for Iceland. But generally, by ingesting a drug that gives the individual, especially during initiation, an insight or journey into the central core of a cultural milieu and its symbols, the individual emerges reborn, his values demonstrated by the ancestors or spirits (Furst 1972).

A long tradition of communication with spirits would "cue" people to the feelings that initiate such experiences. For the Icelanders Anderson studied, the dead do not leave the presence of their living relatives after they die, but may linger for various periods. Their spectral appearance is generally considered to be benign and at times comforting. Their arrival is often described as bringing love or to help erase tension or grief and give purpose. These apparitions are often regarded also as guardian spirits or angels that also come in dreams and speak to the dreamer. One might speculate about the environmental history of the Icelanders and the seeing of apparitions. Not all are positive, certainly not in dreams. For example, there is Olaf's dream from the *Laxdaela Saga* by an unknown author about 1245 CE. Olaf has a dream of retribution where his own son will die in payment by a woman who appears in his dream. It is probably an early example of a hypnopompic hallucination, as she lingers before him as he awakes.

Obviously the landscape of Iceland is consistent with the generally bleak and monotonous ones reported by some of Zubek's (1969) researchers. The history of sparse population and isolated farms and fishing settlements might be contexts to promote the sensory conditions creating hallucinations. There is also a cultural foundation for such beings in Sami and Norse history that Anderson considers of some importance. It is also a type of "bereavement hallucination," a type of experience where people feel the presence of a dead person. The definition of the type is quite diverse and, like that for hallucinations in general, it is difficult to define or produce categories (Ratcliffe 2020).

Maslow (1964) produces his own dichotomizing in his contrast of religion and science, of superstition or religious experience and plain empiricism. He argues that the latter, defined as either science or empiricism, creates the danger of relativism or nihilism and equates such a view with Nazi or communist scientists who would come to work for Americans. This is not the expression of an amoral or nihilistic attitude but one of survival choices, and the system that would use such men and women, capitalism, is the ideology in history, which has the fewest scruples or moral principles. Capitalism is successful, primarily, because it has abandoned the collective and given the individual free reign to exploit god, man, animal, plant, and planet to the nth degree. Traditions of sustainability have been the enemy of capitalist and communist development (as in the USSR) (see Caldararo 2014). Even laws are a questionable limitation to free trade, whether they be tariffs or prohibitions on certain products or services.

My problem with attitude is its inherent progressivism in the case of both Maslow and Freud. Is there a goal for humanity? Is there one for bacteria or elephants? The anthropocentric nature of such arguments undermines Maslow's otherwise empirical and "holistic" approach. In a more contemporary context, and as opposed to a progressive trend, we can view these responses to possession, feeling of presences, and hearing voices in a uniformitarian fashion. If we see human consciousness as a social adaptation as I have argued, then what we see in the ethnographic record reflects aspects of this adaptation. Also, we have seen it in many religious movements of the last two centuries, especially among the evangelical movement. The manner in which the human capacity for perceiving the world in hallucinations, visions, and voices and the presences of other beings can be enhanced and modified by social training, as Luhrmann (2012) found among some religious sects. In her book *When God Talks Back*, she reports on techniques where people are taught to visualize the presence and voice of god, and in concert with others this becomes amplified. While political uses of such approaches to human response have taken place, certainly the cults of personality of the last century provide a laboratory for them. Albert Speer and Leni Riefenstahl have left a certain record of their development in one instance (Speer 1970). It is chilling to imagine how such a process could be unleashed on the world with today's technology and the internet. Robin Fox's book *The Violent Imagination* argues that our creativity may be the source of humanity's ultimate destruction. This is certainly not an original prediction, as H.G. Wells wrote in his *Outline of History* in 1922 that all history has been a race between education and catastrophe. In his review of Fox's book, Ashley Montagu (1989) suggests that our ability to create and to be devoid of most instinct has led to a consciousness that is capable of folly, an ability that abuses our educability so that we can be taught what is sound and unsound, true as false and without the capacity to distinguish them.

A stage of "testing" may appear where the community questions the validity of the experience, as in the case of Luther, Christ, or Mohammed. Luther's father questions whether his vision is an angel or a devil (Bainton 1955, 32), as his choice of profession as a priest means he disobeys his father and abandons the family. This question reverberates, however, in Luther's life, where doubt and certainty balance a tortured idea of self-righteous power. In Maslow's (1962, 1964) view, however, the self-actualized person is most likely to produce social change and engage in social experimentation. I am not sure this is true, but qualifying its "most likely" is perhaps correct, as I think that many self-actualized people can also be the most effective exploiters and regressive, destructive people and leaders. It depends on how they view themselves as "self-actualized" and how they use or if they want power as an expression of their "actualization." Maslow identifies the self-actualized person with social improvement, or as he puts it, being a "helper" to others, in terms of social facilitation and the "bodhisattvic path." He also equates "normative zeal" with scientific objectivity to form a "higher form of objectivity," the Taoistic.

Maslow rewrote the 1964 text for the 1970 republication as a new edition. In it he redefines some of his attitudes toward human nature. Where he had placed primary emphasis on the individual experience in 1964, in 1970 he somewhat reversed himself, shifting focus on the role of the community as the only real and effective vehicle for actualization. In this process, he is aware that this outcome depends on the nature of the community as well as the limits of human nature—that is, how well, he asks, a human nature does society permit? A better question, I think, is what is good for the individual and society. This is a question at the crux of the human debate on the nature of man and society. There have been a vast number of theories on good and the good society, from the Pythagoreans and Plato to Lenin, St. Augustine, Confucius and Buddha, and Hitler. It is obviously an area of research that requires more investigation.

Boksa (2009) finds that survey studies in various countries indicate that 7–30% of children and adolescents report experiencing hallucinations. One complication is the perception of voices versus noise or tinnitus. Distinctions between forms of tinnitus as reported by patients vary considerably, from humming, hissing, and other "white noise" only heard by the patient to sounds audible to others. The demarcation between what is called objective tinnitus, which includes such types of "noise," and auditory hallucinations is subjective. Usually it is said that auditory hallucinations are associated with psychiatric illness, but this is not accepted by all researchers (Traynor 2018). Nam (2005) found clear distinctions of test results from the examination of patients with tinnitus and those suffering from auditory hallucinations by hearing tests and auditory brainstem responses (ABR).

Hallucinations are reported in alcohol abuse as delirium tremens (Junghanns and Wetterling 2017); they appear in borderline personality disorder, which could last for extended periods (Yee et al. 2005), also as delirium in some organic disease, in Alzheimer's disease (mostly visual), patients with Lewy body dementia, and Parkinson's disease (PD; often reported also visual and sometimes tactile). But not all patients with these conditions report hallucinations. REM behavioral disorder has been seen to be a harbinger of Parkinson's disease, and a behavioral paradigm developed from studying patients with dementia with Lewy bodies and PD proposes damage or interference of the resting state of the brain, the default mode network, where people often seem to be thinking or "mind wandering," in a self-referencing state. I have mentioned before that psychedelics, including LSD, psilocybin, and ayahuasca, have been found to affect this network, apparently by reducing activity (Virdi 2020). This then results in false images that are uncontrollable (Lewis et al. 2015; Phillips et al. 2021). An additional problem with Parkinson's is that visual hallucinations appear to be a "complex multifactor effect of different risk factors, mainly of dysfunctions of the visual system" (da Silva 2013). However, when da Silva (2013) studied a group of normal young individuals, it was found that a predisposition to visual hallucinations (while also due to a multifactor effect "strikingly similar" to the risk factors in Parkinson's disease, proneness to hallucinations) was also predicted by a specific personality profile. But da Silva's statements should be recognized as referring to a theory called the "Continuum hypothesis." In this view psychosis-like experiences are found as a continuum from mild to extreme in the general population. What is normal falls on the mild side of the line or curve, and what is illness falls on the extreme or pathological end. This seems a reasonable theory, especially if we consider that human consciousness is molded and limited by culture, and cultures have evolved under the selective pressures of human survival. Then we might be led to consider that the modal perceptions that are reinforced and sanctioned by any particular culture will fall along that continuum at any specific time in our evolution and that the continuum is also constantly changing (Fig. 3.2).

Ayahuasca Archetypes or Vision Categories

Benny Shannon's List	Psychedelic Times Staff	Other
Animals	Otherworldly beings	flower
Otherworldly beings	Animals	womb
Cities	Palaces	place of light
Palaces	Human Beings	infinite creation
Birds	Serpents	insects healing
Felines	Birds	rides & becomes snake
Artistic objects	Angels	Fluorescent liquid*
Celestial scenes	Divine Beings	
Divine Beings	Felines	
Landscapes	Forests	
Human Beings	Cities	
Royalty	Landscapes	
Forests	Flowers	

Fig. 3.2 Ayahuasca archetypes or vision categories. *note, "fluorescent liquid" is a substance reported by Harner (1968, 1973) and called "the hyperdimensional trypamine" by the McKenna brothers, see McKenna (1993). Shannon, Benny (1997) "A cognitive-psychological study of ayahuasca," *MAPS Newsletter*, https://maps.org/news-letters/v07n3/07313sha.html. Based on Dr. Shannon's personal experiences and those of 19 subjects. Also his more comprehensive analysis of indigenous experiences and interpretation in Shannon, Benney (2002) *The Antipodes of the Mind*, Oxford University Press. Psychedelic Times Staff, (2017) "Universal archetypes of Ayahuasca dreams and making sense of your own visions," *Psychedelic Times*, March 14, https://psychedelictimes.com/the-universal-archetypes-of-ayahuasca-dreams-and-making-sense-of-your-own-visions/

It might be thought that these categories are lists of images without specific definitions. Confusion could result from the separation of "Divine Beings" and "Otherworldly beings" or "Angels." Some felines are divine creatures, and etc. However, we will not consider these strict genera but rather simply often related identifications by specific subjects grouped together by the staff and Dr. Shannon without rigid guidelines. Often in the Anthropological literature (see Levy-Bruhl, 1966) we find birds and other animals as messengers of divine creatures, so that complicates the situation.

"Other" includes Hewitt (2019) report on a group of women. In Shannon's 2002 book he also mentions seeing gems in one of his first experiences with the drug as well as a dragon and then going through a long period of historical analysis. See Karsten (1935) for detail on the Jivaro images which are mostly similar to those above.

Sacks (1985) writes of patients hearing songs or voices that increase in intensity and then disappear. A cross-cultural survey of the hallucinations of people diagnosed as schizophrenic found that about 70% had auditory or visual hallucinations (Sartorius et al. 1986). Could then hallucinations be a species of perception distortion, as in tinnitus and hearing? This is a compelling idea, as some treatments for auditory hallucinations, as in hallucination-focused integrative treatment (HIT), use multiple modalities to produce control, as in some training methods to teach the person with tinnitus to ignore the persistent ringing in their ears (Jenner et al. 2006). The category of schizophrenia is variable and research into cross-cultural equivalency has been hampered by this variability, as is true also in the genetic associations (Mullins and Huang 2020).

Mogar and his associates had contacts with researchers at the International Foundation for Advanced Study in Menlo Park, where, by 1965, over 400 people had volunteered to take the drug and be part of a study of its effects (Mogar 1965a). But by the time the FDA revoked all permits for research at the Foundation only about 350 subjects had been fully processed and their experiences analyzed (Harrison 2013). The Foundation had been set up by Myron Stolaroff (an engineer and psychologist), who was an associate of Stanislav Grof and had a number of conversations with LSD discoverer Albert Hoffman. Stolaroff published a number of books and articles based on the research at the Foundation (e.g., Harman et al. 1966). He and one of his collaborators at the Foundation, Dr. Charles Savage (who had a prominent part in the Napa State Hospital Symposium), wrote an article in 1965 during the height of the LSD hysteria in the media attempting to clarify results of use of the drug and plead for patience and caution (Savage and Stolaroff 1965). They especially were concerned with how often subjects were being given the drug, dosage, and the therapeutic and experimental context. Mogar and Savage published some of the work they did together and Mogar (1965a) gave assessments.

A neutral or laboratory setting produced the usual oceanic and evolved concentration on perception, both visual and auditory. But even under these conditions standard objects and events could take on remarkable features. People seemed to view tactile information, especially their own, with awe and the ability to separate objects became difficult but not disturbing. Grof relates how movement of air was interpreted as images, or simple characters, like folds of a towel, translated by the viewer into an image of an elf.

Grof's subjects describe a geometrization of all images, where concentration by the subject on an object, or a blank wall, could result in a world of perceived images and edges, leading to edges. This was noted among subjects of the Mogar Lab, but also by some of the subjects at Humboldt State in the Sensory Deprivation Laboratory experiments. Edges often become halos and lead to other changes; this is true also of peyote and especially afterimages of visual stimulation or the change of two-dimensional surfaces to three and the surface again transforming (Kluver 1928/1966, 62, 68–9).

Much of what Grof describes as well as has been the common experience of users of LSD, appears as a merging of the senses, or synesthesia, and their re-separation (normal condition). They "see music" or "taste colors." There are some rather normal adjuncts to this, however, where people with one sensory loss, as in deaf individuals, experience music as vibration. So once in the 1970s I went to a musical event put on by a punk rock group. The venue was the Deaf Club, which was literally a room in a building that housed people who were deaf as well as some related offices. The punk rock band's theme was always, "faster, louder, shorter." Or the songs should be sung and played at a breakneck speed and as loud as possible (their amplifiers turned up to maximum) and the songs should be shorter than usual (less than three minutes). When I arrived I had thought the name of the venue was a joke or put on. So I was surprised to come to experience the presence of many of the building's residents, of all ages, enjoying the music. In conversation during the night I learned they had been renting the space to various community groups and the punks had rented it to practice, when they decided to put on an event. The police arrived at some point, but since there was no door charge and the non-profit of the deaf organization had provided the legal basis for selling alcohol, they left without any trouble. Another example appears in Humphry Osmond's (1970) experiment with LSD when one of the researchers and his wife had a disagreement. Osmond experiences this conflict as a darkening of light in the room and a distinct bitter taste. So one might theorize that emotion felt is translated into two other senses, light and taste.

This idea of the "merging of senses usually separate " or synesthesia was an area of research in the 1970s and 1980s. The work included clinic studies of people who experienced these sensations and who were examined for physical bases (tumors, genetics, etc.) of the variation in perception, as well as experimental study, especially in cats (Stein and Meredith 1993). These studies focused especially on certain areas of the brain (superior colliculus) where unimodal processing of sensory information takes place. Information from multisensory neurons contributes to orientation interpreted in different sensory maps to form integrated processing (King 2004). Today a considerable body of information has been gathered from pathological human examples (Cytowic 2002, 2003). The examples from pathology provide insights into the evolutionary history of the organization of sensory information in vertebrates, birds, and mammals especially. This same phenomenon of synesthesia has been reported for mescaline by earlier workers, for example, Rouhier, Dixon, Kluver, and Havelock Ellis in the combination of colors and music or taste.

Creativity, Problem-Solving, and Perception

However, of interest also to Grof was the emotional element added by subjects to these modifications of perception. The change in normal experience can be enjoyable, in a novel way, disturbing, often magical, or creative. This emotional variation or change in intensity of perception can add a new dimension for individuals that parallels that noted above for the deaf and punk rock. Grof reports subjects on LSD experiencing music "really" for the first time. These interpretations of the subjects were seen as potential insights into character or personality, as when Grof considered a subject's seeing female images on his palm as a result of his feeling of excessive masturbation. Intensive colors or images and memory of detail are also a character of some deprivation experiments (Zubek 1969). Stafford and Golightly's (1967) collection of essays on LSD as a problem-solving drug appears early in the scene, but has an effect that promotes the idea Leary and others (many Behaviorists I knew) espoused, that LSD could clean the slate of the mind's social conditioning and allow people to start over with their lives, and that the drug, as the microdosing computer engineers I met believed, could increase creativity and drive innovation.

Many of these "psychodynamic" narratives Grof relates, as in the case of the psychiatrist who relates the scene of his childhood community, appear to be both reflections or memories of the past that have been valued to some degree as important to the subject, and modifications that either show a failure of the subject to understand their past or a confusion of consciousness at that time. The case of the woman I related and her injured father are an example of the latter, but the psychiatrist's is an interpretation of the past in which events and roles are reinterpreted in light of the experience of a lifetime. The elements of "secrecy," "mystery," and "hypocrisy" which he finds uncovered in a "symbolic satire" demonstrate the evolution of a mature character able to reconstruct past values.

Grof juxtaposes the unconscious with the conscious and relies on the comparison with dreams and dream interpretation to formulate his own means to "decipher" the LSD state and the experience of reinterpretation he calls the LSD "language." While I was not convinced of this "language," it was clear that much of what people experienced with LSD was clothed in their past experience and development. We must be careful with our interpretations and the assumptions on which they are organized. These assumptions, Freudian or not, may only be valid for individuals and not cultures, and meaning may be tied to particular principles of a culture. For example, for the Pokomam of Guatemala, Reina (1966) reported that dreams were held to be real actions undertaken by the soul in sleep. But the information of the dream is to be read in reverse—a person who dreams they die or some other person dies means they will live a long healthy life.

Dream interpretation plays a central role in some cultures, in others it must not be shared, especially where dreaming is considered an ill omen. For example, Eggan (1966) shows how the Hopi place significance on dreams and their interpretation, so that a "bad dream" invokes a group discussion of the dream and a probing of the dreamer's situation that can be helpful. She relates how for a Hopi in crisis, the dream contains a "dimoki," the bundle of dream thoughts "richly populated with cultural images that act as a rudder to push a demanding self back into the coercive tide of social process" (Eggan 1966, 263). Comparing this to Grof's (1976, 133) referrals of subjects' descriptions of their visions in terms of Western art and media seems forced and questionable. We might note that Sharp's collection of dreams from the Yir Yoront of Australia (43 men, 8 women) supported Lincoln's (1935) findings that the dreams of people in the same culture and society will "likely show some clear regularities in manifest content" (Schneider and Sharp 1969). In a reflection of the social system, dreamers were most often victims of violence (56% of the time) but the conflict involved actual intergroup fighting the men experience at the hands of the mother's brother and elder brother. But we have to keep in mind not only Grof's theoretical scheme (which he often embellishes with his own art interpretations, as in his 1976 work, p. 133), but also the fact that his subjects included both patients with psychological problems and volunteers without objective pathological expression. We have to also consider a professional cultural influence as well as group dynamics, especially in a clinical setting or academic one. This may explain how the Harvard psilocybin project of Leary and Alpert, which had become somewhat a close knit group bordering on spirituality, morphed into a more chaotic scene controlled by a Michael Hollingshead, who had brought LSD to the group for the first time (Stevens 1988).

Laughlin (1976) shows in his book of 260 dream texts from indigenous people in Chiapas that the dreams were considered real experiences; they often also contained information on future events and the behavior of a variety of deities. Each person's infancy and childhood, and certainly adolescence, were constructed in the landscape of a unique institution of culture that appears as family life. But Grof's tendency to jump from his patient's responses to interpretation of normal volunteers presents a problem of experimental design lapse. Morgar (1965) was concerned with this problem and suggested it might introduce bias in results. He found that volunteers were "growth-oriented" while patients were "deficiency-motivated." Rosalind Cartwright (1977, 2010) saw in dreams aspects of health and illness that could be keys to healing. Her studies of dreaming and the quality of sleep led to ideas of interjecting a form of control into the dream by her patients. One might say this is similar or parallel to the use of the concept of lucid dreaming, but it appears from Cartwight's work that the training she offered allowed the patient to think about their nature and to conceive of the dream as participation with waking self-healing. For her, the mind was a dynamic organ, constantly working and reforming information; of memory she said: "Memory is never a precise duplicate of the original; instead, it is a continuing act of creation." Yet the ability to process and benefit from a reassessment of painful and negative experiences, Cartwright found, required the ability to emphasize, to "accurately transpose oneself into the experiences of another." Likewise, the individual must be able to re-experience events and to feel the context as positive or negative with regard to their own needs and relations with others. Here dreams are a self-operating means of accomplishing this task.

Opposed to this theory is the idea of random stimulation from the "dream generator" of the brain stem produced by Hobson and McCarley (1977) and a modification of this idea by Francis Crick and Graem Mitchison (1983). In both cases the idea is presented that dreams are meaningless and random stimulation, but Crick and Mitchison also argue that this is useful in allowing the brain to unlearn unimportant experiences. Recent research has regarded both theories and Freud's in a more integrative paradigm (Boag 2017). It is interesting that Louie and Wilson (2001) found that rats apparently replayed activities experienced when awake in dreams. This demonstrates a parallel in memory and learning in a basal mammal and indicates important aspects of uniformity in cognition as well.

Grof (1976, 212) seems to adhere to a theory in which the manifestations of individual experiences are drawn from early life, but this is neither a strictly Freudian nor a Jungian derivative, and he rejects the idea that differences between different practitioners' interpretation are due to their influence of patients. He places this problem in a criticism of interpretation of different uses of theory. In some ways this view is reflected in Roberto Assagioli's psychosynthetic view that human consciousness and experienced life are not fully integrated, but characterized by levels of unconscious qualities of experience (Whitmore 1981). In this way, like Grof's various paradigms of prenatal, birth, and postnatal experience, as well as aspects of development create an unintegrated being. Reintegrating these fragments in a functional way was a continuous narrative in Mogar's Lab.

One would have to rely on Freud's means of interpretation from psychoanalysis and the familiarity of the analyst with the subject. This has been a concern of critics of Freud for decades, how realistic and authentic are the interpretations from psychoanalysis? What is the nature of influence? The cultural context is vast in dream interpretation. In India this is often mediated by sages by reference to the distortions of dreams and their images "seen" by the mind. These distortions are sometimes placed into context by ideas of the Ayurveda and the different streams of consciousness created by the body (Ramaiah and Rao 1988). In one nineteenth-century Western view there was a strong tendency to believe that dreams produced the opposite of reality, a mirror image of veracity and so—if one found an event in dreams to result in one outcome, the dreamer was told to expect its opposite (Perkins 2001).

The second group of psychodynamic experiences Grof notes are those he characterizes as in the process of concretization of fantasy, dramatization of wishful thinking (daydreams), screen memories, and complex mixtures of fantasy and reality. These can be explained as follows:

a. *Concretization of fantasy* often is defined as the ability to separate realms of ideas of self from reality—as when someone performs as family member yet is a cult participant and takes on the role of a spiritual element, or as a member of a social group where the person performs as a mysterious founder. This "double life" can often be experienced as a continuous interplay of reality engagement and fantasy daydream, as Jung (2014) described. Grof also associates Jung's idea of healing at a distance, or forms of linkage in which people can affect others, or acausality (Jung 1960). Wallace (1958) in his study of Iroquois dreams constructed a theory of unconscious wish fulfillment. There is some evidence, however, that daydreaming may rely on the same neural foundations as dreaming in sleep (Domhoff and Fox 2015). This foundation is active when we are inactive, "doing nothing," and is referred to as the "default mode network" (mentioned earlier), the brain showing itself without interacting with the outside world (Wamsley and Stickgold 2010). A dynamic relationship is possible between the experiences of the day and the dream, with a result that the "archetypes" on which collective memory is based can become modified. Furst (1972, ed. Note page 82) suggests that the similarity of shaman experiences in initiation and entering and traveling in the spirit world, indicate some common language of consciousness that may be a product of psychedelics or biology. Roger Ivar Lohmann (Bulkeley 2019) has suggested this from his experiences with the Asabano people of Papua New Guinea, a process he calls "autonomic culture updating process," as when colonial influences come to overshadow traditional ones. Levy-Bruhl (1966) noted that some indigenous people first dream of conversion and then act on it.

The separation of the experience and its duality is considered dangerous in some cultures, whereas in others, the ability of some individuals to cross the barriers of reality into worlds of spirits or other beings is accepted, for example, as described in many Melanesian societies (Radcliffe-Brown 1932). In fact, illness, related to spirit or soul loss, can be caused by the failure of the individual to return from such a journey.

In Japan the *kami,* which are powerful spiritual beings, can appear in a daytime vision or dream at night. A night dream is considered easier for them. In such *reimu,* or divine dreams they can appear in many different forms, a beautiful woman, an old man, and so on. In such cases the deity may speak or leave an object as in Greek incubatory oracles. Sometimes the *kami* is not seen, but instead its messenger is visible. Sometimes dream can lead to trance in which a dialogue takes place between the individual and the deity or messenger, as in the case of Nao, where Blacker (1975) relates the deity, Ushitora-no-

Konjin, lodges itself, as if a possession, in her stomach (or speaks from her stomach as if some food or water had been the vehicle of possession). The deity's purpose here is to impart some information so the world can be saved. Dreams in Japan were traditionally seen as of divine origin and of four kinds: (1) healing dreams, (2) incubatory dreams brought on by sleeping in a certain holy place in quest of inspiration or information, (3) prophetic dreams, and (4) initiatory dreams. In these, as in many other culture dreams, the dreamer is convinced that the apparition is an objective fact and not a product of his or her imagination by certain signs. Sometimes dream gifts, actual objects or songs, tales, or information are given. In other cases, there is no discernable link between the "gift" and the actions of the dreamer. An example is the case Blacker (1975) tells of the Japanese mother whose child falls ill with an incurable disease. She goes to doctors and healers of all kinds, follows directions and goes on pilgrimages, and still nothing happens. Then one night she dreams of the goddess Kishibojin in a radiant image and when she awakes the child is healed.

In contemporary society this is often considered a type of impairment of symbolic thinking, a pathology of identification and is associated with ideas of melding realities of people who become so engaged on the internet that it is more rewarding than the life they lead otherwise (Toronto 2009). While many people have lived in close communication with ancestors and deceased family (Vansina 1985), this virtual world is not that different. An interesting aspect of wish fulfillment and our next category, daydreams, is the fact that some people lack the ability to create images of events in their minds, the pathological condition of aphantasia, which we will discuss later on. This condition would certainly subvert the authority of any theories of language evolution or development where images are necessary as a means of inferring meaning. Aphantasia affects the ability of the affected individual to recall past events, imagine the future, and dream. This, like the ability of blind people to learn language, requires a concept of symbol that lacks form as image.

b. Perhaps the "dramatization of wishful daydreams" does not need explanation. But it does relate to a complex of Freud's work on dreams where dreams undergo changes over time, and with their repeating, become edited, transforming by condensation, displacement, symbolization, and dramatization. In the means of this process the individual can recast the wish fulfillment into goals of desire or pleasure, revenge, or creative reorganization (Michael 2015). The creative element can be as a discovery, as in the famous case of the benzene ring dream of August Kekule, though now in question (Browne 1988).

c. *Screen memories* is a concept also derived from Freud by Grof that was described in an 1899 paper by Freud. It contains a most interesting analysis of a college-educated man who is likely to be Freud. The concept involves the idea of the creation of phantasies derived from our early years and related to aspects of child sexuality. The interpretation of the child is stored in memory of events the child experiences but cannot understand due to its age and developmental state (the brain, as we know, is still in process of complete growth and differentiation). These memories become locked in a form of amnesia that return to partial consciousness and form confusing and ill-defined images that are not associated with any linguistic context due to the developmental incomplete state of experience. Freud argues by use of a Greek myth:

> The assertion that a psychical intensity can be displaced from one presentation (which is then abandoned) on to another (which thenceforward plays the psychological part of the former one) is as bewildering to us as certain features of Greek mythology—as, for instance, when the gods are said to clothe someone with beauty as though it were with a veil, whereas we think only of a face transfigured by a change of expression.

Grof makes the statement in his 1967 edition that if the results of LSD use were only the psychodynamic, they would be a proof of Freud's psychoanalytic theory. Grof argued in the 1976 edition that the psychodynamic expressions in human subjects required a modification of Freudian theory. While the psychoanalytic theory has attracted a number of negative critiques (Popper and Nagel as being untestable), more recent views have considered clinical and experimental data (Erwin 1980; Grunbaum 1977, 1980).

Grof argued that LSD opened up a new principle in psychoanalytical thinking. He considered this to be defined as specific memory constellations systems of condensed experience. So experiences of life at different times, charged with varying emotional content, were related due to similarities of place, people, psychological content as if constellations, that is, linked in unique ways for the individual (COEX systems). These constellations could be seen as molded in three-dimensional features, with the deepest layers associated with the earliest experiences of the patient. The more superficial were of later life. All of the experiences and memories were negative in some fashion, humiliation, danger, illness, failure, and so on. These all had their own defense mechanisms built for them. While Grof describes in detail this negative COEX system, his mention of a positive one built on pleasant experiences is perfunctory, and his choice of words, "pleasant" versus "pleasure," is significant. His explanation is that the negative systems are more frequently expressed and come in greater variety.

It seemed strange to me that Grof had built up a system of negative associations as the special feature of this new principle when Freud had certainly covered this field with negativity. Yet it also seemed that Grof was, as Freud was, as interested in the phenomenon of human consciousness as in healing. The case of Renata, who had such recurring torturous hallucinations of a sexual nature, was found to resist clarity of her fundamental experience that caused her psychological crises and their repeated cause of her hallucinations. So, as opposed to other cases, like the woman I described and her injured father, a "cure" was elusive. Grof interprets this was a reduction of her COEX system over a series of LSD sessions where she relives the initiating traumatic experiences. Since each following an early child abuse was a repeat of the type of trauma, he theorizes the release was, in each case, only specific to the multiples. One might argue that since the experiences she had with subsequent lovers, doctor's examinations, X-ray rooms, and so on all differed slightly, you could interpret these differences as part of the COEX.

In the end, most of Grof's examples do not clear their psychopathological condition but only reduce the symptoms to some extent. He interprets this as a realization of the trauma of birth as a continuing pathological source. He does not explain why everyone does not have this, yet it is assumed he agrees with Freud, that everyone creates a variety of accommodations (e.g., repression, etc.) to make life "work." However, we might challenge this idea as unsupported by the fact that we know that both the mother and the fetus are bathed in a variety of hormones during the birth experience, one that works to reduce pain and produce pleasure is oxytocin, but beta-endorphins, in general are also present. So the birth experience should be pleasurable for the fetus unless the mother is not producing the hormones. There is evidence that the type of delivery can affect the amount of endorphins present (Karakaya et al. 2018).

Another aspect of this that seems to undermine Grof's belief in the trauma of birth, and perhaps Freud's as well, is the great variety of ethnographic contexts concerning childbirth. For example, my own experience where a group of hippies in Northern California who lived in a commune, or series of communes, had come in contact with the Food Conspiracies in San Francisco and I had some contact with them. This led me to be at one of their houses, or communes of houses, in a remote valley. In the process of work for the food collection, I was invited to stay the night and share a meal with them. I have outlined the Food Conspiracies in the Bay Area in an earlier work (Caldararo 2019). I described this event in an earlier section of this book. There had been general eating of and smoking of hash and marijuana as well as use of LSD and other psychedelics. It was not the only event like it that I had been at. The point being that the birth was made pleasant by community involvement and ritual. I recall studying belly dancing from a number of Egyptian and Berber women and learning (as I had read in books) that it had its origin in preparation for birth and that a number of rituals were associated with creating a pleasant atmosphere for the mother and the arriving child. The rituals of birth in most indigenous people are so oriented, and the idea of birth trauma seems strange in this context. I was present for my own daughter's birth and was surprised by the way the medical staff took charge, even though we had presented them with a protocol for how we wanted the birth to transpire. This was before there was a change in how hospitals addressed birth in family contexts.

Many parties in the communes in San Francisco and Berkeley shared drugs and often were attended by as many as 30 or 40 people. Few of these were attacked by the police, though police might have been present; the only one I knew of in the period 1966–1972 was when the house I was living in was raided by police on Oak Street after a large party. The police came not because of drug use, but due to a midnight stroll several people took to the beach through the park after the party. A police car had come across five or six members of the commune at dawn with a child at the beach chanting and drumming while watching the sun come up. The police searched and detained them. When the police were given the people's address, they came to the house, where the front door was unlocked and entered some time before. Finding marijuana, they arrested everyone present. I had stayed over at my girlfriend's apartment and arrived around 9 am to get ready to go to class, finding the apartment empty and in complete disarray from the police search. The presence of a child, drugs, and hippies as well as some African Americans seemed to be enough to justify arrest. And one can imagine how the criminalization of drugs has negatively affected thousands of peoples' lives since. Feeling safe is a central factor and the threat of arrest is certainly a negative factor.

How people see the world and who they are in it is a central factor in outcomes. This is true of the Harvard project of Leary and Alpert in contrast to the members of so many households in the Bay Area in the 1960s and 1970s. But theory and belief have strongly affected choices in regard to treatment of psychedelics. As in the cases of people who believed in the methodology and theory of Primal Scream therapy (Janov 1970), the individuals I came to know did not seem to be "healthier" or cope better with the world after treatment and the method came under some criticism (Pathis and Younes 2015). The duality of birth and death is central to Grof's approach, as it was to Freud's, and we see it as an essential part of Huxley's interpretation (1954). The so-called birth trauma has been tied to psychological stress of all kinds in recent years, including PTSD (Ayers 2017). The idea of the fetus experiencing trauma during birth that could affect later life was first suggested by Otto Rank (1924/1993) and renewed by Wilfred Bion (1977). Grof (1976, 97–8) reports that his patients experienced many of the typical movements of the fetus during birth in his sessions. I never saw this, in private, or heard it discussed by Mogar's associates. But the relation of the passage from the "oceanic sensation" to a reliving of life experiences, especially those of alcoholics, can be seen as a pattern. So Grof's reports of mixed prenatal experiences and birth trauma with both psychological and physiological memories (he calls these Rankian) seem logical.

Efforts to link the birth trauma to psychopathologies seem indistinct and vague. Everything can be attributed to the birth experience, yet given the fact that there is no specific association and that the fetus brain is about 20–25% developed at the time of birth, with most growth taking place after birth (Gilmore et al. 2018), long-lasting effects seem unlikely. Yet Roheim (1945, 1952, 1968) has argued for the validity of many of the Freudian ideas from his ethnographic research. But this view conflicts with the general worldview of most indigenous religions, where the eternal return is simply a process of rebirth, of transitions of form and rites of passage which direct and structure cycles for individuals. Fear of death or pain in birth is not universal. Van Gennep (1960) demonstrated that this positive view involved an ideology where humans were part of nature, with cycles of ontogeny, development, aging, and rebirth. These were situated within cycles of the natural world, of seasons, and punctuated by the movement of stars and appearance of plants, animals, and greater variations. For many Melanesians, the transition of death to life is one filled with perceptions, and a transformation (Codrington 1891). This is discussed by the Blair brothers in their documentary and also in a 2010 book that covers the series of documentaries they made of various Indonesian islands (Blair 2010). The theory is not incompatible with either the idea of the "Blank Slate" of human consciousness or Anthropology's theory of the Psychic Unity of Mankind of Adolf Bastian, which has become a foundational element in modern Anthropology (Caldararo 2012). So in this regard, Mogar and Grof (1976) do not part company; both recognized that most subjects experienced an "oceanic state of consciousness" and frequently a "cosmic unity" (Grof 1976, 105). So the difference might be Grof's tendency to attribute this feeling to an intrauterine experience and rebirth and we might consider Grof's (1976, 94) assumption that the lack of this experience or its fragmentation and distortion might be due to the pathologies of various clients. The nature of the set and setting and the theoretical orientation of the experimenter or therapist have been mentioned above as factors as well.

In a more expressive form, some like Sacks (2012) have argued that the patterns seen in hallucinations, both pathologically derived like in migraine or in artificial means as in psychedelic drugs, are found in the art of indigenous people everywhere and in religious modern designs. A number of ethnologists and art historians have noted similarities of patterns of this kind, for example, see Grieder (1982). This is very different from saying that meanings are the same. The patterns appear universal as biologically derived, but if a person hallucinates a white picket fence we cannot assume it has the same meaning as such an image perceived by another person (see Hellie 2013). That image is both culturally influenced and a product of the individual's ontology and development. This perspective was expressed by Wallace (1966) of records of psychedelic experiences, both indigenous and through recent experiments.

We face the possibility of another phenomenological problem. Does the theory determine the interpretation of symptoms, so analysts "see" birth trauma in everyone? I did not experience this, nor did I see it in the early years of LSD use. Later, however, as Leary's ideas became more popular in the media, it was reported increasingly. The main problem with this approach of Leary and Grof is the fact that it overrides the individual discovery of self suggested by Korzybski that Mogar found so compelling a feature of his subjects. One might argue that reliving a birth trauma should be part of such discovery, but the theory implied that everyone had a trauma and it was significant to their cure or discovery. Yet this seems forced; does everyone "experience" the birth trauma alike or at all? It seems to me there is no evidence that everyone does. Some women have relatively "easy" births and only a few report traumatic lingering or lifelong repercussions. This process of self-discovery, however, can be vague and ideological. In Aldous Huxley's experience he becomes dissociated, the "Not-self" first (Huxley 1954, 35). Yet Huxley (1963) made it a requirement for achieving a status of being "fully human":

> [T]o be fully human, the individual must learn to deconstruction himself, must be able to cut holes in the fence of verbalized symbols that hems him in. (Aldous Huxley 1963)

But what of everyone else? Are people inside the fence of verbalized symbols proto-human, or subhuman. This idea of the "verbal fence" holding back an authentic experience with reality and the true self would seem at first similar to Mogar's position, but the difference is in Huxley's constant reference to structures that determine his progress and end in his experience of "Hell." He is hemmed in by traditional Western concepts of what "mind" should be and is not. In paleoanthropology some scholars call the hominids of the mid-Pleistocene (600,000–200,000 BP) by the term "prehuman" to indicate the lack of fully developed language, with the ability to abstract only slightly present, and a lack of complex social behavior. I am not in agreement with this term (see Caldararo 2019) but the question of human cognition has baffled most scholars from fields as diverse as Neurology to Sociology and we are no closer to understanding if we have become fully human yet, that claim is certainly filled with hubris.

The role of trauma in the development of hallucinations and delusions is gaining new attention because of soldier injuries and other forms of PTSD, including spousal and child abuse. Particular focus in the last two decades has been on African American and Latinx populations. The number of hallucinations reported for African Americans with psychiatric conditions has been greater than for those patients deemed "white." Some diagnostic confusion may have entered into these figures, though Adebimpe et al. (1981) also reported similar differences in a restudy. They note problems of defining hallucination categories with other symptoms as described later by ffytche (2013). A larger sample of African American patients showing psychotic symptoms found that the content of delusions and hallucinations demonstrated cultural and racial themes different from the general population (Whaley and Hall 2008). This also supports the idea of trauma-associated and culturally derived origins.

A rare case of autoscopic hallucination in an African American female was reported by Gajaram et al. (2021). This is a condition where the individual sees themselves as if in a mirror and differs from heautoscopy, where the individual sees themselves as a doppelganger in two places at one time. Autoscopic experiences are seen in generalized disorders of the central nervous system (CNS), during epileptic seizures, near-death experiences, meningitis, space-occupying lesions, brain tumors, migraine, delirium, post-traumatic brain lesions, MS, some infectious diseases like typhus, some medication side effects, and altered psychological states. This term seems to cover a wide category of phenomenological experiences, as sometimes people do not recognize themselves, but as in some folklore where the hero or shaman discovers they are fighting themselves, seeing themselves die, sometimes ripped apart by demons, then reborn (Campbell 1949; Eliade 1964), some trigger of the therapist's cue or that of memory evokes the realization. In other cases there is the "test" by the subject of the doppelganger, usually of agency, the demonstration of movement of a part of the body, followed by that of the doppelganger or not (Blanke and Metzinger 2008). Experience of this condition is associated with damage to parts of the cortex or epilepsy. In my experience with psychedelics and in observing others, on LSD, peyote or related drugs, this has happened but was short-lived and changed into some other scheme rapidly. It seems to me this is also related to the failure to exit problem seen in some lucid dreaming cases (as discussed elsewhere). If one cannot discern reality from the dream, in some cases of autoscopy (sometimes called heautoscopy), one sees the doppelganger but cannot tell which is real. The patient may attempt a "test" by hurting themselves, or the doppelganger, to achieve unity (Sacks 2012).

Near-death experiences produce REM dream-like hallucinations and the individual is paralyzed, as in sleep paralysis, but Nelson (2010) found a common condition of reduced blood flow to the brain and eyes, inducing alterations in brain function and producing narrowed vision interpreted as moving through a tunnel. Stimulation of the angular gyrus of the brain of a patient with severe epilepsy invariably caused out-of-body experiences (Sacks 2012) while stimulation with theta bursts seems to reduce subjective recollection (Yazar et al. 2014).

In a study of patients and non-clinical volunteers, with a large proportion of African Americans (>66%), it was found that trauma was a significant factor in the appearance of hallucinations, especially repeated exposure (Rosen et al. 2017). The authors of the study remarked, "tactile hallucinations and religious delusions were significantly correlated with history of unwanted sexual experiences and, for tactile hallucinations, with past physical and sexual assault." There is evidence of over-diagnosis of Black patients as schizophrenic over other segments of the US population and this may relate to descriptions of the effects of trauma (Moran 2014).

When addressing other populations we have the added aspects of language and culture and, additionally, culture shock. Latino patients displayed a number of auditory hallucinations, phones or doorbell ringing, children's voices, and visual hallucinations of animals and relatives (Mischoulon et al. 2005), though these are not unusual in the general population. Over 83% of a Spanish-speaking Caribbean Latinx sample were female and were found to report hallucinations in a study by Geltman and Chang (2004). Caribbean individuals have been found to report more hallucinations that other segments of communities, but the nature of this may be related to a cultural acceptance of such experiences. It has generally been found that Latinos in general report more experiences with spirits and angels than other members of the American population (Fortuna, n.d.). Command auditory hallucinations were also common among Asian American patients (Lee et al. 2004). Similar effects of religious beliefs and cultural concepts affect the nature and form of delusions and hallucinations in many Asian patients, especially Chinese (Yip 2003). In a large sample of Chinese patients, most reported not telling their doctors of their hallucinations. Other than a few objects noted, animals, flowers, and cloth, no notable responses were discussed (Tan et al. 2004). The problems associated with the cultural validation of seeing spirits, ghosts, gods, and ancestors complicates the issue of phenomenology and pathology. Wallace (1966) notes the greater feeling of acceptance of the Euro-American population in the pre-World War II period than after. We have touched on this regarding Anderson's (2005) study of ghosts in Iceland.

Another curious aspect of Grof's work and theories is the Jungian framework he often uses. He argues (1976, 72) that certain kinds of events that have powerful effects on the subconscious of patients are due to specific sensitivities in the deeper levels of unconscious that are "inborn and transpersonal in nature." He describes these in various forms and creates several theoretical categories for them, for example, reincarnation and reliving past lives, though these categories often bleed into each other, as in his ideas regarding phylogenetic dreams, reincarnation, and reliving past lives and reliving collective unconscious events. He suggests that some of these "factors" when brought to the surface due to LSD therapy have "the form of ancestral, racial or phylogenetic memories, archetypal structures or even past-incarnation experiences." He sees a link between certain traumatic experiences of childhood and the birth trauma. He speculates that variations in factors or in expression of form of trauma may be due to the time period of the event and critical periods of development in the child.

Early childhood trauma, like the loss of a mother, was a special area of study for Bowlby (1953) and he traveled around the world and collected case histories before describing how damaging the experience was for motherless children. Today research into birth trauma include the emotional effect on the mother, father, and other related individuals regarding the birth and not just the infant and his or her adaptation to it (Beck 2015; Huang et al. 2019). Birth trauma, or childbirth trauma, often refers to extended psychological negative conscious or unconscious feelings the mother has regarding the birth and the child (Greenfield et al. 2016).

Jung (1933) differed from Freud (1966) in the nature of the unconscious. For Freud, it was a repository of repressed biological and psychological stimuli. For Jung, it was divided into a personal unconscious, much like Freud's, layered with traumatic experiences, painful memories, and biologically induced stimuli that were repressed by socialization. But then there was a deeper stratum, one made up of the collective experiences of past ancestors, the archetypal repository. In this stratum could be found a variety of materials, some adaptive in the evolution of human consciousness and others damaging but filed as a racial memory. These can be seen as "[t]he form of the world into which [a person] is born is already inborn in him, as a virtual image" (Jung 2014, 188).

Grof (1976) draws a picture of a significant trauma an individual experiences and the family structure that can magnify and institutionalize the event in a dysfunctional family, so that it becomes a constant frame for the individual, a "macrotrauma," in his jargon. Such an all-encompassing growth of pathological identity distortion is seen in many of Laing's (1959) patients, especially Marie, who spent her life attempting to eradicate her existence. But Grof (1976) separates two types of central trauma released by the LSD therapy. One is the single event that traumatizes the individual, either in early childhood or as evoked as a kind of "archetype" that frames and seems to freeze the individual into a character armor that is alien or incompatible with his or her personality. To Laing (1959) he seems to imply the "archetype" is really more of an image of reality perceived by the child but not understood as described by Freud (1961, 492). This "role" or personification of self, to Laing, becomes alien and can be seen by the pathological case to be attacking the real self or controlling it.

The search for origins of "archetypes" can become both mundane and circular. Here, Barron (1967) finds most are derived from current images and concepts of the popular press. Wolfe (1968) agrees, finding that many images reported by Ken Kesey's group appeared to be from comic books of the 1930s and 1940s. But then Barron (1967) notes that these contemporary images are often derived from earlier ones, mixed and redrawn by generations into the fabric of each social context. Obviously there is the possibility that the artists producing the comic books were influenced by images and ideas of their time, which may reflect earlier ideas and so on. Subjectivity is rife here and the circularity is common in related experiences, as in near-death perceptions. Yet even here there are parallels in the ethnographic literature, as when people dream they enter heaven or a similar world with gods (Levy-Bruhl 1966). In fact, some of these near-death perceptions are very similar to those produced by certain drugs, for example, DMT (Martone 2019). Thus we face a conundrum, are the images from near-death and dreams the product of drug-induced brain chemistry, or is there a mechanism in memory and sleep that produces them, or are they derived from authentic spiritual contact?

Lincoln (1935) noted the community nature of dreams, dream interpretation, and function. Radcliffe-Brown (1932, 177–9) reports a similar condition, with dreams being an identifier of the shaman, yet the community experiences dreams as well and the acquisition of dreams is seen as a power. In healing Melanesian shamans, the dreaming-man, or *tatua qoreqora*, communicates with spirits, often ghosts, to find lost souls or the cause of illness. The professional dreamer is expected to find in dream the answer, and so often this person comes to the house of the ill person and sleeps, dreaming in a journey and often to the abode of the dead Wizards, who can be engaged to find lost items—in both cases they are paid a fee (Codrington 1891). This is different from the nature of prophecy, where a wizard or diviner will go into trance and be possessed by a *tindalo* or ghost of prophecy to find out about future events. He sneezes to begin and show the *tindalo* has entered him and then shakes and otherwise convulses and then speaks in a strange voice, not his own. So here we have the combination in one society of what Bourguignon (1972) has noted a separation of dreaming and trance. But while ghosts, as supernatural beings, may appear in dreams, they can also be seen in daylight for Melanesians (Codrington 1891).

Sometimes ghosts as supernatural beings seem more like visions, as they can be experienced at any time. Though the relation of sleep to the event might be misinterpreted by the ethnographer. Therefore, the visualization of personal images in the conscious or unconscious (trance, dream, hysteria, delirium) seems to have a well-established role in human life. It seems also to be a cultural product, one molded by enculturation and ontogeny. But perception is individual, even if molded by the cultural cosmology. The "Brownian Motion" often seen by people when fixated on an image, especially the sky, was often remarked, but not considered by most people as threatening or evidence of illness. Yet if fixated on, it can result in some degree of concern, as when using a psychedelic. As Leibowitz (1965) noted, the basis of visual perception is retinal excitation, so as light hits the rods and cones of the eye they are excited to "fire" and record the event. As this takes place in a chemo-electrical fashion in the translation from the neuron to the visual center of the brain for each rod or cone, the exhaustion of the excitation works like an "on/off" switch, so we have a dilemma here. This is because the sky or the air between our eyes and a surface does contain atoms of gases and particles. So are we "seeing" the firing of the rods and cones or the presences of atoms? Many subjects of psychedelics believed they were seeing a physical presence, atoms.

In Jung, the archetype is more of an evolutionary and social construct. This realm of thinking assumes some kind of psychological persistence of behavior as a "racial memory." Grof (1976, 167–8) accepts this concept uncritically, and Freud also considered the idea. For Grof (1976), it was a process of development of the COEX system. Once the "core experience" takes place, other similar experiences are coded to it as well as others that may not be intended by other actors to be traumatic, but are interpreted so by the individual. This is why the release of the core experience of trauma by the LSD therapy can lead to the unraveling of an entire false self or oppressive personality trait.

One might say, in reference to Kelly's (1963) *Theory of Personality*, the constructs of the individual under the influence of the LSD reexamination, finds that the traits, linked or identified with the core experience, have not the power predictive of personal goals, and are not consonant with feelings of identity. This triggers a reconstruction of personality into one more compatible with goals and feelings. For the COEX complex of Grof, the added yearly, daily, hourly insults the individual endures (interprets as such) builds up the energy of the basic theme to form a kind of screen of reality, or as Laing describes, a prison of perception, similar perhaps to some theories of the consciousness of women we will discuss below. These become integrated, as Grof notes, in a web of interpreted reenactment of the core experience. But he has designed a system in which this process takes place that he calls Basic Perinatal Matrices (Grof 1976, 102–3). These are the stages of birth. He then characterizes these in terms of what he perceives as the environment the fetus experiences as pleasure or pain. Then within this matrix individuals relate their birth in concepts of their lives, often interpreted as the struggle of heroes, torture, and so on. This would seem less forced to me if Grof had proposed this as a series of stages that the fetus might have such physical experiences and that individuals on LSD might fit into their LSD experience their own interpretation of the feelings they had in this manner. Also concerning is Grof's (1976, 152) idea that if the LSD "session terminates" in a particular Basic Perinatal Matrix, it can determine the outcome, as in whether the patient has succeeded in resolving pathological problems. If it is "terminated," a form of ending of the LSD experience, in one of the early stages of BPM, he seems to be saying that the person may be even worse off than before. He suggests that the patient will stabilize, even if terminating in the intense BPM I stage. However, the mechanical format he has fashioned seems too culture bound and straightjacketed. Nevertheless, Grof (1976, 149) does seem to leave open the possibility that this system is variable by suggesting the sequences are variable, often incomplete, as well as the content.

It seems to me that Bourguignon (1972) has a more elegant perception on this, where she argues that culture forms the dream and hallucination (vision) and gives it shape in Native theory as well as individual experience. She refers this to Hallowell's (1966) "cultural constitution of the behavioral environment." She also mentions, in this context, Fabian's (1966) theory of dreams among the Jamaa Movement of the Congo, where dreams may be divided into human dreams and those that are communications from the supernatural world, from god via "mawazo." This creates a distinction, as these are considered not dreams, but a god's communication. For the Jamaa, to find the meaning of dreams is a social task, one that links all members to each other and the supernatural. However, one respondent argued that there was a tendency for people to compete as dreamers, claiming to receive special "mawazo." Like Hallowell, Fabian finds that charismatic leaders have a theory of dreams that they make "deliberate use, of a potential source of ideas and orientation in a charismatic situation." The set of concepts, definitions, and rules of application on which these are based define the role of the charismatic authority. This applies to visions as described by Hallowell (1966) and as seen when charismatic leaders use visions during speeches or performances as a means of punctuating their legitimacy and connection to spirits. Since such leaders and their movements are often found to develop in the context of political, religious, and economic stress from outside, they can be also considered to be revitalization movements that often incorporate new ideas from outside as a means of adapting indigenous culture. In the example of the Jamaa as well as Christ, the outside sources were forms of colonialism, for Jamaa European colonialism and for Christ Roman power and Greek culture. For the Jamaa, dreaming has special significance and they dream often and follow interpretation with action (Fabian 1966, 545–6). Patai (1990) has shown in the history of Judaism how often dreams and visions have played roles in redefining social and political action. Martin Luther used his visions and dreams in much the same way, to achieve legitimacy and to be examples of a paradigm.

Grof (1976, 78–9) describes how the LSD therapy shatters this complex, in a chaotic fragmentation that the patient can later describe as pieces of events, including the core experience, and all those subsequent that reinforced it. This process of the emerging COEX system, via the disintegration of the attached mosaic of subsequent trauma, is seen, felt, and re-experienced. In many sessions, both in the clinical setting and in private homes, and so on, I noted how people sometimes went through something like this "re-emerging of past archetypes of disease" with vocalizations and often reenactment of the core experience or parts of it. But "archetypes" in the sense, to me, seemed like fragments of their own history, perhaps made even more vague and strange by being the visions of childhood. But related to this is Grof's comment on how the setting or people present can set off a patient into changes of course in the patient's experience during the LSD therapy session. This is something I did see, how people jumped from one focus of present experience to others, or to past experiences. This back-and-forth focus sometimes related to the setting of the room or people in it and comments or music, but often seemed to have no clear relation to anything that was present or spoken. Questions by therapists, or in the private setting, other people, could resolve issues or clarify content, but sometimes this did not occur. Mental chaos, confusion, or simply a period of mute quiet could follow any outburst or focus of intense attention.

Grof's (1976, 91) claim that seemingly inappropriate and/or exaggerated responses of patients to environmental stimuli could be related to "the dynamics of the governing COEX system" may be a result of his intensively studied patients and their background. In my experience, people often had what seemed intense and meaningful mental images and "seen experiences" but could not remember them during or after the session. Once a person seemed shocked and started screaming hysterically, got up, and appeared ready to run out of the room. Seconds later she sat down and was talking about a song she wrote. When asked what had just happened, she seemed surprised as if nothing had taken place.

I was struck in the clinical setting how Mogar and his associates dealt with this situation in comparison, say to the Psychedelic Rangers or Grof. In the clinical situation, the physicians and psychologists would mainly observe and, at times, ask questions about what was being experienced, if the question seemed appropriate. They had a well-developed, but not rigid, protocol of general non-intervention. At the point where there seemed to be a severe and painful passage, a question of a neutral type would be introduced. In the current context, researchers like Nutt and Carhart-Harris (2020) call their staff that engage patients "guides" and their role seems quite similar to that established by Mogar and his associates. The Psychedelic Rangers also had a protocol of non-intervention, and as I had no idea if they were influenced by Mogar or Mogar by them, I asked one and his response was, "Mogar who?" The Psychedelic Rangers, however, varied in their interventions, as their purpose was only to interfere in an extraordinary context. If called, they would come to a home and attempt to "talk down" the affected person. This method involved trying to make contact between the person, their friends (if present) or family (usually absent), or some kind of symbolism that might create stable links to the present, like beliefs, loves, likes, and so on. I should make clear here that the Rangers were not promoting LSD use or any other drug.

Many books and articles have reported on the phenomenon of proselytism among LSD users. I find this word rather provocative, and though many people I knew who had taken LSD or peyote thought others should do so too, and some people established organizations, one might say, churches after the experience, I am not sure this is all linked together. Some people simply wanted other people to see and feel what they had, some gathered friends to do so, but I did not personally come into contact with people who felt their experiences drove them to recruit others to form organizations like a religious body. The idea that LSD did convince some people that they could be positively changed is supported by such a body of evidence that it requires no argument. But the conviction that taking LSD drove people to join such churches or organizations is blatantly false, as many failed to do so. Blum et al. (1964b) reviewed this tendency early in the 1960s and Stevens (1988) has summarized some of the examples. This issue regarding people like Tim Leary and Ginsberg appears contradictory, especially in the reports many people gave and Leary's own comments. There was certainly a group of people who often acted in concert to a limited extent, as in the Trips Festival and Human Be-In.

Grof's description of conflicts with his patients under LSD therapy also seems to reflect the history of treatment many of his patients had and not the nature of the LSD experience. Grof's method and role seem to have been quite invasive while Mogar's colleagues' were more observational. When problems developed, like the Psychedelic Rangers, Mogar's method was to do less and allow the subject to act out or to suggest a slow "coming down procedure." This entailed peaceful interaction built on the responses of the subject, where the practitioner would ask questions of what the subject was experiencing and if that was not calming, then describe beautiful or calm situations or concepts that the subject had written in answer to the interview questionnaires. This seemed to work well in most cases I was aware of or had experienced myself. I remember one especially difficult case where the Psychedelic Rangers had responded to a person who was quite distraught and had done some things (endangering himself) that scared his friends. After a long period of exchange with the Psychedelic Rangers where their theme had been a holistic world, he had arrived at a calm state and was stable. The last interaction had been about what he wanted out of life. He had finally said in a sad tone, "Everyone wants to get something out of life, than just life, so what is left of life?" The answer had been, "You are, we are." To which he remarked, in what seemed like another phase of beginning panic, "But what IS left of life, how much if we take so much?" "There is," said one of the Psychedelic Rangers, "no end to it, you do not have to worry." He then smiled. The facility with which the Psychedelic Rangers always seemed to have the right formula intrigued me. I often asked them where they had learned how to do it. They only answer I ever got was, "From life."

Nevertheless, Grof (1976, 89–90) states that patients often attempted to drive him into roles that were contained in the individual patient's COEX system, and that he resisted these efforts. This is similar to Laing's description of his schizophrenic patients attempting either to act out situations that they interpreted as what the therapist wanted or to act normally as if there were no problems at all. One Psychedelic Ranger once said to me that there was an invisible mirage around people on LSD, one that contained echoes of voices from the past, present, and future. Her opinion was that to help one had to avoid disrupting the mirage and ignore the echoes but not the voice of the person. This sounded a lot like the scene in *Ulysses* where the hero is tied to a mast to avoid being affected by the voices of the Sirens.

Darold Treffert (2010, 2015) has recently defined parameters for penetrating internal worlds. He expresses two different types, one associated with the abilities of savants, and the other, cases where people "know things they never learned." This is a variety of the former but in average people. But I would suggest that it can also be simply an incompatibility of the enculturation form in which the individual is molded in childhood that makes up the family structure and social and cultural milieu of action. I think some psychedelics can trigger this construct. The person reacts to this milieu as if imprisoned and no amount of rewards or punishments can create a homeostasis. This would seem to be most likely where two parents come from different cultural backgrounds and there is a confusion in the learned pathways of personality development.

This problem has been present in LSD research. How are the responses that are interpreted as Freudian or as universal culturally constructed or artifacts of the process of interpretation to be clarified? One would assume that cross-cultural research might shed light on this problem. Lerner and Lyvers (2006) studied responses of individuals who had used LSD and psilocybin from Israel and Australia. While neither specific ethnic backgrounds were defined nor the socio-economic status, the results indicated significant effects of pre-drug characteristics and attitudes. De Rios and Smith (1977) questioned the idea of drug "abuse" in traditional societies and suggested that the interpretation of experience in the context of what is forbidden in the West distorts comparisons. De Rios and Smith (1977) also challenge the concept of abuse in the West. They claim psychedelic drug use is more common in less complex societies (though they credit a personal comment by Michael Harner for the idea; see also de Rios 1984), but one might argue that this is a confusion they introduce, as psychedelic drug use is quite common today and increasing, though past suppression began only in the early twentieth century with opioids, marijuana, and peyote. There is little evidence that past complex societies suppressed drug use of this kind, and in fact we have considerable evidence that it was not in the cults of Dionysus and others (Carod-Artal 2013). De Rios and Smith seem to be conflating modernity with complexity, since both Aztecs and Mayans, who had complex societies, utilized psychoactive plants (see Furst 1972). Usually this is associated with specific values of achievement. For example, do drug users achieve expected levels of status and material productivity in societies where altered states of consciousness are allowed or institutionalized? This is a difficult problem, as not all societies define success in single modes of achievement or material wealth, number of children, or enemy killed. Also, drug use and acceptance seem to change, as in tobacco use in the twentieth century in America became negatively sanctioned at the end of the 1990s. Bourguignon (1973) conducted research on an ethnographic sample of 488 societies and found some 90% had one or more institutionalized and culturally patterned forms of altered states of consciousness. These vary considerably, as do the degree of institutionalization. For example, in America trance has a significant role in religious life for many Protestants, especially Baptists. Weil (1972) argued that there was a natural human desire to alter consciousness, whether by chemical or by physical means. Schultes (1972) produced a compendium of plants used as hallucinogens and their localities and use in the Western Hemisphere.

D'Andrade (1961) drew on a sample of 64 societies from the Human Relation Area Files to determine if there were any uniformities of dreaming and social organization, institutions, or economic status. He found that there was an association with post-marital residence and subsistence economy. Textor (1967) studied a sample of human societies and found there were differences between societies using dreams to seek and control supernatural powers and those that do not. Those seeking such control tended to be in North America, in non-fixed settlements, with simple agriculture or incipient food production and an average population less than 200. Also, they had few complex institutions and little class stratification or hierarchy. For D'Andrade (1961), the element of male transfer in matrilocal groups seemed to be explained by male anxiety of isolation and powerlessness. Beatrice Whiting (1963) and Barry et al. (1959) attempted an analysis of causal chains of child rearing and social conditioning to find latent content in dreams to support ideas of modal personality. The terms "latent" and "manifest" are often found in the literature of dreams, with "manifest" referring to those elements of dreams or whole dreams that are clear or understandable to the dreamer and others (see Freud 1961, 135).

Zinacantecans claim to recall dreams with great detail, but Laughlin (1976) found there was no agreement on the kind of dreams that were recalled. Some thought only good ones, others only nightmares, and a few only "true dreams." But Laughlin also cautions us on the use of dreams as sociological materials. As opposed to D'Andrade (1961), Whiting (1963), and others, he does not find the dreams particularly informative about sociological analysis and quotes Wolfram Eberhard's (1968) conclusion in analysis of Taiwanese dreams where the structure of the family would not include any babies if one were to look to dreams as sources.

The lack of women's similarly structured response to transfer out of their natal group in patrilocal residence was not noted. One wonders if this was a result of a lack of interest on the part of the researchers who produced the original studies D'Andrade drew on or if it was not of interest to him. This question plagues almost all areas of human research. If we are not interested in what happens to women and how they think about their status, we have then only half the story of what it means to be human. Richard's (1956) study of the girls' rite, the Chisungu, is one of the few detailed and situated studies that took place before missionaries and colonial policy masked originality of female worth. Ardener's (1956) sketch of female Bakweri rites of the woman's mermaid world where nothing manmade, imported or traded by men is allowed, gives a glimmer of an alternative world. Women of the Bakweri work in the forest, and natural lands are considered near wild and have a secret language used in healing. McKenna (1992) goes farther, he argues that the central deficit in modernity is the lack of a female principle in the Judeo-Christian-Islamic tradition. Its god, Yahwah/Jehova, is not coupled with a goddess as in most religions. Patai (1990) has argued that there was such a principle, represented in different form over the history of the tradition, including that of the Shekina. But this aspect of the religion has not survived in any significant form in the modern tradition. There has been some argument over the past 2,000 years concerning Mary, but the variation in Marian Cult ideology and function does not provide a framework for female empowerment (see Carroll, 2022).

What is missing from a full understanding of human nature and its potential is not just fuller accounts of alternative lives like that of the Bakweri that women have had, but evidence to unveil the philosophic contrasts of dualities, male–female, day–night, and so on, which appear as if sometimes starkly contrasted by unique conditions. For example, we see in the status of intersex people plagued with similar dualities (Carroll, 2022). This is especially true of those individuals whose condition is due to androgen insensitivity syndrome (AIS). These individuals can look entirely female yet have an X and a Y sex chromosome. In complete AIS, they appear entirely female; male genitalia fail to develop. In partial AIS, they can have testes, usually undescended, but can appear very female. Two individuals have recently made a significant impression on the way many people think of intersex. Susannah Temko and Emily Quinn (https://www.youtube.com/watch?v=stUl_OapUso&t=38s) both appear as normal beautiful women, yet they both were born intersex (https://www.youtube.com/watch?v=Vaq4Ij0qmog). In complete AIS, the individual appears completely female and creates a "female habitus" or body with all secondary sexual characteristics. In partial AIS, the individual has different numbers of male traits. Variation depends on the mutation that prevents an androgen from being fully functional during the development of the fetus and child. What is remarkable is not that it occurs, but that the failure of the functional androgen allows, in some cases, full female habitus to take place. Thus, what it means to be female does not depend on the presence of an X or Y chromosome, but on hormonal presence, yet also the caveat appears when the complete AIS individuals find that they do not have functional reproductive organs, usually only a vaginal area. This is curious, as they have no testes, and one would assume the development of ovaries would take place. Their status, once discovered, as shattering as it is to them personally, also unfolds within a family and social context.

Another type of intersex that is seldom encountered or documented is Pseudovaginal Perineoscrotal Hypospadia. This is a condition where the individual is born with a microphallus, labia-like scrotum, a blind-ending vagina and undescended testicles and Wolffian duct, though the exact physiology varies in different cases. The external genetalia appear female but are either incomplete or missing internally. In some cases at puberty the individual begins to receive normal amounts of testosterone and often undergoes behavioral changes (Bartsch, et al. 1987). In some cases, as among the Sambain people, at puberty physical development of male genitalia takes place with the development of a functional phallus but small. These individuals are called Kwolu-aatmwol and are not considered full males (Herdt 1981; Bergsma 1979). A variety of causes have been discovered for these in neonates (Zdravkovic, et al. 2001).

But to continue the initial thread, if women do not dream of the kind of images of conflict noted for males which D'Andrade's data suggests, is it due to the lack of a struggle for social power characteristic of male roles in society or to the lack of such struggle for women? Is the context of women in a patrilocal family not also powerless and isolated? Should we not expect a young woman to have at least unusual dreams as a result or do they but they are not collected? D'Andrade also looks at childrearing practices as a factor, but does not find it useful. Yet, as one is growing up, the question of what a person can expect does condition their responses, and if males find conflict a constant problem with the matrilineal males in their new location, then that struggle could be a foundation for dreams of power and control, especially as these are qualities associated with being male. For females, this is not the case, and yet should we not expect dreams of isolation and loss? Perhaps we might consider it would not be if they are not expected and the Native theory does not call for them. In the sample of dreams by males and females produced in this text from a variety of sources over time and across cultures, one can see that there are significant differences in female and male dreams. Some researchers have noted this, as in Goodison (1995). Surveying the literature, it would seem that the reason for so many dreams of houses and homes might be due to enculturation.

A considerable debate exists today over this issue of gender identity and expectation of conditioned role acquisition in transgendered individuals. A division between trans and cis males and females (trans-male to female or female to male vs. cisborn as male or female) lies on the boundary of what can one be if not born as a socially recognized gendered person. Some feminists have argued that transgendered males to female cannot really be female, as they did not experience the conditioning of being female (Burkett 2015). Thus, they are exposed to the privilege of being male for some years and then become female-gendered later at some point in life. The central issue here, summarizing most reports, is the vulnerability of women to the violence of men and the potential for rape and pregnancy.

The problem of gender was one I was interested in during my undergraduate years. This became a focus of my study of LSD in 1966–1967: why were so few women involved in the studies, and why were their responses so less emphatic than the males? I was quite interested in animal studies at the time as well, and especially the process of castrating male rats and then administering estrogen to determine the effect of gender as genetic or hormonal. Theories were legion on this subject, especially due to the variation in gender identity already known at the time.

But recent studies of rats and LSD have produced some interesting outcomes. Palenicek et al. (2010) administered 200 mg/kg LSD to male, oestral- and pro-oestral-phase females (EP), metoestral- (MD females) and dioestral-phase females and found that in the males the drug produced inhibitory locomotor effects, but in the pro-oestral-phase females and MD females locomotor and exploratory behaviors were not affected and EP females had increased rearing after. But this does not inform us as to the reason for so few women involved in the studies. Given Darlington's (2002) study, this appears to be mainly bias and neglect.

I wrote in my notes of the sessions I attended, some laboratory and some not, "After the LSD experience, since your conditioning has changed, you will not respond as before to the interaction of friends or exhibit your social role, at least not to the extent of its prior configuration." I think I wrote this down during one of the talks given, not a quote, but a summary. I have mentioned this problem before in relation to my own use of LSD among friends and my expectation that our presentation of self would be modified in some objective and noticeable manner. Blum et al. (1964a, 72) found that 62% of those who used LSD in their experiments and continued to do so changed their habits of social life to spent more time with others who had also experienced the drug. But the architecture of self seemed to be unchanged to all attempts at examination, of friends or myself. So in the consideration of females taking psychedelics I also expected some significant association that would be expressed. One wonders, certainly as Margaret Mead (1954, 1970) discusses male and female roles and responses to psychological tests, that the realization of being a female in a society, especially one that celebrates masculinity and depreciates and exploits females and femininity, why the female individual does not find this oppression questionable in more cases. Certainly we have the feminist revolt, and the sanction of women who do rebel or question the reason for their subjection, as in Elizabeth Gould Davis (1971), Betty Freidan (1963), Germaine Greer (1971), de Beauvoir (1949), and so many others. Even when we tally the victims who rebelled against their condition, the numbers seem so small. Hrdy (1981) attempts to set human gender in a rational biological context, yet ever here the subjugation of women, while plausible, lacks an analysis of why a thinking being can be so degraded. Greer (1971) gives a reasonable explanation of this, but unlike de Beauvoir (1949) accepts many standard biological limitations. Mind control, brainwashing, and identification with passivity and the inculcation of limits as Freud assumed still leave one adrift. Yet acceptance is framed in cultural reinforcement (both positive and negative so that identity is constructed on an awareness that begins at birth). If one does not find contradictions or alternatives, one's rebellion can even seem irrational to the rebel. Manon Garcia (2021) places this in a context that seems parallel to Ardener's (1975) silent or "muted" populations.

Aside from physiological universals due to the effects of various psychoactive substances, like increased pulse, sweating, or decreased heart rate and sleep-induced conditions, de Rios and Smith (1977) found some essential uniformities. These included spiritual feelings, animation of plant and animals as communicative entities, death and resurrection or rebirth, and paranormal phenomena. A point first noted by Harner (1972) and supported in de Rios and Smith's work was the reduction of use and positive regard of hallucinogens as societies become more complex. However, other psychoactive agents like alcohol increase in use and value. Blum (1964) found that in most societies where hallucinogens were used, they were limited to men and this was supported by de Rios and Smith's work. We are not informed if there was any association with social organization, as in matriarchy and the status of women. But it appears in human social evolution that women have been both muted and limited in attaining access to the spirit world via psychedelics. It seems that the fact that women contain a passage to the spirit world through their birth of children is a factor. This condition creates a status that is partly charged with spiritual power or liminality and the liminality of women is well known cross-culturally (Douglas 1966).

Similar to Jung's idea of collective unconscious, Freud also related some notion of a similar type under the term "archaic remnants." In Lecture 13 of the *Introductory Lectures* (1966, 199) Freud discusses this idea as an extension of the recapitulation of the phylogenetic history of each organism as described by Haeckel (1866). A modern conception of this idea is epigenetics, where heritable changes in gene expression take place as a result of DNA methylation, histone modification, and non-coding RNA (ncRNA)-associated gene silencing. This mechanism seems limited, given current evidence (Lind and Spagopoulou 2018), only to gene regulation and rarely constitutes transgenerational inheritance (Skvortsova et al. 2018). This is a much different idea than what Jung or Freud proposed, but one might argue that these changes could theoretically preserve experiences and they could be transmitted. But at present this is in the realm of science fiction. Other means of generational effects are supported, however. Recent research into emotional trauma (Curry 2019) seems to extend Bowbly's findings on motherless children into changes in a child's biology due to the emotional trauma of the parent. It would seem that the only real evidence might be differences in enculturation due to different rearing techniques, over generations. The outcome of interethnic marriages does not provide significant data on this issue, for example, familial patterns of aggression, alcoholism, and so on in one or the other parent broken by an interethnic marriage. Current studies are limited and only address issues of child welfare (Pearce-Morris and King 2012).

I have become rather unmoved by new claims of cures in psychotherapy in general. They remind me of the response of Warren S. McCulloch, Professor of Psychiatry, to a lecture given by mathematician and computer scientist John von Newmann gave in 1951 at the Hixon Symposium. Von Neumann was describing the nature of automatons as machines that could be programed to do things, like make other automatons and repair them. McCulloch's comment related to the problem of healing mental illness:

> Unfortunately for us in the biological sciences—or, at least, in psychiatry—we are presented with an alien, or enemy's machine. We do not know exactly what the machine is supposed to do and certainly we have no blueprint of it. In attacking our problems, we only know, in psychiatry, that the machine is producing wrong answers. We know that, because of the damage by the machine to the machine itself and by its running amuck in the world. However, what sort of difficulty exists in that machine is no easy matter to determine.

It seems in the years since the Symposium, with all the discoveries of neurotransmitters and oxygen uptake in MRI or other instrumentation, we are little advanced in our ability to cure. A number of critiques have appeared in recent years that reinforced my opinion and experience that treatments for psychological problems were often useless, damaging, or themselves a form of entertainment some people became addicted to and thus exploitative. Some studies have supported this idea (Eisner 2000) and received mild criticism. Lilienfeld (2002) produced a balanced review of a number of critiques of psychotherapy, including Eisner's, and cited an early meta-study of techniques and practice (inter-operator error). Meta-studies have been interesting in that they give a baseline for regarding claims of cures. Cuijpers et al. (2008) reviewed 53 studies of treatment methods and found little difference between them in effectively treating depression. Wierzbicki and Pekarik (1993) found that dropout rate of their review of 125 was related to the socio-economic status and definition of "dropout."

A study of meta-studies was inevitable and one by Brown (1987) looked at the six meta-studies published up to that date and identified a number of deficiencies. Another using a network approach found some differences among methods and over "waitlist control condition," which is not a true control, as the control population does receive some treatment (Barth et al. 2013). Other research with psilocybin-assisted therapy has also claimed success (Davis et al. 2020). The authors found in a randomized clinical trial that the psilocybin-assisted therapy was effective in producing sustained anti-depressant effect in patients with major depressive disorder. Assessment was based on the GRID-Hamilton Rating Scale (GRID-HAMD).

Yet Mogar (1965a) reported significant positive results, especially when other treatment methods had failed, and Unger (1964) reported on the successes that he considered resulted from LSD therapy in over 1000 cases. The nature of cure, as in cancer treatment, depends on the view of the patient, their family, and the therapist. If a five-year length of life is "success," then when people report a regression after some years of improvement, it should be seen in positive terms (Insel and Scolnick 2006). The caveat here is the nature of human variability and what is sometimes called "operator error." Not every practitioner utilizes techniques in the exact same way and interpretations of "cure" in both the patient and the therapist may differ as to the goals and stability of treatment outcomes. Efforts to address these problems show promise (Medau et al. 2013).

References

Ackerknecht, Erwin H., (1943) "Psychopathology, primitive medicine and primitive culture," *Bulletin of the History of Medicine*, 14, 3–67.

Adebimpe, V.R., H.E. Klein and J. Fried, (1981) "Hallucinations and delusions in black psychiatric patients," *J. Natl. Med. Assoc.* June, v. 73, n. 6, 517–520.

Anderson, Robert (2005*) The Ghosts of Iceland*, Independence, KY, Cengage Learning.

Ardener, Shirley (1975) "Introduction," in *Perceiving Women*, (ed.) Shirley Ardener, pp. vii–xxiii.

Ardener, Edwin (1956) *Coastal Bantu of the Cameroons,* London, Oxford University Press for the International African Institute.

Aviram, Liat and Nirit Soffer-Dudek, (2018) "Lucid dreaming: intensity, but not frequency, is inversely related to psychopathology," Frontiers in Psychology, Mar. 22, 9, 384,: 10.3389/fpsyg.2018.00384.

Ayers, Susan, (2017) "Birth trauma and post-traumatic stress disorder: the importance of risk and resilience," *J. of Reproductive and Infant Psychology*, v. 35, n. 5, 427–430.

Bainton, Roland H. (1955) *Here I Stand, A Life of Martin Luther*, New York, Mentor Book.

Barron, F. (1967) Motivational patterns in LSD usage," in R.C. Debold & R.C. Leaf (eds) *LSD, Man and Society*, Middletown, Wesleyan University Press, 128–139.

Barry, H., III, Bacon, M. K. & Child, I. L. (1959). Relations of child training to subsistence economy. *American Anthropologist*, 61, 51–63.

Barth, Jurgen, Thomas Munder, Heike Gerger, Eveline Nuesch, Sven Trelle, et al., (2013) "Comparative efficacy of seven psychotherapeutic interventions for patients with depression: a network meta-analysis," *PloS Medicine,* May 28: https://doi.org/10.1371/journal.pmed.1001454.

Bartholomew, Robert; Wessely, Simon (2002). "Protean nature of mass sociogenic illness". *The British Journal of Psychiatry*. **180**: 300–306. https://doi.org/10.1192/bjp.180.4.300.

Batson, G. and M. Mead (1942) *Balinese character: a photographic analysis*, Special Publications of the New York Academy of Sciences, v, II.

Baudrillard, J. (1981) *Simulacra and Simulation,* Los Angeles, Semiotext.

Beck, Cheryl Tatano, (2015) "Middle range theory of traumatic childbirth," *Glob Qual Nurs Res*, Jan–Dec., https://doi.org/10.1177/2333393615575313.

Belo, Jane (1960) *Trance in Bali,* New York, Columbia University Press.

Bickerton, Derek (1990) *Language and Species*, Chicago, University of Chicago Press.

Bion, Wilfred R. (1977) *Two Papers: The Grid and Caesura*, Rio de Janeiro, Imago Editora, reprint, London Karnac 1989.

Blacker, Carmen (1975) *The Catalpa Bow, London*, George Allen & Unwin.

Blair, Lawrence (2010) *Ring of Fire: An Indonesian Odyssey*, Paris, Editions Didier Millet.

Blair, Lawrence and Lorne Blair (1988) *The Dream Wanderers of Borneo*, PBS/C.

Blanke, Olaf and Thomas Metzinger, (2008) "Full-body illusions and minimal phenomenal selfhood," *Trends in Cognitive Sciences*, v. 13, n. 1, 7–14.

Blum, Richard (1964) *Drugs and Society*, v. 1, Stanford, Ca. Jossey-Bass.

Blum, Richard, Eva Blum and Mary Lou Funkhouser, (1964a) "The institutionalization of LSD," in Blum, Richard, Nevitt Sanford, Eva Blum, Mary Lou Funkhouser, Joseph J. Downing, et al., (eds.) *Utopiates: The Use and Users of LSD-25, A Publication of the Institute for the Study of Human Problems*, Stanford University, Atherton Press, 124–141.

Blum, Richard, Nevitt Sanford, Eva Blum, Mary Lou Funkhouser, Joseph J. Downing, et al., (1964b) *Utopiates: The Use and Users of LSD-25*, A Publication of the Institute for the Study of Human Problems Stanford University, Atherton Press.

Boag, Simon (2017) "On dreams and motivation: comparison of Freud's and Hobson's views," *Front. Psychol.* 6 January, https://doi.org/10.3389/fpsyg.2016.02001

Boksa, Patricia (2009) "On the neurobiology of hallucinations," *J. Psychiatry Neurosci.*, 34, 4, 260–262.

Booth, William, (1988) "Voodoo science," Science, v. 240, n. 4850, 274–7.

Bourguignon, E. (1972) "Dreams and altered states of consciousness in Anthropological research," in *Psychological Anthropology*, Francis L.R. Hsu (ed.) Cambridge, MA., Schenkman Publishing Co.,: 401–434.

Bourguignon, E. (1973) *Religion, Altered States of Consciousness and Social Change*, Columbus, OH, Ohio State University Press.

Bowlby, John (1953) *Child Care and the Growth of Love*, Harmondsworth, Penguin Books.

Brown, Joseph (1987) "A review of meta-analyses conducted on psychotherapy outcome research," *Clinical Psychology Review*, v. 7, n. 1:1–23.

Browne, Malcolm W. (1988) "The benzene ring: dream analysis," *The New York Times*, Aug. 16, section C, page 10.

Bulkeley, Kelly (2019) "The cultural dimensions of dreaming," *Psychology Today*, April 19:https://www.psychologytoday.com/us/blog/dreaming-in-the-digital-age/201904/the-cultural-dimensions-dreaming.

Burkett, Elinor (2015) "What makes a woman?" *The New York Times*, June 6th, https://www.nytimes.com/2015/06/07/opinion/sunday/what-makes-a-woman.html.

Caldararo, Niccolo (2014) *The Psychic Unity of Mankind*, Saarbrucken, Scholars' Press.

Caldararo, Niccolo (2012) *Evolutionary Aspects of Disease Avoidance*, Saarbrucken, Scholars' Press.

Caldararo, Niccolo (2019) *An Ethnography of the Goodman Building*, The Longest Rent Strike, New York, Palgrave/Macmillan.

Campbell, Joseph (1949) *Hero with a Thousand Faces*, Cleveland, World Publishing Co.

Campbell, Joseph (1972) *Myths to Live By*, New York, Bantam Edition.

Carhart-Harris, Robin L., Suresh Muthukumaraswamy, Leor Roseman, Mendel Kaelen, Wouter Droog, et al., (2016) "Neural correlates of the LSD experience revealed by multimodal neuroimaging," PNAS, April 26, v. 113, n. 17:4853–4858.

Carod-Artal, F.J. (2013) "Psychoactive plants in ancient Greece," *Neurosciences and History*, v. 1, n. 1, 28–38.

Carroll, Michael P. (2022) *The Cult of the Virgin Mary*, Princeton, Princeton University Press.

Cartwright, Rosalind (1977) *Night Life*, Hoboken, Prentice-Hall

Cartwright, Roslind (2010) *The Twenty-Four Hour Mind*, Oxford, Oxford University Press.

Chandler, Arthur and Mortimer Hartman, (1960) "LSD-25 as a facilitating agent in psychotherapy," *Archives of General Psychiatry*, 2 (3) , 286–299.

Chaudhury, Suprakash, (2010) "Hallucinations: clinical aspects and management," *Ind. Psychiatry J.*, Jan–Jun, 19, 1, 5–12.

Codrington, R.H. (1891) *The Melanesians*, New York, Dover Publications, 1972 edition.

Crick, Francis and Graeme Mitchison (1983) "The function of dream sleep," *Nature*, 14 July, 304, 111–114.

Cuijpers, Pim, Annermieke van Straten, Gerhard Andersson and Patricia van Oppen, (2008) *J. Consult Clin Psychol.* V. 76, n 6:909–922.

Curry, Andrew (2019) "Parent's emotional trauma may change their children's biology. Studies in mice show how," *Science*, July 18, https://doi.org/10.1126/science.aay7690

Cytowic, Richard E. (2002) *Synesthesia: A Union of the Senses*, (2nd Ed.) Cambridge, Mass. MIT Press.

Cytowic, Richard E. (2003) *The Man who Tasted Shapes,* Cambridge, Mass., MIT Press.

Darlington, Cynthia (2002) *The Female Brain,* London, Taylor and Francis.

D'Andrade, Roy (1961) "Anthropological studies of dreams," in *Psychological Anthropology*, F.L.K. Hsu, (ed.) Homewood, Ill., Dorsey Press.

Darwin, Charles, (1871) The Descent of Man and Selection in Relation to Sex, Chicago, W.B. Conkey Company, Revised, Second Edition, 1874.

da Silva, Ksenija Maravic (2013) "The Neuropsychology of visual halluncinations in Parkinson's Disease and the Continuum Hypothesis," in *Hallucination: Philosophy and Psychology*, (eds.) Fiona Macpherson and Dimitris Platchias, Cambridge, MA, MIT Press, pp. 105–120.

Davis, Alan, Frederick S. Barrett, Darrick G. May, et al., (2020) "Effects of Psilocybin-assisted therapy on major depressive disorder," *JAMA Psychiatry*, 4 November, :https://doi.org/10.1001/jamapsychiatry.2020.3285

Davis, Eliszabeth Gould (1971) *The First Sex,* New York, G.P. Putnam's Sons.

de Beauvoir, Simone (1949) *The Second Sex*, New York, Random House.

de Rios, Marlene Dobkin (1984) *Hallucinogens: Cross-Cultural Perspectives*, Albuquerque, University of New Mexico Press.

de Rios, Marlene Dobkin and David E. Smith (1977) "Drug use and abuse in cross cultural perspective," v. 36, n. 1, Spring, 14–21.

Devereux, George (1961) "Shamans as neurotics," *Amer. Anth.* V. 63, 5, 1088–1090.

Doblin, Rick (1991) "Pahnke's 'Good Friday Experiment,': A long-term follow-up and methodological critique,'" *Journal of Transpersonal Psychology*, v. 23, 1:1–28.

Domhoff, G. William and Kieran C.R. Fox (2015) "Dreaming and the default network: a review, synthesis, and counterintuitive research proposal," *Consciousness and Cognition*, v. 33, May, 342–353.

Douglas, Mary (1966) *Purity and Danger: an Analysis of Concepts of Pollution and Taboo,* Harmondsworth, Penguin.

Durkheim, Emile (1915) *The Elementary Forms of the Religious Life,* London, George Allen & Unwin.

Eberhard, Wolfram (1968) "Social interaction and social values in Chinese dreams, " *Journal of Sociology*, National Taiwan University, 4:21–43.

Eggan, Dorthy (1966) "Hope dreams in cultural perspective," In *The Dream and Human Societies,* G.E. von Grunebaum and R. Caillois, eds., Berkeley and Los Angeles, University of California Press.

Eisner, D.A. (2000) *The Death of Psychotherapy: From Freud to Alien Abduction*, Westport, CT, Praeger.
Eliade, Mircea (1964) *Shamanism*, Bolligen Foundation, Princeton, Princeton University Press.
Erwin, Edward (1980) "Psychoanalysis: how firm is the evidence?" *Nous*, v. 14, n. 3, Special issue on Psychoanalysis, Sept:443–456.
Fabian, Johannes (1966) "Dream and charisma, 'theories of dreams' in the Jamaa Movement (Congo)," *Anthropos*, 61, 544–560.
Fabrega, Horacio Jr., (1997) *Evolution of Sickness and Healing*, 172–181.
Ferriar, J. (1813) *An Essay Towards a Theory of Apparitions,* London, Cadell and Davies.
Ffytche, Dominic H. (2013) "The hallucinating brain: neurobiological insights into the nature of hallucinations," Chapter 3, in *Hallucination: Philosophy and Psychology*, (eds.) Fiona Macpherson and Dimitris Platchias, Cambridge, MA, MIT Press, pp. 45–64.
Fortuna, Lisa (n.d.) "Working with Latino/a and Hispanic Patients," *American Psychiatric Association: Best Practices,* https://www.psychiatry.org/psychiatrists/cultural-competency/education/best-practice-highlights/working-with-latino-patients. Accessed January 11, 2022.
Freud, Sigmund (1966) *The Complete Introductory Lectures on Psychoanalysis,* trans. James Strachey (ed.) New York, W.W. Norton.
Freud, Sigmund (1961) *The Interpretation of Dreams*, Trans. And Edited by James Strachey, New York, Science Editions.
Freud, Sigmund (1962) *Civilization and its Discontents*, College Edition, New York, W.W. Norton.
Friedan, Betty (1963) *The Feminine Mystique,* New York, W.W. Norton.
Fromm, Erick (1951) *The Forgotten Language: An Introduction to the Understanding of Dreams, Fairy Tales and Myths,* New York, Grove Press.
Furst, Peter T. (1972) *Flesh of the Gods, the Ritual Use of Hallucinogens*, New York, Praeger.
Gajaram, Ganya, Tiffiney Lake, Dung Nguyen, Sukhjeet Sangha, Ayodeji Jolayemi, (2021) "Autoscopic hallucinations in an African American female patient with schizophrenia," *Cureus*, Feb. 23, 13(2): e13510. https://doi.org/10.7759/cureus.13510.
Galouye, Daniel F. (1964) *Simulacron-3,* New York, Bantam Books.
Garcia, Manon (2021) *We Are Not Born Submissive*, Princeton, Princeton University Press.

Geltman, David and Grace Chang, (2004) "Hallucinations in Latino psychiatric outpatients: A preliminary investigation," *General Hospital Psychiatry,* 26(2):153–7

Gilmore, John H., Rebecca Knickmeyer Santelli and Wei Gao, (2018) "Imaging structural and functional brain development in early childhood," *Nat. Rev Neurosci,* Feb. 16, 19, 3, 123–137.

Goldsmith, S.K., T.C. Pellmar, A.M. Kleinman, et al., (2002) *Reducing Suicide: A National Imperative,* Washington, D.C., National Academies Press.

Goodison, Lucy (1995) *The Dreams of Women: Exploring and Interpreting Women's Dreams,* New York, W.W. Norton.

Greenfield, Mari, Julie Jomeen and Lesley Glover, (2016) "What is traumatic birth? A concept analysis and literature review," *British Journal of Midwifery,* v. 24, 4, https://doi.org/10.12968/bjom.2016.24.4.254

Greer, Germaine (1971) *The Female Eunuch,* London, Granada.

Grieder, Terence (1982) *Origins of Pre-Columbian Art,* Austin, University of Texas Press.

Grof, Stanislav (1976) *Realms of the Human Unconscious: Observation from LSD Research.* New York, E.P. Dutton.

Grunbaum, Adolf (1977) "How scientific is psychoanalysis?" in *Science and Psychotherapy,* (ed) Raphael Stem, L.S. Horowitz and J. Lynes, New York Haven Publishing.

Grunbaum, Adolf (1980) "Epistemological liabilities of the clinical appraisal of Psychoanalytic Theory," *Nous,* XIV, 3, Sept: 427–442.

Haeckel, Ernst (1866) *Generelle Morphologie der Organismen (General Morphology of the Organisms)* Berlin, G. Reimer.

Hallowell, A. Irving (1966) "The role of dreams in Ojibwa culture," in (eds.) G.E. Von Gruebaum and R. Caillois, *The Dream and Human Societies,* Berkeley, University of California Press: 267–292.

Harman, WW, McKim, RH, Mogar, RE, Fadiman, J., Stolaroff, MJ. (1966) Psychedelic Agents in Creative Problem-solving: A Pilot Study. *Psychol Rep.* 1:211–27.

Harner, Michael (1972) *Hallucinogens and Shamanism,* Oxford, Oxford University Press.

Harrison, John (2013) "Love is the answer, an appreciation of Myron Stolaroff (August 20, 1920–January 6, 2013)," *MAPS Bulletin Special Edition,* 44–47.

Hellie, Benj (2013) "The multidisjuntive conception of hallucination," in *Hallucination: Philosophy and Psychology,* (eds.) Fiona Macpherson and Dimitris Platchias, Cambridge, MA, MIT Press, pp. 149–174.

Henning, W.B., (1951) *Zoroaster: Politican or Witch-Doctor,* Ratanbai Katrak Lectures at Oxford, Oxford University Press.

Hines, Kevin, (2013) *Cracked, Not Broken*, Lanham, Rowman & Littlefield.
Hobson, J. A., and McCarley, R. W. (1977). The brain as a dream-state generator: an activation-synthesis hypothesis of the dream process. *Am. J. Psychiatry* 134, 1335–1348.
Hrdy, Sarah Blaffer (1981) *The Woman That Never Evolved*, Cambridge, MA., Harvard University Press.
Huang, Deqin, Ling Dai, Tieying Zeng, Haishan Huang, Meiliyang Wu, et al., "Exploring contributing factors to psychological traumatic childbirth from the perspective of midwives: a qualitative study," (2019), *Asian Nursing Research,* v. 13, 4, 270–276.
Hudson, Charles (1979) *Black Drink: A Native American Tea*, University of Georgia Press.
Humphrey, Nicholas (1986) *The Inner Eye*, Oxford, Oxford University Press.
Hunter, Monica (1961) *Reaction to Conquest*, 2nd edition, Oxford University Press.
Huxley, Aldous (1963) "A philosopher's visionary prediction (about hallucinogens, " *Playboy*, November.
Huxley, Aldous (1954) *The Doors of Perception, and Heaven and Hell*, New York, Harper Colophon Books.
Insel, T.R. and E. M. Scolnick (2006) "Cure therapeutics and strategic prevention: raising the bar for mental health research," *Molecular Psychiatry,* v. 11, 11–17.
Jacobs, Andrew (2021) "Psychedelics gain mainstream traction," *The New York Times*, May 10th.
Janov, Arthur (1970) *Primal Scream*, New York, Dell.
Jenner JA, Nienhuis FJ, van de Willige G, Wiersma D. (2006) "'Hitting' voices of schizophrenia patients may lastingly reduce persistent auditory hallucinations and their burden: 18 month outcome of a randomized control trial," *Can J Psychiatry*. 51:169–77.
Jung, C.G. (2014) *Collected Works*, volume 7, Princeton, Princeton University Press (original Bollingen Series, XX, 1953 as Two Essays on Psychoanalysis.
Jung, C.G. (1960) "Synchronicity: an acausal connecting principle," *Collected Works,* vol. 8, Princeton, Princeton University Press.
Jung, C.G. (1933) *Modern Man in Search of a Soul,* New York, Harcourt Brace.
Junghanns K, Wetterling T. (2017) [Alcohol withdrawal and its major complications]. *Fortschr Neurol Psychiatr*. Mar;85(3):163–177.
Karakaya, Burcu Kisa, Ozlem Morloglu, Rahime Bedir Findik, et al., (2018) "Evaluation of maternal and fetal stress hormones during the process of birth," Gynecology Obstetrics and Reproductive Medicine, v. 24, n 2, https://doi.org/10.21613/GORM.2017.753.

Keitt, Andrew (2005) "The miraculous body of evidence: visionary experience, medical discourse and the Inquisition in Seventeenth century Spain," *The Sixteenth Century Journal*, v. 36, 1, Spring, 77–96.
Kelly, George A. (1963) *A Theory of Personality*, New York, The Norton Library.
King, A.J. (2004) "The superior colliculus," *Current Biology*, v. 14, n. 9:R335–8.
Kleitman, Nathaniel (1963) *Sleep and Wakefulness*, revised edition, Chicago, University of Chicago Press.
Klemperer F. (1992) "Ghosts, visions, voices," *BMJ*; 305:1518–9.
Kluver, Heinrich (1966) Mescal: The Divine Plant and Its Psychological Effects, Kegan Paul (originally published in 1928).
La Barre, Weston (1975) "Anthropological perspectives on hallucination and hallucinogens," in *Hallucinations: Behavior, Experience and Theory*, (eds.) R. K. Siegel and L.J. West, New York, John Wiley, & Sons, 9–52.
Laing, R.D. (1959) *The Divided Self*, Harmondsworth, Pelican Books.
Laughlin, Robert M. (1976) *Of Wonders Wild and New: Dreams from Zinacantan*, Smithsonian Contributions to Anthropology, n. 22, Washington, D.C., Smithsonian Institution.
Leary, Timothy and Frank Barron, (1955) "Changes in psychoneurotic patients with and without psychotherapy," *Journal of Consulting Psychology*, v. 19, n. 4, 239–245.
Lee, Teresa M.Y., Siow Ann Chong, Yiong Huat Chan and Gangaharan Sathvadevan, (2004) "Command hallucinations among Asian patients with schizophrenia," *Can J Psychiatry*, Dec;49(12):838–42.
Leibowitz, Herschel W. (1965) *Visual Perception*, New York, The Macmillan Co.
Lerner, Michael and Michael Lyvers (2006) "Values and beliefs of psychedelic drug users: a cross-cultural study," *J. Psychoactive Drugs*, June, v. 38, 2, 143–7.
Levy-Bruhl, Lucien (1966) *Primitive Mentality*, (originally published in 1923) Boston, Beacon Press.
Lewis, Simon J.G., James M. Shine, Daniel Brooks and Glenda M. Halliday, (2015) "Hallucinogenic mechanisms: pathological and pharmacological insights," Chapter 6, in *The Neuroscience of Visual Hallucinations*, (Eds.) Daniel Collerton, Urs Peter Mosimann and Elain Perry, New York, Wiley, pp. 121–150.
Lienhardt, Godfrey (1954) "The Shilluk of the Upper Nile," in *African Worlds*, D. Forde (ed.) International African Institute, London, Oxford University Press.
Lilienfeld, Scott O. (2002) "The rumors of my death have been greatly exaggerated," Book Review, *Scientific Review of Mental Health Practice*, Fall-Winter, v. 1, n. 2:
Lilly, John (1972) *The Center of the Cyclone*, Berkeley,Ca, Ronin Publishing.

Lincoln, J. S. (1935) *The Dream in Primitive Cultures*, London, Cressett Press.
Lind, Martin I. and Foteini Spagopoulou, (2018) "Evolutionary consequences of epigenetic inheritance," *Heredity*, v. 121, 205–209.
Lohmann, Roger Ivar (2019) *Haunted Pacific*, Durham, NC, Carolina Academic Press.
Louie, Kenway and Matthew A. Wilson, (2001) "Temporarily structured replay of awake hippocampal ensemble activity during rapid eye movement sleep," *Neuron*, v. 29, 145–156.
Luhrmann, T.M. (2012) *When God Talks Back, Understanding the American Evangelical Relation with God*, New York, Knopf.
Martone, Robert (2019) "New clues found in understanding near-death experiences," *Scientific American*, Sept 10, https://www.scientificamerican.com/article/new-clues-found-in-understanding-near-death-experiences/
Maslow, Abraham H. (1961) "Peak experiences as acute identity experiences," *American Journal of Psychoanalysis*, 21, 254–262.
Maslow, Abraham H. (1962) *Toward a Psychology of Being*, Princeton, van Norstrand.
Maslow, Abraham H. (1964) *Religions, Values, and Peak-Experiences*, New York, Viking Press, edition with new editorial introduction and preface, 1970. Originally published as 35th volume in the Kappa Delta Pi Lecture Series
McKenna, Terence (1992) *Food of the Gods*, New York, Bantam Books.
McKenna, Terence (1993) *True Hallucinations, Being an Account of the Author's Extraordinary Adventures in the Devil's Paradise*, New York, HarperOne.
Mead, Margaret (1954) *Male and Female*, New York, Morrow & Co.
Mead, Margaret (1970) *Culture and Commitment*, New York, Columbia University Press.
Medau, Irina, Ralf J. Jox and Stella Reiter-Theil (2013) "How psychotherapists handle treatment errors," *BMC Med. Ethics*, v. 14, Dec. 9th, https://doi.org/10.1186/1472-6939-14-50.
Meduna, Ladislas J. (1950) *Carbon Dioxide Therapy*, Charles C. Thomas.
Meggitt, M.J. (1962) "Dream interpretation among the Mae Enga of New Guinea," *Southwest Journal of Anthropology*, v. 18, n. 3, 21–229.
Metzner, Ralph; Sophia Adamson and Julie Holland, ed. (2001). *Ecstasy: the complete guide; a comprehensive look at the risks and benefits of MDMA*. Rochester, Vt: Park Street Press.
Michael T. (2015) *Freud's Theory of Dreams*, Lanham, Rowman & Littlefield.
Mischoulon, David, Isabel T. Lagomasino and Chris Harmon (2005) "Atypical Psychotic Symptoms in a Hispanic Population: Diagnostic Dilemmas and Implications for Treatment," *Psychiatry (Edgmont)*. Oct; 2(10): 38–46.

Mogar, Robert E. (1965a) "Search and research with the psychedelics," ETC: A Review of General Semantics, v. 22, n. 4, Special Issue on the Psychedelic Experience, Dec.:393–407.

Mogar, Robert E., (1965b) "Current status and future trends in psychedelic (LSD) research," Journal of Humanistic Psychology, Oct. 1, v. 5, n. 2, 147–166.

Mogar, Robert E., and Charles Savage, (1964) "Personality change associated with psychedelic (LSD) therapy: a preliminary report," *Psychotherapy: Theory, Research & Practice, 1*(4), 154–162.

Montagu, Ashley (1989) "Origin of the specious," *The World & I*, April, 416–422.

Moran, Mark (2014) "Overdiagnosis of schizophrenia said to be persistent among Black patients," *Psychiatric News,* 29 Dec 2014, https://doi.org/10.1176/appi.pn.2015.1a17.

Mota, Natalia B., Adara Resende, Sergio A. Mota-Rolim, Mauro Copelli, and Sidarta Ribeiro, (2016) "Psychosis and the control of lucid dreaming," Frontiers in Psychology, v, 7, March 9th, https://doi.org/10.3389/fpsyg.2016.00294

Mullins, Niamh and Hailiang Huang, (2020) "Genetic architecture of bipolar disorder in individuals of Han Chinese and European ancestries," *JAMA Psychiatry*, December 2, 2020. https://doi.org/10.1001/jamapsychiatry.2020.3639

Naish, Peter (2013) "Hallucinations in hypnosis," in *Hallucination: Philosophy and Psychology*, (eds.) Fiona Macpherson and Dimitris Platchias, Cambridge, MA, MIT Press, pp. 121–146.

Nam, Eui-Cheol (2005) "Is it necessary to differentiate tinnitus from auditory hallucination in schizophrenic patients?" *J. Laryngol Otol.* May, 119, 5, 352–355.

Nelson, Kevin (2010) *The Spiritual Doorway in the Brain: A Neurologist's Search for the God Experience*, New York, Fenguin/Plume.

Nichols, David, Richard Yensen, Ralph Metzner and William Shakespeare, (1993) "The Great Entactogen-Empathogen Debate," Newsletter of the Multidisciplinary Association for Psychedelic Studies (MAPS), v. 4, n 2, 47–49.

Nicolai, C.F. (1803) "A memoir on the appearance of spectres or phantoms occasioned by disease with psychological remarks," *Nicholson's Journal of Natural Philosophy, Chemistry and the Arts,* VI, 161–179.

Nutt, David and Robin Carhart-Harris (2020) "The current status of psychedelics in Psychiatry," *JAMA Psychiatry*, June 24, https://doi.org/10.1001/jamapsychiatry.2020.2171.

Oliveri, M. and G. Calvo, (2003) "Increased visual cortical excitability in ecstasy users: a transcranial magnetic stimulation study," *J. of Neurology, Neurosurgery and Psychiatry,* v. 74, n. 8: 1136–1138.

Olson, David E, (2021) "The subjective effects of psychedelics may not be necessary for their enduring therapeutic effects," *ACE Pharmacology & Translational Science,* v. 4, 563–567.

Opler, Marvin K., (1959) "Dream analysis in Ute Indian therapy," in *Culture and Mental Health,* ed., Marvin K. Opler, New York, Macmillan.

Osmond, Humphry, (1970) "On being mad," in Aaronson, Bernard and Humphry Osmond, (eds) (1970) Psychedelics, The Uses and Implications of Hallucinogenic Drugs, Garden City, Anchor Books, 21–28.

Padosch, Stephan A., Dirk W. Lachenmeier and Lars U. Kroner, (2006) Subst Abuse Treat Prev Policy, v. 1, doi: 10.1186/1747-597X-1-14

Pagondiotis, Costas (2013) "Hallucination, mental representation, and the presentational character," in *Hallucination: Philosophy and Psychology,* (eds.) Fiona Macpherson and Dimitris Platchias, Cambridge, MA, MIT Press, pp. 361–380.

Pahnke, Walter (1963) *Drugs and Mysticism: An Analysis of the Relationship Between Psychedelic Drugs and the Mystical Consciousness,* Thesis, Harvard University, https://maps.org/images/pdf/books/pahnke/walter_pahnke_drugs_and_mysticism.pdf.

Palenicek, Tomas, Zdenek Hlinak, Vera Bubenikova-Valesova, Tomas Novak and Jin Horacek, (2010) "Sex differences in the effects of N,N-diethyllysergamide (LSD) on behavioural activity and prepulse inhibition," *Prog. Neuropsychopharmacol. Biol. Psychiatry,* May, 30, 34(4) 588–596.

Parfitt, Will (2003) *Psychosynthesis: The Elements and Beyond,* PS Avalon.

Patai, Raphael (1990) *The Hebrew Goddess,* Detroit, Wayne State University Press, third edition.

Pathis, Lawrence and Helena J. Younes (2015) "False memories in therapy and hypnosis before 1980," *Psychology of Consciousness: Theory, Research and Practice,* v, 2, n. 2: 153–169.

Pearce-Morris, Jennifer and Valerie King (2012) "Well-being of children living with interethnic parents: are they at an disadvantage?" *J. Fam. Issues,* May, 24, v. 33, 7, 898–919.

Perkins, Maureen (2001) *The Reform of Time,* New York, Pluto Press.

Phillips, Joseph R., Elie Matar, Kaylena A. Ehgoetz, Ahmed A. Moustafa, Glenda M. Halliday and Simon J.G. Lewis, (2021) "Evaluating a novel behavioral paradigm for visual hallucinations in dementia with Lewy bodies," *Aging Brain,* v. 1, https://doi.org/10.1016/j.nbas.2021.100011

Pollan, Michael (2018) *How to Change Your Mind: What the New Science of Psychedelics Teaches Us About Consciousness, Dying, Addiction, Depression, and Transcendence,* New York, Penguin.

Press, Michele (1987) "American Scientist Interviews: Wade Davis," *American Scientist*, v. 75, July–August, 412–417.

Radcliffe-Brown, A.R. (1932) *The Andaman Islanders*, Reprint edition, New York, The Free Press of Glencoe, 1964.

Ramaiah, G. Sundara and S.D.A. Joga Rao (1988) "Buddhist interpretation of dreams," *The Tibet Journal*, v, 13, n. 1, Spring:20–7.

Rank, Otto (1923) *The Trauma of Birth*, New York, Dover Books, reprint 1993.

Ratcliffe, Matthew (2021) "Sensed presence without sensory qualities: a phenomenological study of bereavement hallucinations," *Phenomenology and the Cognitive Sciences*, v. 20, 601–616.

Reina, R.E. (1966) *The Law of the Saints*, Indianapolis and New York, The Bobbs-Merrill Co.

Richards, Audrey I. (1956) *Chisungu: A Girl's Initiation Ceremony Among the Bemba of Northern Rhodesia*, London, Farber & Farber.

Roheim, Geza (1945) *The Eternal Ones of the Dream*, New York, International Universities Press.

Roheim, Geza (1952) *The Gates of the Dream*, New York International Universities Press.

Roheim, Geza (1968*) Psychoanalysis and Anthropology: Culture, Personality and the Unconscious*, New York, International Universities Press.

Rosen, Cherise, Nev Jones, Eleanor Longden, Kayla A. Chase, Mona Shattel, et al., (2017) "Exploring the Intersections of Trauma, Structural Adversity, and Psychosis among a Primarily African-American Sample: A Mixed-Methods Analysis," *Front. Psychiatry*, 19 April 2017 | https://doi.org/10.3389/fpsyt.2017.00057.

Sacks, Oliver (1985) *The Man Who Mistook His Wife for a Hat*, New York, Harper & Row, Perennial Library Edition.

Sacks, Oliver (2010) *The Mind's Eye*. New York, Knopf.

Sacks, Oliver (2012) *Hallucinations*, New York, Vintage Books.

Sagan, Carl, (1977) *Dragons of Eden*, New York, Random House.

Sanz, Camila, Frederico Zamberlan, Earth Erowid and Enzo Tagliazucchi (2018) "The experience elicited by hallucinogens presents the highest similarity to dreaming within a large database of psychoactive substance reports," *Front. Neurosci.*, v. 12, n. 7, 22 Jan. https://doi.org/10.3389/fnins.2018.00007

Sartorius N, Jablensky A, Korten A, Emberg G, Anker M, Cooper JE, et al. (1986) "Early manifestations and first contact incidence of schizophrenia in different cultures" *Psychol Med.*; 16:909–28.

Savage, Charles and Myron J. Stolaroff (1965) "Clarifying the confusion regarding LSD-25," *Journal of Nervous and Mental Disease*, v. 140, 218–221.

Schneider, Robert A. (1986) "Mortification on parade: penitential processions in Sixteenth and Seventeenth Century France," *Renaissance and Reformation*, New Series, v. 10, n. 1, 123–146.

Schneider, David and Laurison Sharp (1969) *The Dream Life of A Primitive People: The Dreams of the Yir Yoront of Australia*, Anthropological Studies, number 1, Ward Goodenough (ed) American Anthropological Association, Ann Arbor, Michigan. University Microfilms.

Schultes, R.E. (1972) "An overview of hallucinogens in the Western hemisphere," in Flesh of the Gods, (ed) Peter T. Furst, New York, Praeger Publishers: 3–54.

Seth, Anil (2021) *Being You: A New Science of Consciousness,* Faber.

Skvortsova, Ksenia, Nicola Iovino and Ozren Bogdanovic (2018) "Functions and mechanisms of epigenetic inheritance in animals," *Nature Reviews Molecular Cell Biology*, v. 19, 774–790.

Smith, Robertson W. (1894) *The Religion of the Semites*, New York, Edition, 1972.

Speer, Albert (1970) *Inside the Third Reich, Memoirs,* Trans. Richard and Clara Winston, New York, Macmillan Co.

Staford, P.G. and B.H. Golightly (1967) *LSD—The Problem-Solving Psychedelic,* New York, Award Books.

Stein, Barry E. and M. Alex Meredith (1993) *The Merging of the Senses*, Cambridge Mass., A Bradford Book, MIT Press.

Stevens, Jay (1988) *Storming Heaven: LSD and the American Dream*, New York, Harper and Row.

Suzuki, Keisuke, Warrick Roseboom, David J. Schwartzman and Anil K. Seth, (2017) "A deep-dream virtual reality platform for studying altered perceptual phenomenology," *Scientific Reports,* 22 November, v. 7, 15982 (2017). https://doi.org/10.1038/s41598-017-16316-2.

Tan, C.S.H., V.S.Y. Lim, D.Y.M. Ho, E. Yeo, et al., (2004) "Charles Bonnet syndrome in Asian patients in a tertiary ophthalmic center," *Br. J. Ophthalmol.*, Oct., v. 88 (10) 1325–1329.

Tedlock, Barbara (1987) "Dreaming and dream research," in *Dreaming: Anthropological and Psychological Interpretations,* (ed.) Barbara Tedlock, Cambridge, Cambridge University Press, 1–30.

Teeple, Ryan C., Jason P. Caplan and Theodore A. Stern (2009) "Visual hallucinations: differential diagnosis and treatment," *Prim Care Companion J. Clin Psychiatry*, v. 11(1) 26–32.

Textor, R.B. (1967) *A Cross-Cultural Summary,* New Haven, Conn., HRAF Press.
Tiffin, John and Nobuyoshi Terashima: Paradigm for the Third Millennium, (2005) (eds.) New York, Routledge.
Toronto, Ellen L.K. (2009) "Time Out of Mind, Dissociation in the virtual world," *Psychoanalytic Psychology, 26*(2), 117–133. https://doi.org/10.1037/a0015485.
Toffelmier, G. & K. Luomala (1936) "Dreams and dream interpretation of the Diegueno Indians of Southern California," *Psychanalytic Quarterly,* 2, 195–225.
Traynor, Robert M. (2018) "Heard but not seen: tinnitus and auditory hallucinations," *ASHAWire,* https://doi.org/10.1044/leader.AEA.23122018.20
Treffert, Darold (2010) *Islands of Genius: The Bountiful Mind of the Autistic, Acquired, and Sudden Savant,"* London, Jessica Kingsley Publishers.
Treffert, Darold (2015) "Genetic memory: how we know things we never learned," Sci. Amer., January, 28, https://blogs.scientificamerican.com/guest-blog/genetic-memory-how-we-know-things-we-never-learned/.
Unger, Sanford (1964) Mescaline, LSD, Psilocybin and personality change," in Solomon, David (1964) (ed.) LSD: *The Consciousness—Expanding Drug,* New York, Putnam, 121–122.
Vallat, Raphael and Perrine Marie Ruby (2019) "Is it a good idea to cultivate lucid dreaming?" *Frontiers in Psychology,* 15 Nov, https://www.frontiersin.org/articles/10.3389/fpsyg.2019.02585/full.
Van Gennep, Arnold, (1960) *The Rites of Passage*, Chicago, University of Chicago Press.
Vansina, Jan (1985) *Oral Tradition as History*, Madison, University of Wisconsin Press.
Virdi, Jasmine (2020) "Psychedelics and the default mode network," *Psychedelics Today*, Feb. 4th, https://psychedelicstoday.com/2020/02/04/psychedelics-and-the-default-mode-network/.
Wagstaff, G.F. (1981) *Hypnosis, Compliance, and Belief,* Brighton, Harvester.
Wallace, A.F.C. (1966) *Religion, An Anthropological View*, New York, Random House.
Wallace, A.F.C. (1958) Dreams and the wishes of the soul, a type of psychoanalytic among the Seventeenth Century Iroquois," *Amer. Anth.*, v. 60:234–248.
Wamsley, E.J. and R. Stickgold (2010) "Dreaming and offline memory processing," *Current Biology*, v.20, (23) R1010–3.
Weil, Andrew (1972) *The Natural Mind: Another Way of Looking at Drugs and the Higher Consciousness*, Boston, Houghton-Mifflin.

Wellington, Jack, Alexander Wellington and Grace Wellington (2021) "Meduna's mixture: surreal ecstasy or perplexing abreaction—psychiatry in history," *British Journal of Psychiatry,* v. 219, n. 2, 447.
Whaley, Arthur L. and Brittany N. Hall, (2008) "The cultural/racial dimension of psychotic disorders in African American patients," *J. of Black Psychology,*https://doi.org/10.1177/0095798408316362.
Whiting, Beatrice (1963) *Six Cultures: Studies of Child Rearing,* New York, John Wiley.
Whitmore, Diana (1981) "A psychosynthetic view of dreams: levels of the unconscious," *Self and Society,* v. 9, n 3, 108–116.
Wierzbicki, Michael and Gene Pekarik (1993) "A meta-analysis of psychotherapy dropout," *Research and Practice,* v. 24, n. 2:190–195.
Wilbert, J.(1972) "Tobacco and shamanistic ecstasy among the Warao Indians of Venezuela," In P. T. Furst (Ed.), *Flesh of the gods. The ritual use of hallucinogens.* New York: Praeger, 55–83.
Wolfe, Tom (1968) *The Electric Kool Aid Acid Test,* New York, Farrar, Strauss.
Yazar, Yasemin, Zara M. Bergstrom and Jon S. Simons, (2014) "Continuous theta burst stimulation of angular gyrus reduces subjective recollection," *PloS One,* Oct. 21, https://doi.org/10.1371/journal.pone.0110414.
Yee L, Korner AJ, McSwiggan S, Meares RA, Stevenson J. (2005) Persistent hallucinosis in borderline personality disorder. *Compr Psychiatry,*; 46:147–54.
Yip, (2003) Traditional Chinese religious beliefs and superstitions in delusions and hallucinations of Chinese schizophrenic patients," *Int J Soc Psychiatry,* Jun;49(2):97–111. https://doi.org/10.1177/0020764003049002003.
Zubek, John P. (1969) *Sensory Deprivation: Fifteen Years of Research,* New York, Meredith.

4

A Thesis on LSD Research in the Laboratory and the Street: Sensory Deprivation, Surveys and the Mogar Laboratory, Creating Cures

The problem of what people report and what researchers expect them to feel, see, and describe is significant, yet the reason I decided to write up some of my findings for the student newspaper in 1969 was due to the increased media coverage and the impressions that the expected Leary/Alpert paradigm was producing (Caldararo 1969). It seemed at every level, people of my generation were being confronted with ways of experiencing reality that the drug had opened for an individual interpretation; their personal inner journey seemed to be in danger of being stolen.

This article for the student newspaper, *The Daily Gater*, focused on the fear that seemed to be emanating from every source in the media. Specifically, the article addressed reports in the newspaper that people could damage their chromosomes if they took LSD. Work reported by Hoffmann (2009) did not support these claims. If the idea of safety of LSD is determined by the effect it has on subjects, Cohen (1960), who administered it to some 1000 individuals, found it to be safe, and Levine and Ludwig (1964) reviewing other research determined it to not be dangerous. Vardy and Kay (1983) reported on the similarity of psychological pathology in LSD patients diagnosed as suffering from "LSD psychosis"

N. Caldararo, *A Mental Ethnography: Conclusions From Research in LSD*,
https://doi.org/10.1007/978-3-031-13745-7_4

and schizophrenics in hospitalized settings. However, Cormier (2015) reporting on a large US survey found that users of LSD and similar drugs were no more likely to have mental health conditions than other individuals. The research behind my article was drawn from about 1.5 years of work doing menial chores at the Mogar Lab, work at two psychiatric hospitals in Northern California, and some private survey work. It also drew on my personal experiences and those of several dozen people I knew. So while this section of the chapter deals with seeing as opposed to "context," which was a heading in an earlier chapter, it does pertain to both. The context of the experience was coming under pressure to conform to outside influences. Here I mean, the "experience" as it related to individuals.

One can be diplomatic with Leary and Alpert and say that they were trying to change people's impressions to influence the culture in a way that might result in a better way of life for everyone. But on the individual level, their efforts were contaminating, as if they were telling people what to experience, essentially driving into people's consciousness as they were tripping as individual's memories of Leary and Alpert's concepts came into focus. Stevens (1988) is most harsh on this and one can sympathize with Leary's motives by reading other sources and his later writing. Nevertheless, I saw this intrusion happen many times and it could be just a reference made by someone else, or in just the person's memory and not just their influence, news stories of suicides, war, and jail for using the drug. The issue of chromosomal damage fit in here as a great fear.

I was most concerned with a publication by M.M. Cohen et al. (1968); it seemed simply created for sensational impact. I had been talking to Dr. Mogar about my concerns and he suggested I make a presentation of them. So I wrote up my response to Cohen et al. (1968) and gave a short talk. Comments and criticism I received from this went into molding my article. This article appears in the Appendix. The media took up the sensational ideas in Cohen et al. and finally Dr. Mogar and his associates did write a response that was published in *Science* in 1971 (Dishotsky et al. 1971). My article had focused on presenting information for students to understand what chromosomes were, how mutations (including breaks in chromosomes) happened, and, in general, what they can mean. I added a review of a response to the Cohen et al. (1968) article by Sparks et al. (1968) that found that Cohen's results could not be replicated, and that when Sparks et al. (1968) reviewed the chromosomes of people who had used LSD they did not find any increased mutations or damage to chromosomes. The Dishotsky et al. (1971) summarized 68 studies of LSD and chromosomes and found no support for Cohen et al. (1968). But other sensational books and reports were appearing with increasing frequency in the late 1960s and 1970s; some referred to the use of LSD in counterespionage as a "truth serum" and experiments by the US government, and others were suggested and later documented (Lee and Shlain 1985).

The first part of my original thesis was a treatment of linguistic symbolism, as I thought it related to the individual and as it seemed to be an appropriate background to consider what people were experiencing in the use of LSD. Where do these images come from? Why are they causing difficulties in expressing meaning? Are they entirely biological in nature or is there something else, it related to language production? In 1966 this was considered avant-garde, but today it is quite commonplace. People write entire articles on their own interpretations of their supposed personal archetypes, like reincarnation, channeling, and a host of other similar categories of reliving. Some examples are Davy-Barnes (2014), where he becomes a lion. Struggling with meaning took on heroic stature in the 1960s and 1970s, though the play with language was already part of a literary trend with James Joyce's work.

The internet is filled with literally thousands of such renditions of experience, embellished by the teller. Dobkin de Rios and Janiger (2003) are among a number of writers who refer to Grinspoon and Bakalar (1997), who collected a number of these and attempted a history. Many relate to Jung's work. They describe Jung's interest in LSD and other psychedelic drugs and note that from 1949 to when the drug was made illegal in most countries in the 1960s, more than a thousand papers had been published of clinical research with more than 40,000 subjects. A major problem with this data, aside from the different methods of choosing subjects, setting, and administration of drugs (e.g., dose) is the variety of documentation. In some cases dedicated organizations have attempted to collect this material (as MAPS has), but even in such efforts the original recordkeeping often fluctuated in quality, as de Rios and Janiger (2003) note in the Janiger studies.

An interesting aspect of Jung's regard for psychedelics is his answer to the question, if he had ever taken stimulants or psychedelics. He remarked that taking such drugs was a demonstration of Marxist materialism, that a drug like mescaline is the drug by which you can manipulate the brain so it produces "spiritual" experiences (Jung, Letters, v. II). He argues that using a drug like mescaline (or Hash, alcohol, etc.) is using a poison that forces open the upper layers of consciousness in an artificial way. He recognized that in the case of an aboriginal context, as with the Hopi, this might be different and he suggests this difference. This is similar to my argument that the cultural context is central to the subject being able to have an understandable experience that can be useful. One has to keep in mind that some research contrasts with the idea of regular use of psychedelics by aboriginal populations. Berud Brabec da Mori (2011) found that the use of ayahuasca was not frequently used among the Peruvian Amazonian people he studied.

Jung's juxtaposition of Marxist philosophy and an attempt to create ersatz spiritualism is ironic, in that it makes a moralistic association between the real spiritualism of Native peoples who use drugs and the anti-drug spiritualism of Christianity. On the other hand, while psychologists were experimenting with LSD in the West and attempting to use it as a means of curing illness by the reinterpretation (reliving) of historical events in the lives of their patients, the same approach was used in the Soviet sphere (Marks 2015). Also, of interest, is the fact that the US government saw no contradiction to the use of LSD as a method of counter-espionage. Yet an entire school of counter-culture and cultural studies have grown up since the 1960s, either spoofing the time or glorifying it (Gilbert 2017; Goffman and Joy 2004), and some serious analysis of the use of psychedelics as social change agents have appeared. On the other hand, LSD was investigated by the Mormons as a potential means of religious experience (1967).

Evidence of a breakdown of social conditioning and thresholds of sexuality or acceptance of different ideas (as in "brainwashing") has often appeared, especially since the Korean Conflict. Coercion, torture, propaganda, and advertising with consumer socialization in mind, all seem part of twentieth-century efforts to control populations in one way or another (Dunne 2013). This idea of government interference by the use of drugs has been investigated and evidence well established. What happens in the brain when people have a religious experience (Azari and Slors 2007; Joseph 2001), lose their faith, convert (Dewhurst and Beard 1970), are forcibly converted, or "freed" from the psychological control of a sect? Or what happens when a person changes their anatomy from male to female in the brain (Jordan-Young 2010)? When I worked with the Cockettes (a radical theatrical group from the early 1970s that was made up of heterosexual, bisexual, homosexual, non-sexual, and self-sexual individuals) (Tent 2004), I was struck by the fluidity by which some people were able to move from a male identity to a female one given certain conditions. Women who looked quite feminine could become very "masculine" and vice versa. I went to New York with the Cockettes as a set designer assistant, stagehand, and documentation agent, where I learned a multitude of lessons on gender identity.

The Cockettes were set up in the Chelsea Hotel and several people were housed to a room. There took place the usual drug-and-alcohol treatments with food, good stories, and great sex, as had been the norm in San Francisco. But the general open sex, men and men, women and women, men and women, that took place in these rooms gave a fantastic meaning to the word "orgy" to me. A masculine-looking man could be feminine in performance and vice versa for a woman. But the sexual experience is so diffuse in many people that this should not come as a surprise, especially since attraction to the opposite sex is not only dependent on culture and biology, but on the creative performance of the personality that many people become entranced with and thus come to define "love," "charisma," and perhaps identity. Ernest Becker (1962) referred to this as the aura of meaning a person created for themselves as a projection of their personality. This mirage could become much different in different contexts when one performed different "auras."

But the related concept that alcohol or marijuana or LSD might be avenues to social change on a national or international scale, while claimed at various times in the past, seems overblown. This is sometimes ascribed to ergot mold during the Middle Ages or to effects of disease, as the Black Death (Caldararo 2012). Certainly we can see tremendous effects of Covid-19 both economically and politically. Different elements of conditioning can be modified or relearned by context changes, as

Montagu (1986) discusses in reviewing studies as reported by Gergen et al. (1973), where subjects entered a darkened room where other people were gathered. Within a short time, individuals were reported to engage in touching each other and exploring their bodies, dancing and singing with perfect strangers. When the lights were turned on, a general embarrassment was expressed by most. As with alcohol, social barriers can be reduced, but the idea of permanent change or change on a scale of communities or states is more difficult to establish. While Freudian theory argues that inhibitions are associated with repressed desires and create anxieties and neurosis (Freud 1966), the discharge of these in therapy was seen by many practitioners as a modification that allowed a return to a healthy balance of conditioning (Thompson 1950). But if society is producing illness, then "cure" only becomes coping (Becker 1962).

With LSD the concept of relearning or "imprinting" new patterns of behavior to replace old ones associated with pathological behavior was discussed in the 1960s and 1970s among researchers and users. Borrowed from ethology the idea was discovered by Heinroth (1910), who called it "pragung," German for "impressing," as in making an impression in clay. It was later translated into an English term, "imprinting," by Lorenz (1937).

Some researchers in the 1970s (e.g., Kaiser and Gold 1973) attempted to put the thesis of the use of psychedelics as culture change agents in the context of actors like shamans (Eliade 1964) and religious formulators like Luther, as described by Radin (1937). But for Eliade (1964) the shaman can reach the spirit world via ancestors who are awakened by the means of pain or dreams, hyperventilating, or other extreme circumstances that create the foundation for a vision path. The class of initiators of change as in Maslow's self-actuators (Maslow 1962), or those who exercise conservative repression like prophets (Patai 1990), are sometimes users of drugs or alcohol to gain inspiration, or are simply possessed of a mania for power or chaos (Canetti 1966). In the realm of psychohistorians like Lifton (1970), the protean man, created in the crises of the time, rises to the occasion and the use of drugs is a means of achieving an effective motivation and vision.

All of these considerations place us back at an initial conundrum, where do these inspirations, dreams, visions and images, or voices come from? Why do people search for or desire them? If the "Argonauts of

Inner Space" (newly defined by a number of popular books, e.g., Strassman 2008) [and here I include Native peoples' religious leaders or specialists, individuals who attain some means of spiritual travel] are correct, then these images are derived from some silent and invisible worlds about us. I recall in the 1960s there were a group of communes whose leaders simply took drugs all day and every day. They called this, "climbing Mt. Athos." At the time I did not know that there was a Mt. Athos (the one in Greece), but to them it meant a spiritual journey beyond the knowledge of the living world as we learn it is structured.

A few of them were ex-students of philosophy, one or two were older, once G.I.s or professionals like electricians, and to them the world of the unseen was all about us but the means to reach it was lost to our preformed perceptions. I recalled once listening to a lecture on sight, that some people who lose their sight through trauma or illness and then regain it later in life have to relearn how to see and for some this is too difficult and so they remain blind. This reminded me of the "kaleidoscopic" visions mentioned by Grof's subjects, an experience I had had (before reading it in Grof) and had heard other people talk about, both when they were under the influence of LSD and after. One tries to focus, but the effort simply pushes the scene into some other, more complex form or sense, like from sight to sound (or as one friend under LSD put it, he could see the sound but not hear it).

These were some of the famous "Argonauts of Inner Space" so talked about in the Haight-Ashbury in 1966. They disappeared and I have no idea what could have been their fate. Michal Pagis (2010) studied participants in Vipassana meditation, where people participate in a group of silent members. He came to address the space of their silent gathering in terms of phenomenology, which in some interpretations argues we cannot know what others experience and so the presence of some group together meditating in silence creates a world itself, of unknown links but formed by virtue of their decision to do so "together" in space. Some who meditate have experiences similar to those induced by fasting and psychedelics. Huxley (1954) reports on the meditational experiences of George Russell, who saw strange faces, beautiful landscapes, aurous objects, and wonder in grains of sand. But one has to ask, where did these come from, a cocktail of memories? Where do they go when people travel in the mind? Are these linked to the person in coma, or to the dreamer, or the drug addict who has numerous near-death experiences; do these means (drugs, etc.) open a door of perception or worlds as Huxley suggests; or do they receive signs as fragments from parallel lives? In some cases people attempt to get as close as possible to death by strangulation. Such feats are termed "auto-erotic asphyxiophilia," yet they seem to have other qualities in the proximity to death (Downing and Nobus 2004). When death occurs is it suicide, accident, or murder? That is, can it be interpreted as a journey that failed? Just as the Siberian shaman undergoes tremendous action accompanied by violence and self-harm, does the auto-erotic asphyxiophiliant conceive of death as a means to an end, or is it part of a more complex transit initiated by pleasure that casts the individual in a wider and wider net of self that eventually is peopled by motives, history, and mythology that overwhelms a failed attention to demise? Suicide rates and self-harm in general are up in the United States (CDC 2017) and especially among those over 40 and white, but up by more than 60% among young Americans (Reinberg 2020). What does this tell us about the meaning of life and the success of the culture and society of the United States?

Certainly there is something here that is similar to suicide, or to accidental death by overdose of drugs or alcohol, but also there is the question of experience. In Pagis' group of meditators, is their proximity a vehicle without which they could not sustain a quality of the experience? In the case of chanting Indian monks or *sramanas* or the esoteric movements and rituals of Buddhist monks (Winfield 2017), we see a group ignoring each other and any exterior beings. Their journey is personal, interior, and a singularity.

There is some debate on the biological effects of meditation, trance, and the use of psychedelics (Hove and Stelzer 2018), and ideas of evolutionary aspects are intriguing yet vague. One aspect of drug use, stimulants and depressive agents, things people smoke or do to get "high," the idea of change and of personal satisfaction is quite different from leading the revolution, becoming Pope or giving birth. Perhaps this last has had the most significant effect on humans, as many primitive peoples (as we have termed people in less complex or technological societies than today's) created myths, rituals, dogma, all aimed at containing and controlling the natural power women possess in giving birth, as mentioned above. There is a channel from this world to some other where Native peoples could recognize an opening through to women where babies came with souls (i.e., life). The power of life is creative and women are not just seen as the vessel, perhaps in a patriarchal world, but active performers and agents of that world or worlds. Strange that we find elaborate rituals and religious explanations built around giving birth, but usually, even in some of the simplest societies a male definition underscores the significance of the birth (Fienup-Riordan 1995).

Some Examples from the Mogar Lab and the Caldararo Survey

As I mentioned above, the Mogar protocol was devised to sort out subjects that might undergo detrimental outcomes. A short interview was done by interns who were trained to take certain notes. These were then reviewed by staff: usually graduate students, psychologists, or some of the medical staff associated with the Mogar Lab. I was also collecting potential subjects for a study by Allen Rinker, who worked in association with Dr. Mogar at the time.[1] Mr. Rinker participated in a number of events at the time to explain psychedelics and "hippie culture," as in a "Hippie Press Conference" with George Darling, Reverend Leon Harris, and Leonard Wolf on August 17, 1966. He also participated with Dr. Mogar and Mike Snedcor in a student-faculty conference discussing drugs on campus at San Francisco State on April 19, 1967 (OAC 2021). An MMPI test was then given to some of these individuals, who seemed to be stable candidates for research. Below I have reproduced examples of the notes I took. The subjects below are referred to as part of a subculture; the media at this time (1967) was calling them a variety of names, but "hippie" became a standard, yet this was not descriptive of anything characteristic of them. Most of them lived in large groups in one or several flats in the Haight-Ashbury or the Fillmore. Often several people clustered around a few people who had regular jobs, but some groups lived in abandoned houses, sustaining themselves on welfare, food stamps, or unemployment. While Stevens (1988) claims that people at the time believed LSD made the Haight-Ashbury special, my memory is that it was the music, as most people, in my opinion, did not use LSD, only marijuana. What seemed to distinguish the Haight-Ashbury were ideas (most I met were students), youth, music, and smoking marijuana. From my experience, in 1967 the vast majority were not taking government assistance; they generally distained any government contact and prided themselves as being self-sufficient. By 1968 this began to change markedly, as the image of freeloading "hippies" became the media message. It was not until late 1968 and the beginning of 1969 that this transition became nearly complete, as most of the self-supporting commune people moved out of San Francisco, either to Marin, Sonoma, or Mendocino or beyond.

The atmosphere in the summer of 1967, however, was still quite fluid and the attitude of people adventurous in the extreme, with people leaving to travel to India, North Africa, Europe, and South and Central America. It was a great diaspora. I hitchhiked with a friend to Monterey and Carmel to stay in a commune and meet more people who had relocated earlier. Jimi Hendrix was to play at the Pop Festival and I had been invited to Los Angeles to stay at some communes there and in the desert to the East. There seemed to be two trends taking place in people's minds: one was forming groups and becoming independent and self-sufficient communities; the other was a kind of grifter ethos, where people wanted no ties to anyone and made pains to demonstrate they were not held back by any laws, morals, or ethics. To a certain extent I had come into contact with a few of these in the early Haight-Ashbury and they came to represent most hippies in the media, though the communal type was more typical. There were also people like Emmett Grogan (or "Groan," a moniker I think came to someone speaking with a reporter, but has been repeated as an alias of Grogan by Peter Coyote), whose book *Ringolevio* does capture some of the aroma of the time. I had met Grogan at the Diggers' free store on Haight Street when the police came in and asked for him by name as who was in charge. Everyone then raised their hands, women too, and said, "I am Emmett Grogan." The police were not amused. The personality Grogan describes in his book was a type as well, people who were from somewhere else, had been everywhere, and done everything. It struck a chord with me, as my father had grown up in New York's Harlem and the Bronx. He had the accent and mien of the place. These people projected a fearless, congenial, knowledgeable but not condescending persona; they made up a core of "wise people" who seemed to slip from group to group over time across the Haight, the Fillmore, and the communes beyond. I describe the communes at the time in a chapter of my book on the Goodman Building (Caldararo 2019).

Subject A: Parentheses are introduced for new comments since 1967, brackets are original. I was told to open a general conversation and make notes, beginning with the question, "Tell me a bit about yourself." The Survey Questionnaire used is appended as Appendix B. The first question in the questionnaire was: "Would you like to participate in research concerning the personality effects of LSD usage?" This collection of questions was gone over later by Mr. Rinker with the goal of choosing subjects for his experiments. I do not recall if I was supposed to collect both male and female subjects, but I do recall interviewing females as well. However, I no longer have those notes and they might have been retained by people in the Mogar Lab, though all the records of the Mogar lab were lost when San Francisco State University renovated the old Psychology Building on campus.

The first person, whom I will refer to as *Subject A*, has a middle-class background; this is common to a large number, though not a preponderance, of this subculture. (What I meant here, as I have mentioned elsewhere, is not the media idea of "hippie," but a more amorphous definition of people who were—at least at this early time—more like young Beatniks, thoughtful, creative, and open to new ideas.) He is a male, 21 years old, single, and of Mexican and French ancestry (this point was stressed by Subject B when asked the same question, as opposed to the term "nationality"). He has no religious preference. His is from urban areas. He is a Junior at SFSU, a Botany major, and has no political orientation. His national hero is the first governor of Tennessee, and his greatest hero outside of the United States is I.F. Stravinsky, a Russian composer.

He believes in different levels of reality. He thinks that American culture is responsible for an inability to think under pressure, and also a misguided optimism in its members. He does not believe there will be a thermonuclear war. He does not know if (or what it would be) advertising has any value in our society. The subject states that changes in value emphasis come about as a result of advertising and the mass media. He believes that if we stop having children and stop feeding all the poor people of the world we can solve our population problem. He feels advertising ruined his reason, relates culture change, and gives information. He is in school because of the army. He thinks television has great practical educative value. He doesn't feel that the quality of goods improves by advertising competition, but that it does remove the inconsistencies on the market. He does not believe the prediction of the book *1984* will come about. *The last two questions on the questionnaire he did not answer because they were added to the list after his interview.*

Subject B: He is a 23-year old male, single, and a "WASP" (White, Anglo-Saxon, Protestant—his choice as a descriptive term). In response to religion he states he is a humanist, or a Dewey pragmatist (John Dewey, US philosopher, psychologist, and educator, father to a number of unusual theories on reality). He comes from a suburban area (generally true if we consider his birth, but on origins, his father was a sea captain who was originally from Boston and was quite itinerant). He is in his first year of graduate study in the Social Sciences and Musicology. To the question of politics and political affiliation, he first answered as being apolitical and then revised his statement to be a humanist. He does not want to participate in an LSD study (1).

His national heroes are: Spiderman, Dr. Strange, Red Skull, Chief Thunderthud (these are cartoon characters, as in Dr. Strange a Marvel Comics property). Also, his heroes include the Beatles and the Esso advertising character.

Instead of "levels of reality" he states he sometimes believes in perceptual alternatives. He thinks American culture is responsible for the absence of creative personality traits, that it is contributing to anality (at first I thought he meant "banality") and limits aspirations and values. He also does not believe there is going to be a thermonuclear war. He feels advertising has value as an inane art form, which gives some information but is esthetically and morally disgusting. He states that advertising is a learning experience to most of the immigrants to this country and that it has educational possibilities, but mostly it only creates an exposure to new cultural alternatives. He doesn't believe advertising creates dynamic culture change in our society. He feels the songs and jingles used by advertising in the mass media work as a prolonged Pavlov's dog type of response to products, and that this may create a population of similar generalized responses in all areas of interaction (e.g., politics). He would have birth control pills used more extensively followed by "healthier" attitudes as an alternative to the population explosion. He thinks advertising has conditioned some of our aspirations in relating them to ads by the use of unattainable models, which reflects on personality. However, he feels that mostly advertising has produced models for every situation and we generalize our emulation of these to our personalities. He is in school because the "other life is harder"; it gives a livelihood, the Draft, and is stimulating. He does not think television has practical educative value as it stands, because it does not project real person for self-fulfillment. He thinks advertising improves the quality of products in some "very perverse and limited ways." And he believes 1984 is already realized. (Questions 17 and 18 were also not used here.)

Subject C: Is 23, male, single, Italian on his mother's side, Austrian, French, and English on his father's. He has no religion (formal) now but when he was younger he was Lutheran. He comes from a suburban area, and is a first-year graduate student in Drama Studies. He is apolitical at present but was Republican.

He would not like to participate in the LSD research; he has never had it and never will (but he does use other drugs). He has no national heroes but his mythological heroes are: Aristotle, Apollo, and Jesus Christ. He does test reality and believes in levels of it (this question was an attempt to gather some experiential information on diverse perceptions of events or existences; its failure is by now evident). He states that American culture produces short-sighted (compassion-wise) impatient persons who view materialism as reality. Also he states that it is responsible for a loss of the romantic in the Greek sense of joy. He thinks advertising is unethical and dupes people. He feels we will have a thermonuclear war. He thinks we convince immigrants by advertising, to believe America is all good and we Americanize them to materialism. He feels that advertising, instead of creating dynamic cultural change, emphasizes appearances as reality, and the only change it creates is that in buying habits. He feels that advertising causes us to get away from the real basis of life to the artificial values of materialism. It makes our values shallow and pushes us away from (other) people. To alleviate the population problem he proposes we suggest birth control techniques in sex education and make sex a pleasure act, and possibly promote or at least recognize homosexuality. He feels advertising has caused him to revolt against it and now he only buys by price and volume and necessity. He is in school to learn what he wants to learn. He thinks television has potential educative value but is not used correctly at present. He feels advertising improves the quality of products, and doesn't think the *1984* (the book) society will come about in his lifetime and probably never. From life he wants to practice what he learns, and attain the "good life," one meaningful to himself; he wants a lusty sex life and good friends. His father is a representative for a firm and his mother is a clerical worker.

Rinker would tabulate the answers that people made, giving them a score related to the MMPI if they took it beforehand. He would then ask me questions about particular people or about the questions. Then he would have me or another student call the person and follow up on their drug use and determine if they might be a candidate for a laboratory session.

Becoming Human

The question of the nature of human consciousness was also paramount in my studies in 1967. On this I wrote: "In the genesis of the process of enculturation the social context of a society, of a family however defined, provides the neonatal with its initial views of life and order." This occurs as infancy begins with instruction, verbal and by gesture and inference, and also by the organization of space (type of dwelling, permanent or not) and lifestyle. During this process of becoming human a child comes to learn this schism of his or her social order, and again in 1967: "that vague and uncertain area of behavior which separates the ideal culture forms from the real or observed actions and intentions of people about one." At this point in development the formation of basic language capacity is theorized to take place, in Chomsky's form and also the means of distinguishing aspects of the environment in that of Piaget, Vygotsky, and others, as I have related elsewhere. Hallowell (1966, 269) adds to this scenario the idea that this creates the mechanism for "imaginative processes." Here we have the concept of being able to imagine or recall images to the momentary attention and where an individual can consider such images in different ways over time. This process, the simplest perhaps of a mother holding an object and naming it with a reward to follow, is well known. That this object is, later the non-existing image, subject to manipulation in ways that the mother and child can communicate, yet allows the infant to plan future action or construct fantasy, and later in life become a part of a complex of personality as a favorite recreation or ideology. This ability to imagine is crucial to being human, though one cannot consider whether other animals are capable or do it as well in different ways using different neurological mechanisms (see Macphail 1982 and Caldararo 2017 for animal studies).

As one comes into consciousness as a person who has come to inculcate the precepts of one's society, the contradictions begin to loom, but not on all. And on some the effect is great—they rebel, either politically, morally, or as anti-social deviants searching consciously or unconsciously for a wild or singular existence. This was the social milieu of the 1960s and one might also say of the 1950s with the Beats; Stevens (1988) emphasizes the rebellion aspect and argues that LSD was often used to in a therapeutic fashion to deprogram hippies of "establishment" conditioning. I think this was more characteristic of the 1970s. On the other hand, Leonard Wolf (1968) in his "voices" from the 1960s focuses on enjoyment and self-discovery, which I think was more what I noticed at the time. I think Stevens (1988) and others who have made the same connection are correct that the Beat scene led to "hippie," or counter-culture or whatever one wants to call it. This is consistent with my own interactions with people who called themselves "Beats" or Beatniks" then and later with Beat artists like Jay DeFeo and Wally Hedrick (Caldararo 2004). There were people like the Thelin brothers, who were revolutionaries in the best sense. They wanted to change the world, and as Jane Lapiner recalls in the Digger Docs, there was already a well-developed ethos by 1966 of people who shared everything, who wanted to live in a free society, and the housing, the "crash pads," were part of this culture. I discuss some of this in my book on the Goodman Building as it relates to people in the squats in the Western Addition in the 1960s.

As Jane says in the interview, "somebody told somebody to ..." go to this address and find a place to sleep, food, and so on. The Diggers' free food and store was a physical criticism of a materialist society that was so rich it could develop and use an atomic bomb, fight war in Vietnam, dump food in garbage yard, and build things with a built-in obsolescence. I think a critical mass of awareness came into existence and spread across the nation. People were talking all night, not just on drugs, or about god and love, but about everything. There was a hunger to know and a desire to create something new. That something was, as people often said, "out there," "being born." The disparity between Leary's "Tune in, Turn on, Drop out" and what was happening in the Haight-Ashbury was extreme. The Diggers were doing things. The media and Leary and Kesey et al. were creating a mirage of instant satisfaction, come to San Francisco, drop acid, live for free. The illusion of a revolution as an easy separation from a typical life was certainly attractive and many came. As David Simpson (former Digger) put it, the slogan sounded great, but the reality of encouraging people to come to San Francisco or to drop acid without any preparation of support was "extremely dangerous." The foundation of what was happening, I think, was that San Francisco had a long history as a border town, the Californios, the 49ers, the thousands of women who started businesses after the Gold Rush, the Asian workers and miners, farmers, and craftspeople, and African Americans. It was a union town that had attracted artists, poets, and misfits from around the globe. The milieu that the Diggers fit into, and they were also in the Mime Troupe, was well established as seeing the world differently.

One cannot imagine the Haight isolated from what was going on in the rest of the country, the Vietnam War, the demonstrations, the Civil Rights struggle, and the Draft. All these lent a considerable pressure of daily life and a certain reality to the events in the Haight, especially by the time of the Human Be-In in January 1967. The Draft caused some to go to Canada, others to take up false names, and many others to escape by dropping into the anonymity of the hippie communes in the country. I traveled up and down the coast in 1967–1968 and visited a number of these from LA to Portland and New Mexico. Answers to problems of what happened next after the Be-In saw the development of the communes and collectives, especially the San Francisco Food Conspiracy, which grew to include several hundred households connected to farms and distributors. No banks were used to pay for the transactions that ran to tens of thousands each week. I was part of the Mission District Food Conspiracy and it only suffered one loss when a driver ran off with the cash given him (several hundred dollars). Teaching people what to on farms turned the communes into institutes, and other needs, housing, building, and maintenance especially were taught in places like the Goodman Building, including law. These places, one of which I have written about (Caldararo 2019), became an academy of arts of sciences, partly funded by the San Francisco Art Commission.

One might say that there were two strains that developed, one of Leary, Ginsberg, and Kesey, where you could just use drugs and live off the product of mass society, hoping it would change in example; the other was concerned with how things changed and worked. To discuss how people had to work to get the food and deliver it was often met with, "oh, that's a hang up, man, don't go there or you will never make it." The same attitude was shown when people had illnesses or disabilities that somehow they were responsible for them, as if they willed it. This fit with Leary's Eastern generally (Hindu borrowed cosmology, and reincarnation based on the caste system). But the other side wanted a new world, one free of the kinds of ignorance and excesses and violence of the past. Some of these later become more political (hung up on the game, as Leary and Kesey might put it and how Kesey addressed the crowd at an October 1965 anti-march). But the split was more varied, and some people thought the government had spiked LSD with speed or another drug. Yet the variation was also due to the power of manipulation, for while Leary and others thought LSD could allow people to reprogram themselves, others found (as the CIA had hoped) they could use it to create followers. The power of the leader across human history and of group reinforcement and sanction created communes and "churches" that looked much like the past. Exploitation, violence, and control were clothed in an ethos of futuristic happiness and mission. Only the colonial symbols were missing. Some, nevertheless persevered in attempting to understand why the drug had the effect it did, and in that vein, the empiricist path has continued on, as has a great plethora of alternative lifestyles in a variety of forms.

Helen Perry (1970), in the introduction to her book on the Haight-Ashbury of the time, describes her arrival to a strange new world in the summer of 1967 and the "death of hippie" parade in the fall. This is often taken as the endpoint of what was described as a magic moment by many people, described best by Helen Perry. A sense of sadness and mourning for this glimpse of social bliss was felt by many. I wrote then, "Into this 'gap' youth as ever ventured following the paths of accepted and forbidden behavior to personal happiness, fame, degradation or despair." If drug use was more than escapism (and certainly "escapism" is a form of rebellion), then the search for new meaning was an important aspect as revealed in the often-heard reference to "argonauts of inner space" (Ken Babbs put it at Ken Kesey's funeral as the "astronauts of inner space"; see BBC News, November 15, 2001: http://news.bbc.co.uk/2/hi/entertainment/1657414.stm).

Here the problem of how each social group defines its experiences in linguistic forms subject to a unifying identity has to be kept in mind. Meaning, as Malinowski and other anthropologists suggested, is always tentative in cross-cultural analysis and communication (see his essay in Ogden and Richards 1923). The effects of language development and social context create a web of significance that goes beyond the idea of simple translation of words; it structures thought and symbols.

With regard to Ken Kesey, as with Tim Leary and Ram Dass, the idea of "dropping out" seemed to me to be a defeatist approach to social change. It also appeared to me as a cowardly response that negated the responsibility of the citizen. For young people who had hardly been engaged in society to give up, "opt out" was a surrender before even testing the water. I wrote in the manuscript in 1967, "The transmission of experience is basic to human behavior and when blocks to the orderly or culturally 'logical' integration of information occur, as when what is 'supposed' to happen (in an ideal sense) but does not (and this seems to be the case with the so-called 'opt outs' or 'drop outs' of the present day) a paranoid-type reaction may be expected which places negative associations with information of either a sensitive nature (what occurred to an individual) or to a general information (complete rejection). This is the all-pervasive conflict of 'real' behavior versus 'ideal' cultural forms. No society lacks this contradiction to some extent. The personal reaction to the contradiction is a type of fixation, which creates a selective set for information, or what is popularly called a 'credibility gap,' a 'generation gap' in the gross sense. Cultural fundamentals are questioned or the priorities thereof reordered." I glued on the page of the manuscript at this point an image of Theodor Billroth during an operation in a large auditorium, so characteristic of nineteenth-century teaching of medicine and anatomy (Fig. 4.1). What I meant by doing this was that the body of society was assaulted by a plethora of traumas, some induced by faulty

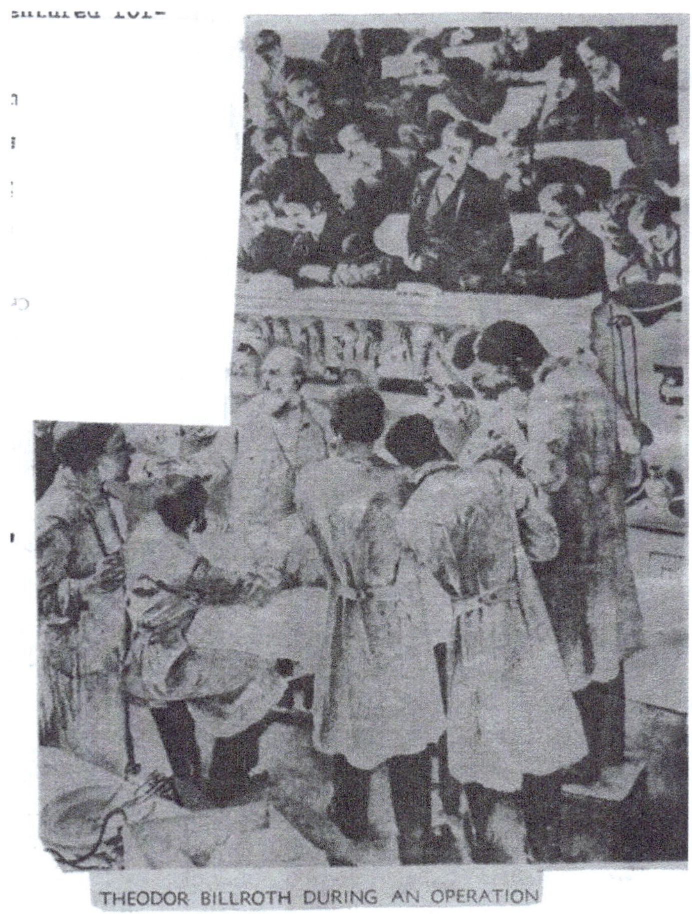

Fig. 4.1 Theodor Billroth during an operation

family life, others by failed education, poor business practice, greed, and corruption of every kind. One might look at the body of the society as hopelessly ill, like that of a person, yet in both cases usually there is a course of treatment. Thus I was hopeful that society could be mended.

Many of my instructors and fellow students, especially those I met at the Mogar Lab, felt that LSD and peyote could be a means of allowing for a "ripping off of the cultural blinders," giving one a true and new view of reality. I was not sure there was a "real reality" or a true one, but it did seem to me that as primates we were limited by our biology in sensing the world, and our culture history further seemed to categorize our perceptions. I took this view, in my 1967 manuscript, to a further point: "Much more, however, may be learned from this on a macro-societal scale. We must realize that historical processes are chemical interactions as are epochs." I was studying general chemistry at the time and geology, so the focus might be said to be logical. Today I would say in lecture to my Biological Anthropology Introduction class, that we live at the bottom of a sea of gases (not an original thought) and as denizens of this sea, with molecules of different elements streaming here and there, viruses, fungi, and bacteria, as an invisible fog of life penetrating us and mutating everywhere, it is hard to speak of us as individuals. (Today I usually refer students to Lynn Margulis and Dorlon Sagan's *What is Life,* for reference especially with regard to the additional life of the inner microbiome.) I went on to say, "One may view every portion of an event as a chemical reaction which may be in any stage of completion. An excellent example here is that of the cyclical pattern of radiations of various animals which G.G. Simpson uses to picture evolutionary processes. A family of animals, say mammals, spreads out into a 'new' ecological niche (usually one not occupied before in their history) and differentiates. Its differentiation is a direct result of chemical conditions of the atmosphere, the vegetation and the species' genetic manipulations (e.g. mutations)." Today I would add, epigenetic mechanisms. This was the kind of view I developed to understand ideas of cosmic unity and so on that were abroad at the time.

A further idea that seemed significant to me was what we think of as history, memory of events, of people in a general sense, as disaster, conquest, journeys, and often mixed with myth. As people, that is, as animals, we situate our species in time and space in a way that contrasts with all other animal life. We presume we are the only conscious beings and only beings conscious of our place in nature and in time. On this I wrote in 1967: "I must note that what I am attempting to clarify in the LSD journey concerning perception and linguistic culture-bound meditation, Aldous Huxley charted years ago." His article "A Philosopher's Visionary Prediction" is a clear statement of the problem. Indeed, we may find that Gordon Wasson was right in his belief that the mind-expanding drugs are responsible for creating the mental capacities which are peculiar to *Homo sapiens*. This is implied in Johns' (1990) compendium of foods and their effects. Thus some have argued that all of human cognition above the ape level, including all philosophy, history, and so on, are the result of drug experiences of our ancestors (Arce and Winkelman 2021; McKenna 1992). Some experimental work could support the idea of psychedelics stimulating "higher states of consciousness," but this depends on definitions and interpretation (see, e.g., Bayne and Carter 2018).

Certainly diet has an important effect on the evolution of any animal, and it may be that the eating of certain psychotomimetic herbs by an early "ape-man" created the beginnings of a significant trend in hominid mental evolution, which led to the *sapiens* phenomenon. The eating of a psychedelic substance in a plant may itself simply create confusion, as it does in most people, and not lead to intellectual development or cognitive evolution. Many animals eat such substances, reindeer in Siberia, caribou, wallaby, bees, goats, rough-toothed dolphins, domestic cats, and dogs (Siegel 2005). We can review the resulting behavior of such animals after ingestion, but we cannot know what goes on in their minds. Human societies have rites of passage where individuals at different ages undergo often extreme pain or suffering. These rituals act to impress different statuses and the general social identity of the group. Such conditions, sometimes linked with psychedelic substances, can produce hallucinations and visions (van Gennep 1960). Again, as I have suggested earlier, the evolution of the large human brain may have been an epiphenomenon, linked to the metaphysics of group membership mediated though spirituality. This aligns with the ideas of Durkheim (1915) of the group as a representation of god (or vice versa) and with ideas of social roles for the brain proposed by people like Dunbar (1998). We can also see it as part of a process where the evolving brain becomes a preadaptation for both complex behavior and complex social life; a parallel in the evolution of the social brain has also been explored for eusocial insects (Caldararo 2017; Lihoreau et al. 2012). If we can understand the recent arguments for a group of drugs, including LSD, peyote and ketamine, for a role in promoting dendritic branching and increases in spine/synapse number in cortical neurons (Olson 2018), then the group ingestion of such "psycho-plastogens" could be regarded as a dietary avenue to accelerated brain evolution, not just increasing brain size, but connectivity. But given euso-cial insect complex behavior, agriculture and husbandry, warfare, and other traits we usually associate with civilization, I do not think that human consciousness evolution necessarily is unique. But the question of consciousness is a black box, yet experiments to probe it have seemed more than crude. Ketamine, for instance, is often associated with out-of-body (OFB) experiences (Wilkins et al. 2011) and DMT with near-death experiences (release, transit to other worlds, etc.) (Timmermann et al. 2018). The brain correlates of out-of-body experiences are related to functional disintegration of lower-level processing at the temporal-parietal junction (Bunning and Blanke 2005). Interruption or distur-bance of such processing to higher levels seems a common feature in such experiences (Barbara 2021). This seems nebulous, and in the case of trauma-induced OFB experiences, the projection of self sometimes is related with a saving action for the person, but one wonders how this projection takes place (Sacks 2012)? What was separated and came back together to produce the unity of mind and body?

Research at Humboldt State was centered on responses from sensory isolation. Historically, the idea was associated with developmental infor-mation where the developing young is deprived of some essential stimu-lation, creating a block to behavioral ontogeny, known in some cases as the "Kasper Hauser" condition (Johnsgard 1967). The experimenters seemed to be attempting to identify psychological states with sensory abnormalities. This related to experiments with rats, for example, and the process where the animal has a sensory field removed (e.g., blinded tem-porarily, or made deaf) so that the experimenter can evaluate the animal's ability to accommodate the lost information about the environment and adapt using other sensory information. In the research setting students were placed in sensory conditions that limited their normal capacity to use combinations of sensory information, like vision and sound, or smell to help orient themselves to various tasks. Often such sensory limits can induce emotional responses, what Grof called, a psychodynamic level of the experience. This was his interpretation also when LSD subjects experienced changes in their sensory modalities (light strobing, or other fluctuations in light intensity or modifications of sound—higher or lower than normal, or the smell of sound, etc.; see, e.g., Munn 1950). Grof interpreted emotional responses of the subjects to abstract stimuli as biographical in nature of the personal past experience of the subjects. It could also be seen as indicative of personality constructs (Kelly 1963).

Here follows my original context for my paper in the form of the construction of a group living situation. I have made a few changes to clarify details or to update information; otherwise, it is as it was:

Due to popular misconceptions and fantasies concerning the nature of the LSD experience and the recent spate of biased research publications on its psychological and physiological effects (and media accounts that draw from this literature), plus the legislative and law enforcement reaction to the drug's use by our nation's youth, I submit this paper. It contains conclusions drawn from one year of research into the literature on the scientific study of LSD. It also contains conclusions and observations drawn from five years of research experience with LSD "users." This research experience includes living with individuals and personal relationships that, in certain cases, extend back to a maximum of ten years. The form of this paper reflects my research history on this subject, and my personal experience with the drug.

At the time this paper was written I was taking a class at SFSU from a chemist named Dr. Shaw. It was a class in general chemistry and one of our assignments was to follow the professor's steps in demonstrating the synthesis of LSD. During the demonstration he kept saying how simple the processes were. He was very enthusiastic about chemistry and I was sorry to have to drop the course, as I was taking too many units at the time. I was living in the Haight-Ashbury with two other males at the time I registered for the class, but halfway through the semester, one of my roommates, Tom Schaftner, met a girl in the park whom he invited home. They had sex and that evening she invited her friends to live with us. The number of people and a couple of children numbered about 10 or 12. It was fluid, as they seemed to meet more people and invite more in, to live with us.

One of my roommates was incensed by the imposition. He first protested to Tom and complained that it was unfair and illegal. That is, too many people in a two-bedroom flat. Tom pointed out that the protesting individual was living in the utility room, which was also illegal. However, since the utility room/bedroom was the only access to the backyard, many of the "visitors" were trooping through the protester's room and had been doing so for hours before he had returned from school. Also, Tom and I held the rental agreement with the owner, so the protester was doubly illegal. Rather than put up with the situation another minute, the protester called his cousins, who lived around the corner, and moved in with them temporarily.

This was a character of the times; people were transient in mass, as was Tom's new girlfriend's "family." Groups of people moved from one part of the country to the West, mainly California and generally to the Bay Area. Of the group, besides the female friend of Tom, there as an ex-Air Force mechanic, a one-time pharmacy school student, a nurse, and several people who were crafts specialists. They were of various mixed ancestries, English, Irish, Scots, Italians, Jews, German, and so on, one Native American and a Jamaican. They came with an already well-developed concept of a new world in the making that drew its energy from begging, selling drugs, and part-time labor. Their idea of future opportunities was defined by possibilities of musical achievements and welfare. It was not a world that was compatible with my own well-defined second-generation immigrant background. As I came from a farm family where hard and sustained work was seen as a way of life, my ideas of cyclical endeavor and rewards were foreign to them.

Once I came home from school (I worked at night at the Post Office) to find all the posters and paintings that had decorated our walls (hallway and living room) removed and replaced with their art. This was a formative moment, not so much of territorial defense, but of identity. I was not so concerned about their presence (my background had a family history of feeding poor and homeless travelers), but I was confused by their presumption to remove what we had put up and change the décor at all. I then spent an hour replacing every wall decoration, chair, rug, or other object to that place it had been. Joey, the main spokesperson of the group, who had been watching the process I was going through, remarked at its end. "Wow, you knew where every thing was. What a Taurus you are, what energy!" Everyone clapped. I never changed anything back again after that, and Joey and I were friends from that day forward.

That aside brings us back to the paper. The first part of which was an involved treatment of linguistic symbolism as it relates to the individual as mentioned above. I had taken a class at UC Berkeley in Linguistics and found it dry, pedantic, but marvelously demanding. Where language came from became a driving curiosity. How did we understand each other and how did that evolve? The class proved that to uncover the answer to that question would be most difficult. I did read Chomsky (1968) and thought I knew something about how language worked. Later I would read Deacon (1997) and Bickerton (1990) and find that little progress had been made.

The nature of experimental information I was able to present in the paper was partly generational, with what I felt was rooted in generational conflict. It seemed to me that there was a differential experiential background in the process of categorization of information by different age groups and/or subgroups within a traditional culture. Part of this feeling was drawn from the "Storms of Youth" I was experiencing as a young person. But also, it seemed obvious that young brains were still influenced and more pliant than those older brains of people over 30 or 40 years of age. Obviously the "don't trust anyone over 30" was a popular theme at the time and had some influence.

Nevertheless, from reading Garrett Hardin's (1966) book on biology at the time (required reading for a class), which had a comprehensive and comparative approach to all life's physiological organization, it did seem logical that learning and adaptation were required to cope with changing conditions and competition. The minds of young people seemed to be required to be malleable for future adaptation, not in a Vitalist sense or the general understanding of Lamark's theory, but a more amorphous approach. I had read Herbert Wendt's *In Search of Adam* (1955), which was a wonderful and enthusiastic journey through ancient biological thought from Egypt to Greece and Persia to China, Rome and medieval Europe, the Renaissance, Enlightenment, and Rationalism. The development of scientific thought and methods was described in the debates of hundreds of minds and laid out how difficult it was for people to understand ideas that challenged their learning, customs, and personalities. But Wendt's journey gave me the tools to organize an approach to the evolution of the human consciousness after some 50 years.

When I read Freud and his argument of the development of human consciousness through ontogeny with the construction of the id, the superego, and the ego, it all seemed quite logical. In fact, it seemed like a rendition of what I had read in the works of Haeckel, where he looks at ontogeny as the recapitulation of phylogeny, that is, in the process of growth from a fertilized ovum the individual develops as a very primitive organism that looks like many simple multi-cellular beings as the zygote divides and multiplies the number of cells and is called the blastomere stage. As the cells divide they become smaller than the original cells and these cells are referred to as being totipotent; that is, they are each capable of developing into a single human being on their own. This is how we get monozygotic twins. This in itself is amazing; you can produce a whole number of individuals theoretically from one fertilization event. Sort of like Jason and the Argonauts, where he seeds the soil and then up jump warriors all alike and armed.

The development of the embryo continues as a zygote made up of many groups of cells we call blastomeres until it has a structure, with an internal area where an inner cell mass is created, a blastocyst. From this mass of cells all the organ systems of the individual human grow and this is true of the nervous system and brain. So as the neonatal comes to experience the world after birth, their brain is developing further, with more neurons being created and these actually swimming into place as the framework of the brain's areas is laid down by cells called glial cells. But from the zygote stage to birth, the individual goes through changes in organization where gill slits appear and are then remade into parts of the jaw. At times it does seem like Haeckel was right: each human goes through a stage of development in evolution that first happened millions of years ago—but not all stages, certainly only some related to mammals and primates, not insects, for example. Yet the most of the whole cascade of genes that determine development and produce proteins needed for growth are conserved across life.

So Freud's idea of the development of human consciousness is similar to Haeckel's idea of the conservation of life's evolutionary mechanisms. It is also similar to Deacon's idea of how the neurological structures in the infant come to be used for the construction of the ability to produce language. So all these ideas of early life, whether Freud's, Bickerton's, Primal Scream, and so on, all build on the basic biology of complex organisms that we are. We possess the language of life, the DNA code, in which the information of evolution is preserved and from which we are constructed and come to perform as social beings. As Deacon notes, each baby goes through the process of learning to use its Chomskyan mechanism; that is, they recapitulate the evolution of language, being conditioned to sounds, images, rewards, and punishments until a system of meaning is created. The amazing thing is that this happens at all and that we can understand each other. This realization "blew my mind" in 1967 when it came to me one night after "dropping acid" in the morning. I was typing away on this manuscript and all of a sudden my fingers melded with the typewriter. I was astonished, yet gazed at the keyboard and my fingers until they separated as I realized it was impossible and I was only hallucinating. Yet the hallucination, like the discovery of the benzene ring, had insight into the idea of how the stream of stimuli we receive is constructed by the brain into categories that produce our own version of primate reality. What Oliver Sacks was concerned with in his book *The Man Who Mistook His Wife for A Hat* is that we can agree on reality at all. In reading Stein and Meredith's (1993) book on the multisensory integration in human sensation I realized that my LSD experience 30 years before was an example of the interruption of this integration.

Sacks (1985) describes a patient with Korsakoff's syndrome who manifests histories of himself that are entirely false and engages in personality changes that are dramatic. These are called "confabulations" or defined as "falsification of memory occurring in a clear consciousness in association with an organically derived amnesia" (Berlyne 1972). Since individuals can present the symptoms of the syndrome from a number of lesions in the brain as well as a history of alcoholism, along with a diet depleted in vitamin B, the exact underlying physical deficits are varied. However, the performance of forms of falsified history is clearly common. They are believed to result from the fact that most patients have short-term amnesia, where they cannot add to their store of memories on a daily basis and so at one point in their history they have good anterior memory of that date to early childhood but nothing from that date to the clinical interview (Barba et al. 1990). In some cases it is believed the deficit in memory forces the patient to attempt to "fill in" the missing information and events.

But the patients often are described as producing momentary confabulations due to their inability to control their responses or make self-corrections. Here the result is often memories out of time with actual events. The other type is fantastical and, in either case, is rare in patients with other deficits or disease, as in Alzheimer, "pure amnesics," and general dementia. The more spontaneous are the fantastical and these seem to be the result of false memories (Kessels et al. 2008). But as in the case described by Sacks, the question then is, where do these false memories come from? Suggestion has been one theory, but that seems more likely in the provoked category, not spontaneous ones (Kessels et al. 2008). Functional problems due to the underlying physiological deficits can be involved, as in the cases Sacks notes of songs appearing in the mind of patients spontaneously and becoming quite prominent, but in these cases they seem to be memories.

There is evidence that dreams are an indication of a less likelihood of dementia in later life. Patients with dementia dream less than controls; that is, they enter REM sleep less often (Pase et al. 2017).

Similar abnormalities like tinnitus is also a spontaneously appearing syndrome that is unclear in origin, but affects many otherwise healthy people. So "things" events, songs, memories of all kinds, perhaps mixed in with novel scenes or themes from TV or movies, can become momentary surface conscious affairs created perhaps by a variety of changes in brain chemistry and these perhaps can explain the hallucinations of LSD.

One has to introduce a number of caveats to ideas of reality. Kelly (1963) argued that reality was built from familiar conditions and responses to others and expected occurrences. Freud (1937) makes a similar observation over his visit to the Acropolis and its unexpected "falsity." Its presence could not be real, as it was unexpected. The unfamiliar, remote placement and lack of correspondence with typical responses of the Aztecs left many of the Spanish conquistadors feeling they were in a dream (Diez del Castillo 1576).

So in 1967 I approached this problem by attempting to deal specifically with the relationships of language, experience, and cognition. I had an argument with Leslie White on this problem about two years later when he came to SFSU to give a seminar in Anthropology. I was frustrated with his use of what seemed to me jargon, "cognition," "language" and symbols, and "abstractions." Morgar (1965) referred to Korzybski (1948) and the idea that an abstraction is a semi-conscious act of "awareness that in our process of abstracting we have left out characteristics." To White I asserted that these terms had become fetish identifiers for how humans regarded their own type of communication. I thought, as I had just read von Frisch on bee language, that we should hold in reserve these concepts for other life forms until we had definitive evidence that they were unique to humans. White argued that we did have enough evidence; "they" ants and others could not abstract or have ideas. I was unconvinced and in class challenged him by saying, "How do you determine that, unless you can be in the minds/brains of an ant or bee?" His response was that he and I could not understand each other due to a generational problem. He was probably right. But I also felt it was due to the dogmatic way people, scientists included, talked about language and cognition.

Mogar (1965) argues that the LSD experience "increases one's ability to recognize and hence respond to fundamental sense impressions, without semantic barriers." That this "freshness of perception" and "feeling of unity" "suggests that the 'is' of identity is temporarily eliminated." This corresponds to the view of many people at the time, and before, like Huxley (1954). But this takes us back to our earlier discussion about synesthesia (the merging of the senses in some people) or in the nature of human awareness as some have described it (see the discussion with Humphrey's Inner Eye concept below). This is distinct, I think, from cultural ideas of self-extension, as in the case of the Zinacantec idea that a person's possessions are representative of him or herself, and have acquired an aspect of his soul. Corn in this case also shares his or her soul, as do the implements and humans associated with it (Laughlin 1976). Thus, the loss of things imperils one's health. The unity of links of earth, corn, self, community, generations is what sustains one. One might argue that the LSD experience and other psychedelics bring out the mental mechanism on which such associations are built by various cultures and how they are inculcated.

Grof (1976) also reports that a number of subjects during LSD therapy undergo muscle spasms, and a variety of other abnormal physiological changes (like nausea, vomiting, cardiovascular variations, etc.). Some of these are typical of ingestion of other psychedelic drugs and some of reports of culturally defined trance as well as a variety of psychopathologies either involving hallucinations or not—for example, rolling of the eyes (Orengo-Garcia 1998; Kawai et al. 2017; Connelly 2015; Hageman et al. 2010; Davis 2001; Kreig 1964).

Grof (1976) maintains that the core experience influences the unfolding of the re-adaptation of the individual's ontogeny in the session by its nature and that the people present at the LSD therapy session as well as the room in which it takes place also are utilized by the past event's structure. This may be why Mogar and his associates made sure that all staff wore white lab coats and the room in which the sessions took place was sparsely furnished and had white walls, ceiling, and flooring tile. This was, however, standard in most of the rooms used at Humboldt State for the deprivation sessions. However, at Humboldt, as at Mendocino State Hospital, there were variations. At Humboldt not all staff wore white lab coats, and the students especially were clearly visible as different from the professional staff. But in Grof's (1976, 80) examples, patients transform the staff present into actors from the past, real or phantoms, and the therapy rooms into past settings of core experience or later related experiences. Also patients often, in Grof's work, seem driven to act out the roles of all individuals present at key traumatic events in their lives. This is something that never came to my attention, either when the therapists in Mogar's group had discussions or Grand Rounds at one of the hospitals. Nor did I ever see this in private settings, though people often did act out events, usually in incoherent and disjointed fashion.

In sessions outside of the lab settings, in private homes and clubs, there were no such limitations. People wore whatever they wanted, though I can recall a couple of houses of people who had communal ideas about the drug who wore different clothing during the sessions, and the rooms were sometimes draped in various color bed sheets or tie-dyed ones or forms of designs thought to evoke themes. There was often no furniture, only rugs and cushions.

Note

1. I was collecting research subjects for Allen Rinker at the same time that I was interviewing potential subjects for the Mogar Lab experiments. Rinker was engaged in LSD research at San Francisco State in an independent group.

References

Arce, Jose Manuel Rodriguez and Michael James Winkelman (2021) "Psychedelics, sociality, and human evolution," *Frontiers in Psychology*, v. 12, Sept. 29: https://doi.org/10.3389/fpsyg.2021.729425

Azari, Nina P. and Marc Slors (2007) "From brain imaging religious experience to explaining religion: a critique," *Archive for the Psychology of Religion*, v. 29, n 1:67–86.

Barba, Gianfranco Dalla, Lisa Cipolotti and Gianfranco Denes (1990) "Autobiographical memory loss and confabulation in Korsakoff's syndrome: a case report," *Cortex*, v. 26:525–534.

Barbara, Vanessa (2021) "I took Ketamine for my depression. Things got pretty weird," *The New York Times*, December 28.

Bayne, Tim and Olivia Carter (2018) "Dimensions of consciousness and the psychedelic state," *Neurosci. Conscious.*, 1, https://doi.org/10.1093/nc/niy008.

Becker, Ernest (1962) *The Birth and Death of Meaning*, New York, Macmillan.

Berlyne, N. (1972) "Confabulation," *British Journal of Psychiatry*, v. 120:31–9.

Bickerton, Derek (1990) *Language and Species*, Chicago, University of Chicago Press.

Brabec da Mori, Berud (2011) "Tracing hallucinations—contributions to a critical ethnohistory of ayahuasca usage in the Peruvian Amazon," in *The Internationalization of Ayahuasca*, (eds.) Jungaberle, Hendrik and Beatriz C. Labate, 23–47, Zurich.

Bunning, Silvia and Olaf Blanke, (2005) "The out-of-body experience: precipitating factors and neural correlates," *Prog. Brain Res.*, v. 150, 331–350.

Caldararo, Niccolo (2004) "*The conservation of Beat art," in Modern Art, Modern Museums* (Eds.) Ashok Roy and Perry Smith, Contributions to the Bilbao Congress, 13–17 Sept, London, International Institute for Conservation of Historic and Artistic Works, 180–192.

Caldararo, Niccolo (2012) *Evolutionary Aspects of Disease Avoidance*, Saarbrucken, Scholars' Press.
Caldararo, Niccolo (2017) *Big Brains and the Human Superorganism, Why Special Brains Appear in Hominids and Other Social Animals*, Lanham Maryland, Rowman and Littlefield.
Caldararo, Niccolo (2019) *An Ethnography of the Goodman Building, The Longest Rent Strike*, New York, Palgrave Macmillan.
Caldararo, Nicholas (1969) "Genetics and LSD" *The Daily Gater*, November 11–12: Page 3 At the time I was using the Americanized version of my first name.
Canetti, Elias (1966) *Crowds and Power*, Carol Stewart trans., New York, Compass Books.
Castillo, Bernal Diaz del (1576) *The True History of the Conquest of New Spain*, trans. Maurice Keatinge, London, Penguin Books edition, 1963.
Centers for Disease Control (2017) FastStats: Suicide and Self-inflicted injury," https://www.cdc.gov/nchs/fastats/suicide.htm (accessed November 27th 2020).
Chomsky, Noam (1968) *Language and Mind*, New York, Harcourt, Brace and World.
Cohen, M.M., K. Hirshhorn and W.A. Frosch, (1968) "LSD and chromosomes," N. Engl. J. Med., Jan 25, v. 278, n. 4:223.
Cohen, S. (1960) Lysergic acid diethylamide: Side effects and complications. *J. Nerv. Ment. Dis*. 130: 30–40.
Connelly, Chris, (2015) "The physiology of trance," *Paranormal Review*, issue 74: 23–24.
Cormier, Zoe (2015) "No link found between psychedelics and psychosis," *Nature*, 4 March, https://doi.org/10.1038/nature.2015.16968.
Davis, Wade (2001) *Light at the Edge of the World*, Vancouver, Douglas & McIntyre.
Davy-Barnes, Malcolm (2014) "Some Jungian reflections on LSD," *Psychedelic Press UK*: https://psypressuk.com/2014/09/24/some-jungian-reflections-on-lsd-by-malcolm-davy-barnes/
Deacon, Terrence W., *The Symbolic Species: The Co-evolution of Language and Brain* (New York: W.W. Norton, 1997).
de Rios, Marlene and Oscar Janiger (2003) *LSD Spirituality and the Creative Process,* Rochester Vt., Park Street Press.
Dewhurst K. and Beard, A.W. (1970) "Sudden religious conversions in temporal lobe epilepsy," *The British Journal of Psychiatry*, v. 117:497–507.

Dishotsky, Norman I., William D. Loughman, Robert E. Mogar and Wendell R. Lipscomb, (1971) "LSD and genetic damage," *Science*, 30 April v. 172, 2981:431–440.

Downing, Lisa and Dany Nobus (2004) "Iconography of asphyxiophilia: from fantasmatic fetish to forensic fact," *Paragraph*, v 27, n. 3:1–15.

Dunbar, Robin L.M. (1998) "The social brain hypothesis," *Evolutionary Anthropology*, v. 6, n. 5, Dec. 7th: 178–190.

Dunne, Mathew W. (2013) *A Cold War State of Mind: Brainwashing and Postwar American Society*, Cambridge, MIT Press.

Durkheim, Emile (1915) *The Elementary Forms of the Religious Life*, London, George Allen & Unwin.

Eliade, Mircea (1964) *Shamanism*, Bolligen Foundation, Princeton, Princeton University Press.

Fienup-Riordan, Ann (1995) *Boundaries and Passages: Rule and Ritual in Yup'ik Eskimo Oral Tradition*, Norman, University of Oklahoma Press.

Freud, Sigmund (1966) *The Complete Introductory Lectures on Psychoanalysis*, trans. James Strachey (ed.) New York, W.W. Norton.

Freud, Sigmund (1937) "A disturbance of memory on the Acropolis," reprinted in *Character and Culture*, reprinted, trans. James Strachey, New York, Collier Books, 1963:311–320.

Gergen, Kenneth J., Mary M. Gergen and William H. Barton, (1973) "Deviance in the dark, "Psychology Today, Oct. 129–130.

Gilbert, Jeremy (2017) "Psychedelic socialism," *openDemocracy*, 22 Sept.: https://www.opendemocracy.net/en/psychedelic-socialism/.

Goffman, Ken and Dan Joy (2007) *Counter Culture Through the Ages*, New York, Villard Publishers.

Grinspoon, L. and J.B. Bakalar, (1997) *Psychedelic Drugs Reconsidered*, 3rd edition, New York, The Lindesmith Center.

Grof, Stanislav (1976) *Realms of the Human Unconscious: Observation from LSD Research*, New York, E.P. Dutton.

Hageman, Joan J., Julio F.P. Peres, Alexander Moreira-Almeida, Leonardo Caixeta, Ian Wickramasekera II and Stanley Krippner, (2010) "The neurobiology of trance and mediumship in Brazil, " Chapter in S. Krippner and H. Friedman, eds, *Mysterious Minds: The Neurobiology of psychics, mediums and other extraordinary people*, Santa Barbara, Ca., Praeger, 85–111.

Hallowell, A. Irving (1966) "The role of dreams in Ojibwa culture," in (eds.) G.E. Von Gruebaum and R. Caillois, *The Dream and Human Societies*, Berkeley, University of California Press: 267–292.

Hardin, Garrett (1966) *Biology: Its Principles and Implications*, 2nd Ed. San Francisco, W.H. Freeman & Co.

Heinroth, O. (1910) "Beitrage zur Biologie, namentlick Ethologie und Physiologie der Anatiden," *5 International Ornithologisches Kongress*, Verh. 5:589–702.

Hove, Michael J. and Johannes Stelzer (2018) "Biological Foundations and beneficial effects of trance," *Behavioral and Brain Sciences,* v. 41, e76, 6 April: https://doi.org/10.1017/S0140525X17002072.

Huxley, Aldous (1954) *The Doors of Perception, and Heaven and Hell,* New York, Harper Colophon Books.

Johns, T. (1990) *With Bitter Herbs They Shall Eat It,* Tucson, University of Arizona Press.

Johnsgard, Paul A. (1967) *Animal Behavior,* Dubuque, Wm. C. Brown Co. Publishers.

Jordan-Young, Rebecca M. (2010*) Brain Storm: The Flaws in the Science of Sex Differences*, Cambridge, Harvard University Press.

Joseph, R. (2001) "The limbic system and the soul: evolution and neuroanatomy of religious experience," *Zygon*, v. 36:105–136.

Hoffmann A. (2009) LSD my problem child. Santa Cruz: Multidisciplinary Association for Psychedelic Studies, originally published in 1980 by McGraw-Hill, Boston.

Kaiser, Charles and Robert Gold (1973) "Perception, psychedelics and social change," *Journal of Drug Education*, v. 3, n 2:141–151.

Kawai, Norie, Manabu Honda, Emi Nishina, Reiko Yagi, and Tsutomu Oohashi, (2017) "Electroencephalogram characteristics during possession trances in healthy individuals," *Neuroreport*, Oct., 18, 28, 15:949–955.

Kelly, George A. (1963) *A Theory of Personality*, New York, The Norton Library.

Kessels, Roy P.C., Hans E. Kortrijk, Arie J. Wester, and M.S. Gudrun (2008) "Confabulation behavior and false memories in Korsakoff's syndrome: role of source memory and executive functioning," PCN Psychiatry and Clinical Neurosciences, 14 April, v. 62, n. 2:220–225.

Korzybski, Alfred, (1948) *Science and Sanity,* Lakeville, Institute of General Semantics.

Kreig, Margaret B. (1964) *Medicina Verde*, New York, Rand McNally.

Laughlin, Robert M. (1976) *Of Wonders Wild and New: Dreams from Zinacantan,* Smithsonian Contributions to Anthropology, n. 22, Washington, D.C., Smithsonian Institution.

Lee, Martin and Bruce Shlain (1985) *Acid Dreams: The Complete Social History of LSD, The Sixties, The CIA, the and Beyond*, New York, Grove Press, revised edition, 1994.

Levine, J., and Ludwig, A. M. (1964) "The LSD Controversy," *Campr. Psychiat.* 5: 314–321.

Lifton, Robert Jay (1970) *History and Human Survival*, New York, Random House.
Lihoreau, Mathieu, Tanya Latty and Lars Chittha, (2012) "An exploration of the social brain hypothesis in insects," *Front. Physiol.* 27 Nov. v. 3, 442. https://doi.org/10.3389/fphys.2012.00442.
Lorenz, K.Z. (1937) "The companion in the bird's world," *Auk*, v. 54:245–273.
Macphail, Euan M. (1982) *Brain and Intelligence in Vertebrates*, Oxford, Clarendon Press.
Marks, Sarah (2015) "From experimental psychosis to resolving traumatic pasts: Psychedelic research in Communist Czechoslvakia, 1954–1974," *Cahiers du Monde russe*, v. 56, n. 1, Jan–Mar:53–75.
Maslow, Abraham H. (1962) *Toward a Psychology of Being*, Princeton, van Norstrand.
McKenna, Terence (1992) *Food of the Gods*, New York, Bantam Books.
Montagu, Ashley (1986) *Touching: The Human Significance of the Skin*, New York, Harper & Row.
Morgar, Robert E. (1965) "Search and research with the psychedelics," *ETC: A Review of General Semantics*, v. 22, n. 4, Special Issue on the Psychedelic Experience, Dec.:393–407.
Munn, N.L. (1950) *Handbook of Psychological Research on the Rat*, New York, Houghton Mifflin.
OAC (Online Archive of California) (2021) "Student-Faculty Conference discussion of drugs on campus, San Francisco State College," Box 1493, sleeve 140307_01 Creator Eddie Murphy.
Ogden, Charles K. and I.A. Richards, (1923) *The Meaning of Meaning: A Study of the Influence of Language Upon Thought and of the Science of Symbolism*, London, Routledge.
Olson, David E. (2018) "Psychoplastogens: a promising class of plasticity-promoting neurotherapeutics," *J. of Experimental Neuroscience*, v. 12, 104.
Orengo-Garcia, F. (1998) "On the anatomo-physiological basis of trance and dissociation," in Spanish, *Actas Luso Esp Neurol Psiquiatr Cienc Afines*, Jul-Aug, 26, 4: 247–253.
Pagis, Michal (2010) "Producing intersubjectivity in silence: an ethnographic study of meditation practice," *Ethnography*, v. 11, n. 2: 309–328.
Pase, Matthew P., Jayandra J. Himali, Natalie A. Grima, Alexa S. Beiser, Claudia L. Satizabal, et al., (2017) "Sleep architecture and the risk of incident dementia in the community," *Neurology*, August 23, https://doi.org/10.1212/WNL.0000000000004373.
Patai, Raphael (1990) *The Hebrew Goddess, Detroit*, Wayne State University Press, third edition.

Perry, Helen (1970) *The Human Be-In,* London, Allen Lane The Penguin Press.
Radin, Paul (1937) *Primitive Religion,* New York, Viking Press.
Reinberg, Steven (2020) "Suicide rate keeps rising among young Americans," US News, Sept 11, https://www.usnews.com/news/health-news/articles/2020-09-11/suicide-rate-keeps-rising-among-young-americans, Accessed Nov 27, 2020.
Sacks, Oliver (1985) *The Man Who Mistook His Wife for a Hat,* New York, Harper & Row, Perennial Library Edition.
Sacks, Oliver (2012) *Hallucinations*, New York, Vintage Books.
Siegel, Ronald K. (2005) *Intoxication: The Universal Drive for Mind-Altering Substances*, Rochester Vermont, Park Street Press.
Sparks, R.S., John Melnyk, and L.P. Bozzeti (1968) "Chromosomal effect in vivo of exposure to Lysergic Acid Diethylamide," *Science,* June 21:v. 160, 3834:1343–1345.
Stein, Barry E. and M. Alex Meredith (1993) *The Merging of the Senses,* Cambridge Mass., A Bradford Book, MIT Press.
Stevens, Jay (1988) *Storming Heaven: LSD and the American Dream*, New York, Harper and Row.
Strassman, R. (2008). "The varieties of the DMT experience," in Inner Paths to Outer Space, 1st Edn., ed R. Strassman (Vermont, VT: Park Street Press), 51–80.
Tent, Pam (2004) *Midnight at the Palace: My Life as a Fabulous Cockette,* New York, Alyson Books.
Thompson, Clara (1950) *Psychoanalysis: Evolution and Development*, New York, Hermitage House.
Timmermann, Christopher, Leor Roseman, Luke Williams, David Erritzoe, Charolotte Martial, et al., (2018) "DMT models the Near-Death experience," *Front. Psychol.* 15 Aug., https://doi.org/10.3389/fpsyg.2018.01424.
Van Gennep, Arnold, (1960) *The Rites of Passage*, Chicago, University of Chicago Press.
Vardy, Michael M. and Stanley R. Kay, (1983) "LSD psychosis or LSD-induced schizophrenia," *Arch Gen Psychiatry*, v 40, (8): 877–883.
Wilkins, Leanne K., Todd A. Girard and J. Allan Cheyne (2011) "Ketamine as a primary predictor of out-of-body experiences associated with multiple substance use," *Conscious Cogn*. Sept., v. 20, n. 3, 943–950.
Winfield, Pamela D. (2017) Esoteric Ritual Remedies: Kukai's cures for Emperor Konin," in C. Pierce Salguero (ed.) *Buddhism and Medicine,* Chapter 23, New York, Columbia University Press:222–225.
Wolf, Leonard (1968) *Voices of the Love Generation,* Boston, Little, Brown.

5

The Indigenous View and Categories of Normality

This chapter investigates the nature of change and expectation in the use of psychedelics. It refers to events and attitudes in the 1960s as experienced by the author and as described in the literature. Specifically it focuses on the aspect of self we call personality, how this is assessed, especially by the MMPI. An examination of cultural differences in dreams is also included. It also discusses how many people interviewed or known by the author saw themselves and psychedelics and how science can describe some of the aspects noted.

I am going to consider "indigenous" in this book as an identity and as a process. We might use the word "endogenous" to mean those things that emanate from inside something or someone. And then we could use the term "exogenous" for those things that come from the outside. But these terms are seldom applied to humans, except in recognition of pathological origins and some other related meaning, like "endogenous virus," though these terms are also applied to kinship and mate choice in groups. The term "indigenous" has been used to mean original, aboriginal, and essentially to a place or person. The antonym would be "foreign" or unfamiliar, strange, alien. All of these are appropriate to the problem of experience and interpretation.

N. Caldararo, *A Mental Ethnography: Conclusions From Research in LSD*,
https://doi.org/10.1007/978-3-031-13745-7_5

There is another essential distinction and that is where an individual takes LSD or peyote or other mind-altering drug alone, in a small social group in a modern urban society, in a medical context with a physician or psychologically trained monitor, versus an indigenous context where an individual consumes a drug in a social context that is constructed culturally for special purposes. These purposes might be, as in the case of the Tarahumare, for healing and might be associated with an end that the ceremony is designed to achieve. Other drugs might have specific purposes, but the effects on the brain are less dramatic, as in the case of tobacco smoked by the Cheyenne to seal a decision (as in a peace arrangement between two men or tribes; see Hoebel 1954, 162).

In recent years ideas of the transmission of ideas (memes) in populations have been attractive (Dawkins 2016) and Sperber's (1975) suggestions about ideas held by a population of individuals in a culture are interesting—how do ideas differ among people in a society, do subgroups form due to similar perceptions of concepts and their variations? This is also similar to Kelly's (1963) ideas on constructs and their variability. The theory of a population of individuals holding slightly different interpretations is attractive both from a practical standpoint (it reflects reality) and from a Darwinian standpoint. Ideas can lead people to non-adaptive acts (self-destruction, castration, war, etc.) and can result in more efficient use of resources, that is, more adaptive.

Thus, the theory so often repeated at the time that LSD allowed a form or re-creation or ontogenic reorganization which provided an opportunity to relearn or unlearn traumatic experiences was tethered into a logical biological system. One takes LSD, as in the case of Grof's subject Richard, and one travels through one's cellular history (some people expressed this as a total body process where all cells participated, or all DNA, but perhaps today we would say the chromosomal histones with their epigenetic role) to produce in neurons a reconditioning of memories. Today's research in memory consolidation, retrieval, and reconsolidation seems to provide some support for this on a biochemical basis (Steinberg 2004). Such "relearning" has an important role in treatments proposed for PTSD (Xu et al. 2009) and related conditions (Rashid et al. 2016).

Combat veterans suffering from PTSD and specific pain have come to the fore to legalize the use of psychedelics for treatment (Jacobs 2021).

But another of Grof's subjects takes this metaphor farther; he experiences the consciousness of all life in his DNA, as if it was a book of life. Often Grof's (1976, 202–3) descriptions border on the metaphysical, as with his description of Tantric "memory" in subjects. But as with his description of subjects who experience the "Universal Mind" version of reality, Grof is left with the difficulty of a fair and accurate reproduction. These kinds of experience often leave the subject in a state where either the pleasure of knowledge is so great it defies verbal definition or the subject's identification with it produces a Buddha or Meher Baba-like condition where any expression is not only inadequate, but also unnecessary—Meher Baba being a guru who at one point in his life stopped speaking as his speech was so often mistaken.

Grof (1976, 127), in my view, mistakes the conception of destruction, and then creation, for violence. He argues that violence is often a part of the LSD experience. This was not my understanding from the Mogar data or my own interpretation of others' experience or my own. In some of the examples in the literature on this subject, for example, Grof's, the described violence is part of an individual's description of their personality, at least that is how it is often interpreted and how Grof (1976, 128) does— though some theories of psychopathology suggest violence relived is violence done again. This is why, in my opinion, some researchers saw LSD as a "truth serum" and therefore the interest of governments. But I think the evidence points more to suggestion and to environmental context and experience than to a prediction of personality or differentiating means of separating truth from lies, or using psychedelics as torture weapons. Drugs that were used by governments and judicial systems or clinical settings were judged not effective (Naples and Hackett 1978). I am not arguing that there is no association between psychedelics and violence. De Rios (1984) argues that there is a historical relation in some New World cultures (Aztec, Inca, Mochica) between organizrd violence, even war and certain drugs.

Two problems present themselves here. One is the realization of actuality. How can the subject recognize the hallucination as not reality, or is it a kind of reality and it has some unexpected and unknown effect on actuality? The Australian Aborigines and a variety of other people believe that the experiences of the soul in sleep take place in an alternative, but very significant reality. The same is true for forms of trance, what happens to the person's presence or awareness is interpreted as a journey. I gave a reference to this regarding dreams and some indigenous ideas, for example, from the Andaman Islands. How can one recognize danger and what kinds of responses are appropriate? As the Yaqui shaman's response to young people in the Haight-Ashbury demonstrated, many indigenous people see adverse events can take place in either "world," so how does one respond? I have to admit, I did not learn from the Yaqui shaman what he was going to do if he came to San Francisco and spoke to people taking STP.

There are methods in indigenous knowledge for how to recognize realities and how to respond to specific danger. The plasticity of the human brain seems to allow different peoples to interpret the experiences of the same plant extract in different ways. Metzner (1968) lists some of these groups for the Mexican province of Oaxaca, as does Wasson (1962). This seems to be true even within the same groups, as where Barbara Myerhoff (1974) is told by her Huichol *mara'akame* (or shaman-priest as she interprets his role) that the hallucinations she has, like all Huichol except the *mara'akame* are for "beauty's sake alone," and while spiritual in nature, only the *mara'akame* can understand them. This seems to me a problem of learning and inculcation of meaning. Metzenich, (2013) reviews the advances in neuroscience that has led to new ideas of brain plasticity and how the brain can constantly "rewire" or reorganize itself.

How different people or peoples come to utilize these hallucinations and build cultural meaning that is adaptive is an aspect of human creativity, opportunity, and accident in my view. Here Korzybski (1948) suggested that "it takes a good mind to be insane" and that "the average person in 1933 must be considered insane." He found it remarkable that humans could advance technologically in fields like science, medicine, mathematics, and engineering and yet act in ways that seemed irrational with misunderstanding, suspicion, bigotry, hatred, and violence, both individually and as whole societies. Perhaps this is due to our ability to split attention and awareness, to be awed by the social hallucination, able at the same time to conduct otherwise rational and logical actions in another set of attention and hallucinations (in Seth's context).

There is a considerable debate among the philosophers of mind concerning the nature of hallucinations. The comparison of hallucinations to "veridical perceptions" (the degree to which one's internal representation of the world accurately reflects the external world) fails the test of phenomenology, and as ffytche (2013) points out, no common definition of hallucination is satisfying. Basing ideas of kinds of experiences on individual cases of introspection seems the ultimate exercise in subjectivity. The theory of epistemic hallucination just argues that hallucinations seem the same as real perceptions and the disjunctivist theory argues that hallucinations are different from real perceptions (Siegel 2008). Blom's (2010) monumental work, *A Dictionary of Hallucinations*, provides a catalogue of types and attempts to address some of the problems of definition. This might be expected from Hebb's (1954) observation on experimental animals and human cognitive variability and complexity. But if, as I have argued here, we can reflect on the ethnographic evidence that people in a small-scale society, without industrial and electronic age interference, could understand not only their own dreams and hallucinations (includes the concept of "qualia," as discussed before), but those of others of their culture as well, then we have a basis to work from. Yet from her survey of the ethnographic literature de Rios (1984) sees greater variability. Culture is the mechanism, the key to the phenomenological lock and yet the confusion and distraction of modern, pluralistic society seems to have broken that key, or at least blunted its facility. Perhaps there is then something to Durkheim's (1915) collective representations that existed in a small-scale society as the epiphenomenon of a low-density living context and extended family interaction that promoted such integration of images and meaning.

Vansina (1985) have applied this idea to larger societies and one can see in Canetti's (1966) discussion of symbols and ideology how it has been extended to modern industrial states. At least we might argue that it can form the basis for the Native Theory concept of dreams.

Goody and Watt (1968) call this situation "dynamic homeostasis," based on the existence of a homogeneous society. This could be seen as parallel to Bourdieu's (1977) "habitus," where the borders of commonality of experience include perceptions of the body and its various extensions. This could be related to Stewart's (1951) Senoi dream theory (see also Dentan 1968), though it has been challenged (Domhoff 1990). A child's life (as all members) includes daily dream interpretation, a certain means of inculcation of values and beliefs. It cannot survive where there has been the creation of a heterogeneous society, which they (Goody and Watt, 1968) define as resulting from literacy. Vansina (1985) disagrees, arguing that such a homeostasis cannot exist, as all societies retain "archaisms," but I think this is a misunderstanding of Goody and Watt's concept, though I think literacy is not the only means to dismember the homeostasis—any separation that creates significant boundaries in the society could result from power accumulation. My and Vansina's criticism would seem to make the idea so rare as to be a special case and perhaps only theoretical. Nevertheless, it seems obvious that if such a state of society existed, it would require people to grow up within a limited community and inculcate these representations from birth; thus, we return to Vygotsky and the social context.

There is a question here regarding literacy. While the earliest graphic expression of meaning from languages we know of were mainly pictographic in their origins, the evolution of writing demanded the abstraction of the literal representation of a house or person to a symbol. This seems like a process of "relational character," as some philosophers describe the "naïve realist" view, and that of veridical hallucination (Nudds 2013). If an image was that of a real thing, like a symbol in early cuneiform, but evolves into a design that had little similarity, then the individual reading it must constantly be replacing one form of image for another, even if subconsciously. This is where Seth's "controlled hallucinations" (I would argue, "continuous hallucinations," not to be confused with the uncontrolled stream of hallucinations of hemianopia or the loss of half of one's visual field, caused by damage to one occipital lobe; Sacks 2012) can fit, for as each person learns to use language and to read, the process is facilitated by the social context, where reinforcement from others permits a limited paring of the specific image that an individual might have from experience, into a general one that can be referenced to the use of others and is subject to constant sanction and conditioning.

The second question mentioned above relates to time. Time seems often to be affected by psychedelics and certain pathologies that produce hallucinations. What time is it? I recall once being at a Fillmore Auditorium musical event where the Grateful Dead and some other bands were playing. During a break I was standing with friends when one stranger who was very "high" on something came over and asked a friend,

"What time is it?" No one could answer at the moment as it seemed the question was not one of what was the time for all people at that place in San Francisco (i.e., relative to time zones), but a diffuse question, "time" eliciting eventually from one person as relative and mundane, "time for the next band," "time for a change in world consciousness," and so on.

Human Be-In, All Is One, Illusion, and Radical Futures

One event in my memory combines these two questions. During the 1967 "Be-In in Golden Gate Park" I was walking with friends, Michael Canright and some other people, to the event. We came to Shrader Street, which bordered the residential area from the Park and the Panhandle. The light was red and we were all coming on the LSD and there was a general stasis where it seemed time had stopped. All of a sudden Michael threw up his arms and shouted, "I can't be killed!" and ran into the street, causing some consternation among drivers, though the light changed as he was in the middle of the street. Time, obviously, is relative to a number of factors, yet under the influence of psychedelics and certain contexts (as in Osmond's [1970] description of "Peyote Night"), time seems to melt, disappear, or blend into a vast soup of vague impressions.

There were often odd events that took place in the Haight-Ashbury in 1966, the year before the Human Be-In, but one often reads of the time as if it had been a constant circus. Several books have promoted this idea, as in Jay Stevens' *Storming Heaven*, where he opens the book with scenes of people dancing, singing, putting on ad hoc plays, and describes it as a rather perpetual gypsy camp. This is strange to my memory, as I do not recall anything like that. The Haight-Ashbury in 1966 was still an integrated, working-class neighborhood where many students found reasonably affordable housing. There was a large Russian immigrant population as well as new transplants, many African Americans, but also other ethnic groups, from the evictions by the San Francisco Redevelopment Agency in the Fillmore District. Now and then there were events put on by the several "houses" of students or former students where they might engage in the behavior Stevens recounts. However, in his defense, I can say that on the day of the Human Be-In there were people from all over who had come to the park, many acting as the strange people they had read about in the media.

To use the term "hippies" would be presumptuous—the word was not what most people called themselves, just like the "Beatniks" who lived in the apartment next to the one I lived in on Oak Street then. They were graduate students at SFSU, but in their dress, manner, and attitude they appeared to be Beatniks to me. They invited me and one of my roommates to dinner one night. I brought my girlfriend on the recommendation of one of the "Beatnik" women. As the dinner progressed they began asking a lot of personal questions, like how often did we have sex, did we do drugs, which ones, did my girlfriend use protection, and so on. Then as the alcohol spread out after the meal, they began to evaluate us as if we were not there. One of the women said, "They seem really uptight to me." Another commented, "Very conservative and close-minded to be sure." To me they were just strange, and since I had spent some time hanging out at UC Berkeley as a high school student, they just seemed like students to me. To my girlfriend, they were Beats. More experienced than I, and a year older, she had had some older boyfriends that she called "Beats."

This kind of generalization is common in most situations. In Stevens' book he repeats many of the identifiers published in the press at the time—for example, the hippies rejected the middle-class society, which had created them. This was not what I knew, as most of my friends were from working-class families, if you classify them by whether people receive a paycheck and punch a time card. Most of them worked, part time or full, though a good number did receive money from home. They were certainly not "dropping outs" but interested in everything, though their draft status (at least for the men) was a gnawing concern. And there was the problem of if you dropped out of school, you could lose your deferment and go to Vietnam.

Obviously, the determination of a danger is based on assessing inputs of information, visual, auditory, olfactory with memory (as also with "phantom limbs," a certain type of hallucination) and training (conditioning) as well as context, and this includes time, as when children born without hands can use phantom fingers to count, thus a useful continuous and consciously controlled hallucination (see Sacks 2012). To return to Michael's run across the street on LSD, it regards the issue of awareness of danger. For myself, at this moment I could assess the light and cars as elements of caution and, in a moment or two, the context of danger was realized. I then also saw my friend dash among cars and wondered if he really could not be killed. Seconds later I was across the street safely and no one mentioned Michael's challenge to reality. Kluver (1928/1966, 74–5) reports this same modification of time with peyote—it can be perceived as sped up or slowing down, just as his subjects reported size increases and decreases; unnatural movements, as in jerky ones, are also reported as well as the unnatural movement of stationary objects and mirror images (Kluver 1928/1966, 80–83). He also notes that some people state they are "beyond desires" when on the drug, not thirsty or hungry or wanting sex, and so on. This is true also in LSD, but mainly I think from my observations, this is due to the fact that people move from one idea or sensation rapidly to another or become so fixed that an operation can take a long time for completion (I recall some people surprised at one moment that they were eating). Also, actual eating, for example, becomes an intense examination of the object, cake, apple, drink, and so on, instead of consumption. Like with peyote, as Kluver reports, a very common experience with LSD is an indescribable "euphoria." An amused state arrives that persists for some time, often accompanied by laughter or giggling (see the results reported by Blum et al. 1964 on euphoria). I recall this especially with marijuana or hash in baked items, where the taste was such a delight that conversation concerning chocolate or nuts or some other taste could take on what seemed hours only to be found to be minutes.

The nature of any interpretation depends on assessments but also on context. Later that day with Michael and the Human Be-In, when thousands of people had listened to bands and talks, the chanting started, which was considered by my friends to be a signal for get more food and search for other friends. I wandered off, meeting a girl I knew, and stood for a moment as she said something about Timothy Leary. I realized that most of the day I had not really listened to other people with any care and my memories of conversations were fragmentary at best. Then two men approached whom she knew slightly who were dressed, in my assessment, as medieval wizards complete with staffs. They said they were looking for food and she said they should come to her house, where there was a rather large food preparation event going on. Seconds later I heard another voice—a man, also wearing a costume and with a staff, asked, "Got a match?" One of the two men looked at him and said, "No we are not queer." The man then said, "You misunderstand, I need a light for my joint." Immediately there was a wave of fear I felt from the girl and the two men, who responded asking him if he was a cop. At this point I was viewing the conversation as if from afar, their voices almost tiny and with a noticeable vibrato. At that moment the beauty of the girl took on an overwhelming quality. I had known her for about a year, we had met in a literature class and been just friends. We had studied at night and had some really intense conversations, unaffected by drugs of any kind. She looked at me and I heard her lips move and air against my face. Then came the words, "Did you hear me? Let's go." I then said, "I'd like to lay in the grass with you." The next thing I knew we were laying in the grass, kissing. The exploration of her face with kisses, her hair with my fingers, led by thoughts through a tempest of scenes of all kinds. I could sense people walking around us. The Human Be-In was over.

This sequence of interactions I wrote down when I returned home, which was only a block away on Oak Street. I was struck by the disjointed nature of the conversation and the lack of comprehension. I also found that most of the memories I had of that day were images and sound but not words. A girl I did not know had joined us at some time (my friend told me) and I had snuggled in the grass with both for some time in a rather joyful but unisexual riot of caressing. But then someone else came by she knew, two girls, and they all left together. I had heard them say something and it sounded inviting, but I had felt rooted to the spot with the mass of people at the time.

These reminiscences emphasize the problems and complexity of interpretation in time and space between different individuals and single individuals in typical modern situations. Mogar (1965) was concerned with this agreeing with Lancelot L. Whyte (1930) that there was too much "investment in language and higher-order abstractions at the expense of nonverbal experience and nonverbal communication." Whyte called this

"Western dissociation," as if it placed those in Western societies in a special category of information processing. One might agree and go so far as to say that people in Western complex societies, or where globalism has substantially transformed their cultures and education, are at a disadvantage in understanding the world and communicating their perceptions. However, as with the discussion earlier on literacy, I think this goes too far. Was the sensuous event I experienced at the Human Be-In due to LSD or the setting? Could it have happened on alcohol, or did it happen at all and was only a hallucination? Luckily, a few days later my female student friend corroborated my memories of the event, though with added detail.

So, we are trapped in semantics? Korzybski might say yes. If so, perhaps we should simply look at behavior. In 1967 I was satisfied with a general approach, this became an exposition of the effects of LSD in altering the established relationships in any particular individual, thus giving one a new perspective both on prior information and on present perceptions. What are these relationships? Some psychologists I spoke to at the time felt LSD modified the structure of the learned penetration of the id, superego, and ego. If these "penetrations" can be described as repression by an adult, training by schoolteachers, or other social interactions that become "ingrained" or habitual parts of one's character (perhaps what Kelly [1963] called "constructions"), then does the relearning process reduce their emphasis in memory?

This idea leads to some rather fantastic ideas, like in psychiatric analysis, where the idea put forth is that there exists an internalized parent and it is the job of the successful therapist to replace or remake this (if "oppressive") "inner eye," as Humphrey (1986) has put it, with a less destructive form (Forer 1969). Like with the construct of the ego, id, and superego of Freud, or the role of repression and internalization of the parent in the process of enculturation theorized by Freudians like Roheim (1945), the nature of this idea is an entirely subjective one. How can it be proven? It is as elusive as the nature of ultimate truth or systems of values. Maslow is critical of the way Freud avoids this question, but then it seems to me Freud hit on it straight on in his book *The Future of an Illusion* (1927/1957). We should be cautious here as the concept of an "inner eye" has been reexamined in the light of new discoveries about how the brain functions. Oliver Sacks' discussion of this feature of human consciousness is more elaborate and detailed than Humphrey's and gives a number of examples from pathological conditions that limit this inner vision that Sacks calls "the (Sacks 2010) mind's eye." But perhaps the "inner eye," "mind's eye" and "self perception" are not related or the same condition as aphantasia or describe variations of a similar one.

Adam Zeman et al. (2015, 2020) have found that some people lack an inner eye, or at least the ability to produce a mental camera of images of experience and fantasy. This condition is termed "aphantasia," and they estimate it is fairly common, with millions reporting the condition or variations of it. In contrast, some people experience extraordinarily strong mental images, now called, "hyperphantasia," which is also rather common. We might imagine that people in the hyperphantasia category would have perceptual experiences in a fairly routine fashion that others might consider hallucinations. The two conditions cause us, as in so many other cases, to reconsider what is normal perception. This brings us to the question of the nature of the inner eye. When silenced, as in meditation or aphantasia, what actually happens to a person's sense of self? Is the inner eye the Freudian "superego" that is implanted by the family during enculturation? Does it allow for governance in society and its loss creates madness and chaos?

The fact that Buddhists who meditate and seem to lose their "egos" do not become chaotic madmen is of interest, but also that people with aphantasia are rather normal. Galton (1880) was surprised by how many people "suffered" under this condition, many of them Galton's colleagues in science. Zeman et al. (2015) found that many people with the condition could experience involuntary images, sometimes as faces, as in dreams. We mentioned this condition earlier as hypnagogic hallucinations. Some people have extremely vivid images but no narrative, the process of "going to sleep" is a complex one and we might say it can leave traces of memory as it "closes down the brain." Investigation of these "faces" and their changes and multiplication in different cases led ffytche et al. (1998) to the discovery of the fusiform face area of the right brain, where use of fMRI allowed its localization and functional identification. When faces are hallucinated, it is stimulated. These images may differ at the same time, with faces in one area, a landscape and with incredible detail, which may suddenly appear to race toward one. In a homologous area of the left hemisphere of the brain, an area is stimulated when people experience lexical hallucinations. Some of the images are of recent memory, others unfamiliar (Sacks 2012).

We might attribute some aspects of extra sensory perception (ESP) to this idea of the mind's eye. Often people imagine events, since we can think about anything with such detail and emotion that it seems to be happening in real time—in other words, "mind travel" or projection in time, and this sensation could easily be mistaken for actual contact of people and events across time and space. Gordon Wasson reported to Metzner (1968) just such an event. While in Mexico he had been asked by a curandero if there was something that bothered him. He made up a concern for this son and was told that his son was in trouble with a girl and being taken into the army. Some time later, after traveling back to Europe he found a telegraph message that his son had had problems with a girl and had enlisted in the army. The problem of separating our abilities to imagine and project thoughts and the actual association of events is summarized by new research in psychedelics and ESP, now called "Psychedelomancy" (Luke 2012). I experienced this once under the influence of peyote and was present several times when other people had similar sensations. I cannot say they were authentic, as there was and still is lacking a means of verifying such associations. ESP in the form of clairvoyance is reported for the use of yage among the Tucano (Lowie 1948) and the Jivaro (Harner 1968). There is sometimes argued a theoretical link between predictions of events and time travel or travel in seconds across great distances on Earth or the cosmos, sometimes called "spooky actions at a distance," a theory that bothered Einstein (Aczel 2001).

To Freud all religious beliefs are illusions created to protect against the feeling of helplessness. If one is to analyze the ultimate reasons for human behavior at base, one does find in every culture a group feeling that is manifest in ritual and dogma, as Durkheim (1915) described. One does not become a nihilist on discovering there is no god or that one's natal religion is false. Usually people convert to an alternative or create a new system more to their liking. The rejection of "what is" does not create the immediate question, "is there nothing?" Rather the questioning individual is faced with a multitude of options and an infinite of possibilities. Alan Watts' (1970) description of his personal experience of this process is of interest here. To embark on such a journal of discovery can be one of rejection and opposition, or to attract disapproval, as often happens to atheists by others in reaction. Agnostics, though considered cowards by some religious people and scholars (note Karen Armstrong and her debate with Richard Dawkins), can find themselves in an ark or ship of inner and outer space.

But this is unfulfilling for Maslow; he criticizes Freudian psychoanalysis as being only a system of psychopathology and cure of psychopathology, of backing away from being a psychology of spiritual life. As noted above, Freud did accomplish this, but what after it? Can psychoanalysts be believers in any religious dogma? Can they see their clients as simply wrongheaded unbelievers who should be cured by a firmer belief or as poor animals suffering because a distant god allows errors from the perfection possible that it called "normality"? Or would psychoanalysis and psychiatrists find themselves duty bound to attack and expose every false prophet and irrational belief that appears in place of a firm empiricism? I once told a class that I believed in nothing, that I was an empiricist and I thought it was difficult for an anthropologist to be a believer. A student asked me why and my answer was that to study and describe the world's cultures, social organizations, and religions with a particular belief system (Christian or Marxist, for example) would violate the cultural relativity necessary to be balanced and as unbiased as possible. Empiricism, the view of reason and proof and cultural relativity, a system of categories and not comparisons, seemed the only honest approach. Maslow (1964) argues that Freudians shield themselves by arguing that religious beliefs are sublimations for biological drives, that is, defenses against instincts. If this were true, then we would be poor learners at that, as crime is low and the plundering horde long gone, or is it? It seems to appear at will during war and conflict, riots and economic crises.

Maslow (1964) also attacks the Behaviorists (like Skinner), who he argues have no answers at all to human problems, but deny all morality and belief on the basis of learning and instinct. Like many scholars of the late twentieth century, Maslow excused humanity by reference to the stress of war (two world wars) economic collapse (Great Depression), and invention of weapons of mass destruction. These are, however, all human-created problems, problems that are at their core driven by human values, the very values he shames the Behaviorists for lacking respect for. He believes we are in danger due to the nihilism and valuelessness of the times, yet it is values that have created the crises.

This brings in the idea of religion as a natural consequence of human biology, of human consciousness. Alexander Fingelkurts (2009) surveys the literature on the topic from two diametrically opposite positions: (1) Is the human brain hardwired to produce a god or gods? (2) Is our brain hardwired to perceive a god or gods? Included in this should be the basic question of people like Lang and Tylor (see De Waal Malefijt 1968), does animatism represent the foundational premise for the evolution of god systems of religion and magic? This idea is partially based on the work of heritability of attitudes, especially twin studies (Olson et al. 2001). One problem with this research is that documented by Damasio et al. (2000), where self-generated emotions can reproduce brain activity of personal life episodes, so it reinforces the idea Freud had that childhood experiences (see Nyhof and Johnson 2017, for example) are the basis for unusual dreams and visions in adulthood and these can be the foundation of Lang and Tylor's concept of the evolution of religion (Tylor 1889). Reinforcing this basis by systemic enculturation processes, myths, rites, and so on can be a cause not only for uniform religious belief but variation. As Mead (1932, 1975, 133) found, there is a lack of specific ideas of parental group religious tradition in very young children (three to seven year olds). Instead she found more diffuse, universal ideas that reinforce both the idea of the Psychic Unity of Mankind theory of Bastian and the Blank Slate concept of Locke, undermining foundations for religious iconography as a biological or development process.

Earlier I was examining the idea of Deism and religion, or acosmic conceptions of reality. One might ask, what happens when one lives without religion or are there societies without religion? Often people point to the Soviet Union, where at the time of collapse, some two-thirds of the population reported being atheists, and recently, some 71% reported being Orthodox Christian believers (Zubovich 2018). Obviously some of the people reporting to be believers now must have reported being atheists in 1990—can people change beliefs so fast or is acknowledging belief or disbelief a social performance of allegiance or membership? What about crime, usually tracts against Communism or atheism argue that without god and religion, man would simply return to bestial life? Soviet Union crime statistics are difficult to determine, even though data has been made available of what was once considered a state secret. The classification of what is a crime has been obfuscated by political considerations in the opinion of some students of the subject (Butler 1992). Yet it has been claimed that the United States, obviously a Christian nation in its founding and institutions, has more people in prison than the Soviet Union at the height of the Stalinist gulags (Gopnik 2012). Many LSD proponents in the 1950s and 1960s predicted either utopian transformations of humanity or a psychotic future—though in a mid-ground were the more agnostic leanings of some of the people at the Mogar Lab who suggested a variety of outcomes if psychedelic experiences were neutral (philosophically that is, with only a blank slate-like effect) or could be uniformly manipulated as some of the early government (CIA) researchers had thought.

What of mental health? This factor is distorted by racism in the United States and by the Soviet idea that mental illness was a product of capitalism. The Soviet system also treated resistance to the Soviet system as mental illness, so comparisons are difficult to make (Petrea and Haggenburg 2014). Perhaps it is an unfair comparison—one could consider the Soviet system to be an ideology not unlike a religion and thus it would have similar stresses inflicted on its population. Studies of atheists and other forms of non-believers, like agnostics, show they have fewer mental health problems than religiously affiliated individuals. This might also be an unfair comparison, as there are so few of the former and so many varieties of religious belief in the latter (Baker et al. 2018).

Even more difficult to understand is the fact that about half of all dreams people have contain at least one element from a specific experience of the subject while awake (Fosse et al. 2003; Greenberg and Leiderman 1966). For Greenberg and Leiderman (1966), this was part of the theory of dreaming where events of the day, "residues," are transferred to long-term memory. Yet given that the hippocampus part of the brain is involved in memory, people possessing a damaged hippocampus still apparently dream (Torda 1969a, b). These dreams were shorter than normal, contained memory of events the subjects had experienced before the brain damage or deficit occurred, yet the subjects had lost the ability to recall recent events when awake. Still the subjects were experiencing in dreams events, which did happen to them yet of which they had no conscious memory (Stickgold et al. 2000).

More recent work on episodic memory and construction using fMRI demonstrates that the hippocampus is only one area involved in this complex process of organizing memories and perceptions into plans in a reconstructive process (Hassabis and Maguire 2009). Numerous others are now known to participate: the prefrontal cortex, parahippocapal gyrus, lateral temporal cortices, temporoparietal junction, thalamus, retrosplenial cortex, posterior cingulate cortex, precuneus, and cerebellum. Recent experiments have indicated that the hippocampus builds associations across stimulus domains and damage to this area severely reduces associative memory (Borders et al. 2017). This exposure of the interaction of so many parts of the brain perhaps explains why damage to the hippocampus would not destroy memory or use of memory. But patients with bilateral damage to the hippocampus were largely unable to construct as new images future experiences (Hassabis et al. 2007).

This information about memory construct is curious in light of how LSD affects the brain. As Carhart-Harris et al. (2016) found, the drug enhances the visual center activity, with some reduction in the parahippocampus and the retrosplenial cortex, but also other area reductions, as in the precuneus. Perhaps the relative enhancement of visual information in relation to the reduced flow of activity in other areas produces the perceived effects of users.

Yet much of this work on dream analysis and pathology, or Western subjects' dreams, is difficult to apply to the experiences of LSD. Many of the comparisons are based on assumptions about the vivid nature of dreams of normal people, which is questionable. As Huxley (1954) expresses in his disappointment with peyote, his dreams in sleep were not very significant and certainly not vivid and detailed. But what is new to him is how color appears in prominent and abnormal significance and everything takes on a greater meaning, as when his books glow. Mogar (1965) makes this distinction between the people who seek an uplifting experience, or a searching mentality for philosophical import, versus those who are selected as patients for treatment with LSD.

Kilborne (1981), in reviewing the work of Malinowski and Lincoln (1935) on the dreams of non-Western societies and isolated indigenous peoples, found their dreams to vary considerably from peoples' experiences in industrialized Western countries. He noted that dream analysis and interpretation by many anthropologists had followed methods of psychologists in approaching dreams as individual, private, and non-social experience. Herdt (1987) among others, emphasizes the public private nature and function of dreams in indigenous context. Yet dream analysis in the West is based on the foundation of the ancient dream books of medieval students of dreams derived from Greek and Babylonian sources. The use of life histories or forms of autobiography is a prominent feature in the former approach. In the latter approach, a "grab bag" of symbols were sought to break the "code" of dream. More recent public private nature and function of dreams in indigenous context. Yet dream analysis in the West is based on the attempts followed Jung (his archetypes we have already discussed) and Durkheim (1915) in his collective representations, or an eclectic approach, as in Goodison (1995). This latter approach is more of a social experience of interpretation. This approach can be seen to meld the life history method with a social context when, as in the work of Dorothy Eggan (1961), the individual's experience is interpreted in a culture personality context where responses are seen as expressions of cultural means and functions. This approach was considered to be most effective where dramatic culture change was occurring.

From Lincoln's (1935) study we find a significant difference between indigenous dreams where the societies are still remote from industrialized and colonial influence (especially missionaries). This idea is reinforced by Kilborne (1981), where he defines the different types of dreams, starting with the "message" dream. These have a certain form that seems to be unique to particular cultures. Here he uses the ancient Greek examples where the dream agent, as the visit of Patroclus to Achilles in the *Iliad*, always enters the dreamer's consciousness through a keyhole. A dream form and a conventionalized narrative, the message, mark the experience. The Greeks did not speak of "having a dream" but of seeing one. The cultural pattern then is that the reality of the dream exists outside the dreamer. Sometimes the dream agent would leave a "dream token" behind that might have some future significance. This differs from the "dream marker" that the medieval European was told to put under the bed so it could be checked to see if he or she was dreaming.

In many North American tribes dreams were directed for the experience of a journey or life change, so the soul undergoes a trip to the land of the ancestors, as in the case of Black Elk (1932), where the dreamer receives special knowledge, either a skill, role, or prophesy. Dream patterning appears to have been characteristic of ancient China and Eastern Asia (Laufer 1931). In some cases, as in the Book of Dreams of Duke of Zhou, the interpretations seem to be linked to ancient Chinese medical models like the Yellow Emperor's. Here the dream of the person's body's self-implication or reference is clear. A dream of a hot situation may reflect on the imbalance of Yin and Yang (Ong 1985). Freud (1961) and other psychologists interpreted some dreams in terms of the body as well, or in the case of some of Jones' (1921) material, people in their dreams are disguised as themselves. While Rivers (1920) first argued that the social form of nightmare was revolution, the same can be seen in illness or personal relationship, where the loved one is perceived as ill, angry, or violent.

But even in his description of pattern dreams of peoples still intact culturally, Lincoln (1935) reports two types of dream one can have, one that is "individual" and significant to the personal, and one that has a "special tribal significance." Malinowski (1929) reports in similar fashion on "true" dreams that are responses to magic and spiritual influence; these cannot be avoided and are not spontaneous. In contrast there are "free" or spontaneous ones that seem to be similar categories to Lincoln's. These latter dreams are considered by the Natives as lies or illusions and they do not put much store in them. While this division of dreams in ethnographic context seems to have some general validity, the nature of the intent may be difficult to always assign, as in the "unsought" dreams, both of shamans and of individuals. It is often part of the shamanic narrative that individuals do not seek to become shamans, but it is forced on them, either by spirits, parents, or the disease experience and calling in dreams (Eliade 1964).

Among the Artic Inuits, many such experiences one might call hallucinations or "daydreams" are common to many in a group, but others are associated with trance (Rasmussen 1930), while a peculiar class of visions and trance is part of a condition known as *menerik*. Shamans in the arctic are often chosen from people suffering from this condition. *Menerik* is often included or described separately from the condition known as *pibloktoq* or Artic hysteria (Gussow 1960). *Pibloktoq* is described as affecting men and women at any time and has a range of symptoms, from temporary madness to depression to hysteria. Attempts to associate it with seasonal lack of sunlight, dietary conditions, and isolation have been suggested (Novakovsky 1924). Temporary madness or periods of unusual or abnormal behavior are reported from many people, after which the individuals return to normal productive lives, as Cora Du Bois (1945) reports of men and women among the Alorese.

Another problem with LSD experiences that is related to researchers is the question of authenticity, conscious manipulation of the experience by the "user/subject," and what the researcher interprets and writes down. In Grof's case he rejects Eva's retrieved memory of her father's brutality on the basis of its improbability, given his own experience and sensibility. The problem bothered Kilborne (1981), especially where he questions Lincoln's argument that culture dreams tended to be replaced by individual dreams as a process of acculturation. In some Native American cultures personal dreams that are culture dreams pertain to the individual's transition in life, while others point to new roles, as in the case of Black Elk. Some of these are one-time visits while others form relationships, as with guardian spirits. But dreams can bring knowledge that is new to change the life of the individual or tribe, yet in some cases, as among the Mohave, dreams occur in the prenatal life, where at the moment of creation the souls of future shamans lived with deities at the sacred mountain, where the child god Matavilya gave powers to the unborn souls (Kilborne 1981). These dreams are forgotten at birth and reappear later, and the shaman dreams from the store of the unchangeable world of the Mohave world at the time when need appears.

This brings us to another dilemma. Kilborne (1981) is concerned with Lincoln's (1935) reference to dreamed songs, and other knowledge, and their acceptance by the group as authentic as dreamed. Thus, among the Flathead (Merriam 1967) songs are acquired from the supernaturals when in contact in dreams. Therefore, the idea of memory is the "remembering right" to the group. Kilborne is critical, as is Vansina (1985) and Goody (1987), of similar and constructed their own activities as a processes elsewhere, but in both their cases, they are not dealing with materials from intact societies, so perhaps the comparison is not valid. Devereux (1951,

1957) argues that dreamed knowledge was often complex and it was necessary to learn it in waking life and then dream it in "condensed or symbolic" form after. This problem also vexes psychiatry, as in the example Grof gives of Dana and her mother. While we might accept the mother's confirmation of the description given by the daughter of events and conditions when Dana was two years of age, there is a methodological problem. The mother's memory would have been of more value had she not heard the daughter's story and description of the room first. The creation of false memories is always a problem, whether they are accidental, as in this case, or planned, as in brainwashing and advertising (Dunne 2013).

On the other hand, it may be just an aspect of variation, as in the dreaming of the Yuman, as reported by Spier (1933). They saw dreaming as of fundamental importance to life; they placed great emphasis in dreams and dreamed frequently and used them in real life. One might suggest from this that there is a learning process to dreaming, that the social milieu also forms a platform to enlarge on the means of dreaming to create a "dreaming society." Dreaming brought success to the Yuman, but not all people dreamed of spirits. A curious reference in Spier's (1933) report is that "handsome" individuals did not dream of spirits. In this interpretation, the information from Spier is incomplete, as being handsome may be an element of attraction or power that makes the aid of spirits unnecessary.

Too much dreaming was also considered dangerous, especially in children, and could lead a man to become "berdache," not transvestites in the Western sense, but transformed men into women, who took the role of the female gender (Lincoln 1935). There also appears to be an element of time travel in the dreams of children, as in the report given by Harrington (1924) of Joe Homer, when as a child he goes to the sacred mountain and meets the god Kumastamxo "at the very beginning." In some cases the dreamer relives lives and events in myth. This relates also to "secret desires of the soul," what Freud might call elements that are repressed from childhood. But in the Native American context this indicates a means of communication between events that took place before being born and lodged in the subconscious later to be "awakened" in dream as knowledge or "a secret desire of the soul manifested by a dream." This was described by Wallace (1958) and can be interpreted as an interplay between the unborn child, the child in development, the subconscious, and the spirit world. The social interaction was also central, as the dreamer would often tell the dream to other members, who would decide on action, as in the case of the individual Huron man who dreams he is taken captive and burned. The council interprets this dream for him and sees in it a possible future event that indicates war. They intervene by having him perform a ritual where he is burned by professional torturers and he seizes a dog as a substitute victim. The social action then blocks the future event, freeing all from the damage of the predicted war.

This sharing of dreams however is not all-inclusive, as some dreams are not shared, as Hallowell (1966) describes—though among some people of Melanesia, dreams are shared and provide a means for public discussion as well as political debate and action (Robbins 2003). Some dreams are the power dreams specific to the dreamer and a spirit or are dreams so terrible their repeating could create real events. This brings us back to nightmares and dreams as individual or general in meaning. There is a contrast here, one of dreaming where changes can be instituted into cosmological events and lives, and the idea that all knowledge is unchangeable. Where the Mohave belief holds a constant eternal knowledge of which small amounts are dreamed over time, they also engaged in modifications, as when rifles were dreamed into the cosmological knowledge. The plasticity of dreamers and dreaming is made most complex by the Australian "dream time" (Roheim 1945, 1952)—a flow of events that is intertwined so that the idea of an arrow of time or even an eternal return is upended and confounded in the Western sense.

Personality, Identity, Stability, Psychedelics, and Change

So how does this fit into the scheme I was attempting to draw together in 1967 surrounding changes in perspectives of individuals experiencing LSD? It seemed to me that people were undergoing distressing transitions that the new perspectives created, not just because this caused a change in identity, who people saw themselves as in relation to their past self-images (Kelly's constructs and the construct relation to other people, places, and experiences) but also a new reality. The new perspective confronts most often with the prior systematic organization of one's definition of oneself in terms of memory, ways others usually respond to your behavior, and you in the stimuli of your overall typical environment. This confrontation occurs most in the ways others are accustomed to respond to your presentation, how the society conditions your identity. After the LSD experience, since your conditioning has theoretically changed, you will not respond as before to the intersection of friends or exhibit your social role, at least not to the extent of its prior configuration; the difference will vary in individuals, of course. Why this change occurs, and how, I will explain in detail later.

At the beginning of Terence McKenna's *Food of the Gods*, he discusses the forms of repression that Europeans utilized to suppress addictions; de Rios and Smith (1977) also deal with this, both in a number of settings regarding abuse and in post-colonial situations in the Americas. One aspect of addiction McKenna remarks on is the idea of possession. The drug or the vine, in the case of some Amazonian peoples, seems to possess the person, and this condition is the way it is sometimes described (Davis 2001). The same can be said for inner voices—one might consider that the production of the superego in Freud's sense is a particular product of a certain family and social structure—the "voice" of the parent internalized. Then imagine that a culture does not create a singular voice, but instead a multitude of parents, ancestors, and heroes. The people of Teotihuacan produced a clay image where the inside of the human is filled with dozens of little humans (Berrin 1993) (Fig. 5.1). This reflects the idea that a person "becomes a mountain" over time, not only by growing up in a family and modeling their behavior in the image of moral and ethical percepts, but by interactions with other humans, animals, ancestors, and in the legends and myths of its people (Haly 1992) (Fig. 5.2). The individual has incorporated past relatives' personalities, accomplishments, and skills, which is similar to forms of reincarnation (Irwin 2017). To Shepard (1978), the same process of inculcation or incorporation of spirit image and personality can happen in some indigenous settings with animals, and yet the duality seen in many European historical contexts with the Roman genius or the apotheosis with a tribal or clan god is very similar to how souls are seen to be entered into by both the Holy Spirit and angels.

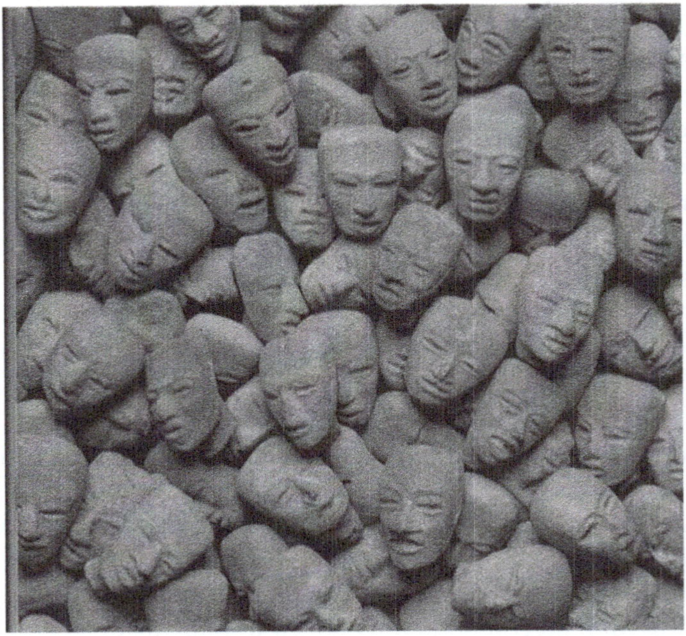

Fig. 5.1 Many voices with each person are set in the torso of the figure below; figurines from pre-Columbian Mesoamerica

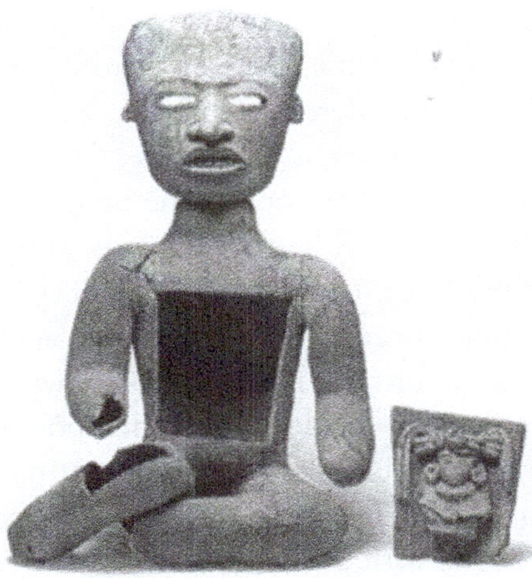

Fig. 5.2 Within the self are held the voices of ancestors, spirits, and knowledge

However, we have to consider the assertion put forward here, as much as in any claim of change of personality or character armor in psychiatry or specific other theories like Kelly's. From a personal and thus very anecdotal example, my use of LSD and peyote did not seem to change my character or personality or affect my values. When I took the MMPI at the Psychology Department in 1966 I was told by the administrator of the test that I had a most stable personality and had scored very high on satisfaction and adaptability as well as happiness. The vocational segment of the testing at the same time had placed me in a class of work that I was not pursuing and was not to in the future. I was curious about psychedelics and especially LSD and wondered, from what I had heard from other people and in the news, what all I would reveal if I took LSD. People had been calling it the "truth drug." So I was surprised when I did take it with friends and we all sat down to await its onset and nothing was happening. I felt nothing. Neither did anyone else. We, being five males of about the same age, then sat down to play cards. During this series of games people began to act strangely to me. Two brothers began to sing ancient sea shanties and one of their long-time friends began to pace the room, speaking in short sentences about his girlfriend, and then suddenly left the building. A short time later I realized that everyone was starting to "come on" to the drug and that I would be soon as well. So I said I was in need of my typewriter and was leaving. One of the brothers then said he was going to make toast and my friend (from high school) just kept drinking beer and got up to use the toilet. I then left and went outside down Oak Street along the Panhandle park to the apartment I was living in with two others at the time (before the onset of our visitors). Arriving home, I went to my room and sat down in front of my typewriter and started to work on examining the experience. I described this experience that then followed a few minutes later. The fact that what I wrote was coherent was disappointing in one way to me at the time, as I expected grand perceptions and insights. Some ideas did come forth and I did experience the oneness and oceanic feeling, and perhaps even a "rebirth" of sorts as I felt myself swirl from a sea as if present at the birth of life on the planet and went through what seemed to me as the evolution of life to the time of the present and then past to a universe of stars and gases. And this feeling was remarkably similar in a variety of people from different backgrounds, consonant with Grof's (1976, 106) but often expressed as so encompassing as to be indescribable. Being nothing, but in all things, knowing all, but understanding it not as facts but as comfort in knowing. A feeling of "indescribable radiance and beauty" is related by Grof (1976, 196) as common among those with their eyes open and who are vocal. This is similar to those reports of Mogar's subjects and others.

However much that experience and the next eight hours or so of interesting and compelling thoughts were to entertain me, I did not reveal any secrets or come to change my personality in my estimation. Some three or four hours after I had arrived, my girlfriend of the time came to the door and my roommate, Tom Schafer, let her in. She had met Michael Canright, my high school friend, on the street with his cousins (the two brothers) and found them quite incoherent and, as she put it, "stupid." What was of interest to me at the moment she came into my room was the uncontrollable desire to tell her everything I had experienced. The next day after I had slept several hours, she summed up my discourse as "a class in evolution." I was quite surprised at that banality, then she said we had had great sex, mutual oral and then intercourse, with each trading places, top and bottom. She said at one point, "You let me fuck you." At first I was embarrassed and then it appeared to me that my memory of the sex was how we had merged into one person, that I became her and she me. I had long questioned her about what it was like to be female, as I was quite taken with the dominance in our world of maleness and femininity. She was my senior by two years and very beautiful, feminine, and yet not at all shy or retiring as many women I knew. When I told her I had experienced us as one and changing bodies, she agreed and yet she said she had wished she had also been on LSD at the time, as she was not aware of the sensations I had experienced.

Some weeks later we both took LSD at the same time and walked to the ocean down through the park. There we began to feel the onset of the drug and she (as a plastic artist who worked in clay) made a number of huge sand sculptures. We then retraced our steps to her apartment and along the way recounted our lives from the beginning. At her apartment we again engaged in sex and with the same nature of a fluid changeableness until the next morning. But, while we had certainly discovered a lot about each other and had a lot of fun, I was unsure anything had changed in myself and she was also unsure, but unconcerned. The idea of personality changes had been studied by Mogar (Mogar and Savage 1964) using the MMPI. They seem clear on this, but was it a characteristic of LSD use or some subset of response, and I was curious if I was missing something in myself.

In pursuit of the idea of personality change or character, I asked my girlfriend to come to my parents' home the next weekend. She had never met them and was anxious at the thought. We did it, however, and after on the way home, she abruptly said, "Why do you go back and see them? They hate you." I was shocked and did not understand. Her analysis of the encounter was that my family did not understand me (I was the first to go to college) and they had spent the evening saying dismissive and cruel things about me. I had simply considered this banter to be how we treated each other, but her perception was interesting. I had taken each of my family members aside and asked if they thought I had changed in any way–none gave serious answers except my sister, who said, "No, why, what are you expecting? What have you done?" She was afraid I had tried heroin or engaged in some other life-ending tragedy. Had my sex behavior with my girlfriend revealed something about me or had I changed at that moment? I asked my girlfriend and she said, "No, you were not macho before and not feminine now." I described the event to my sister and she said, "Our grandmother said once that women whose husbands have a woman's heart could have happy lives; those whose husbands have men's hearts will live a life of sorrow."

I could not see any changes in my girlfriend nor in my friends I had taken the LSD with before, including Michael Canright. I then started asking all the psychology students, grad students, and PhDs as well as the MDs involved in the Mogar Lab about these questions of changes. The general view was that people did not change personality or have other modifications in character unless they were pathological in some way. Here the idea of being sick and not knowing it or knowing it and changing created a dilemma. Did one make changes only if one was pathological in a social sense, or could changes occur if people were dissatisfied, which did not seem to be illness, though dissatisfaction as expressed in depression could be? This has been determined in cases like eating disorders linked to body dissatisfaction (Mangweth-Matzek et al. 2014). This is obviously a complicated question and it relates to concepts of happiness and well-being as well as cultural forms of being (body size, beauty, achievement, etc.). Hine et al. (2012) argue that some 8% of the US population express substantial unhappiness or are troubled with feelings of a dissatisfied life. They associate this with a 1% of the population that these feelings are pathological in resulting in clinical depression.

I was interested in the stability of the MMPI test, but not enough to do any research at the time, though most of the psychologists I talked to thought it was. Some 30 years later a family friend who was an industrial psychologist administered a variation of the MMPI to me, and the results were quite similar to the original, which unfortunately I had not preserved to compare. Some research was done in the 1970s by Leon et al. (1979) on the general population, non-patient subjects, and they found the test results were quite stable. The same results were shown in patients for different psychological conditions, except the authors were able to record improvements in some cases (Greene 1990). Changes in MMPI scores after LSD were noted by a number of researchers (Belleville 1956), though other research showed similar results when several drugs, including alcohol, were compared, but LSD produced the most positive effects (Jarvik et al. 1955).

People changing their sexual orientation is not new, nor is the desire to change the physiological nature of gender. Today this is often termed "gender dysphoria" and defined by the American Psychiatric Association as "a conflict between a person's physical or assigned gender and the gender with which he/she/they identify" (see: https://www.psychiatry.org/patients-families/gender-dysphoria/what-is-gender-dysphoria).

An instructive example of this is that of Ryan Barnes, who apparently was born as a beautiful biological female but found difficulty performing as a typical female in American culture. She had problems with relationships with men and with accepting female roles or identifying with future roles as mother, wife, and so on. She explains in her YouTube videos that this confusion led to her thinking that she might be bisexual but also a transgendered person. She thus decided to take testosterone and attempt to transition to a male identity, which seemed to be more consistent with her desires in freedom and behavior. After a few months on this regime of drugs and changes in clothing and personality, she found that performing as male and the resulting expectations of other people, especially males, was not compatible with her feelings as a person. She also did not enjoy or like the effects of the drugs. She then decided to detransition back to female identity. She was able to get estrogen from a source without extensive counseling and yet felt more consonant with the effects.

This example is but one of thousands one can examine in the literature and on media platforms like YouTube, where people are attempting to understand their sexuality and to perform it in ways that is satisfying. I will discuss gender issues in the chapter on "The Female Exception" (in research). There seem to be several problems with these attempts. Like with Ryan, cultural roles for gender are not necessarily constructed to fit individually developed gender performance needs or the needs of individuals for bonding, sexual satisfaction, and achievement. Tensions in this have been long recognized by anthropologists like Margaret Mead (1954) and Ashley Montagu (1953). We often find disagreement on the effective nature of enculturation in creating acceptable patterns for every person to be of a certain gender, yet the idea of duality of male and female is not entirely reflected in every culture and variations are quite common. And each person makes an attempt at psychological adaptation with the available forms of gender identity. A huge realm of institutions exist in societies to help channel people in this process from rites of passage (van Gennep 1960) to shamans and psychiatrists. Usually social and spiritual worlds are divided up between male and female terrains, based on a real sexual dimorphism; this difference is magnified and extended to where male and female sides of villages exist, houses are divided, and movement is regulated by gender and gender status (young woman versus old woman; see Hunter 1961; Mead 1975, 57). This is associated with ideas of loss of power through contact with unclean objects or people, as in India in the caste system or examples of taboo over gender or concepts of religious power and what is called liminality (Radcliffe-Brown 1939; Douglas 1966).

This brings up another point, how stable are personalities, and also "cures" or therapies? Are we simply helping people adjust to conditions they cannot change (fooling themselves or "settling for less") or is it a constant adjustment people need, constant reinforcing of their conditioning schedule? This thought was depressing and it became clear at the time that Tim Leary and Ram Dass' idea of the use of psychedelics was also not enlightening, as the chanting and Eastern ideas they were using, as in Buddhist meditation, were aimed to "kill the mind," lose yourself, and so on.

This difference perhaps relates to the variation in the number of treatments Grof's patients needed to achieve cleaning of repressions (Grof 1976, 61). The new perspective confronts most often with the prior systematic organization of one's definition of oneself in terms of memory, ways others usually respond to your behavior, and you to the stimuli of your customary environment. Some of Grof's patients needed numerous "trips" and define those with the easiest, shortest, or fewest sessions to be "the hysterics."

One has to ask why this was true? As Korzybski considers sanity to be situational at best, Nettler (1961) sees the dilemma of interpretation in the "health" of a man who behaves badly because he sees accurately versus the "health" of a man who behaves nicely because he has learned the popular (e.g., socially self-delusional) way of seeing falsely. This strikes more than just the evolution of norms of societies, or historical development of institutions that condition people to follow certain culturally defined modes of behavior. It implies that rationality is not an indigenous element in human society, but one foreign and conditional. A subject of Grof's (1976, 122–3) experiences a view of life and attitude that he realizes is his self, his worldview or personality. It is a reference of being able to see one's self as others might see one, but more than that, to also see the cultural context of one's reality. Often individuals reported "stepping out of their skin" and looking at themselves as if they were an unbiased observer. In this stance, judgments can take place and we might call this a form of conscience or reflection. In some cases individuals became quite harsh in viewing themselves, as if they disapproved of their behavior or what they had become. The reflection of regret by people, after the fact, is often a point of discussion of why they did not act otherwise, what drove them to accomplish acts they then wished undone. We see this in history.

Tzvetan Todorov (1984) reviews the horrific slaughter, torture, and brutal destruction of Native Americans by the Spanish conquistadors. The murder and abuse, especially in the treatment of women and children, had no practical meaning or purpose. It was often simply a rampage of hysterical violence, as many of the recorders like Las Casa explain in disgust. Most of the men who were perpetrators of these crimes went on to live somewhat normal and even respectable lives. The capacity for animal irrationality seems to be both ever present and yet socially triggered and responsive. The same could be said for Nazi Germany or the treatment of African Americans by Southern slave owners (Abtheker 1983) and the continued brutalization and discrimination of African Americans and Native Americans today.

References

Abtheker, Herbert (1983) *Negro Slave Revolts,* New York, International Books.

Aczel, Amir (2001) *Entanglement: The Greatest Mystery in Physics*, New York, Four Walls Eight Windows Books.

Baker, Joseph O., Samuel Stroope and Mark H. Walker, (2018) "Secularity, religiosity, and health: Physical and mental health differences between atheists, agnostics, and nonaffiliated theists compared with religiously affiliated individuals," *Social Science Research*, v. 75, 44–57.

Belleville, R.E. (1956) "MMPI score changes induced by lysergic acid diethylamide (LSD-25)," *J. Clin Psychol.*, July, v. 12, n. 3, 279–282.

Berrin, Kathy (1993) "Teotihuacan: City of the Gods," *Triptych*, n. 66, 10–16.

Black Elk (1932) *Black Elk Speaks, Being the Story of a Holy Man of the Oglala Sioux*, As told to John G. Neihardi, Lincoln, University of Nebraska Press.

Blom, Jan Dirk (2010) *A Dictionary of Hallucinations*, New York, Springer.

Blum, Richard, Eva Blum and Mary Lou Funkhouser, (1964) "The institutionalization of LSD," in Blum, Richard, Nevitt Sanford, Eva Blum, Mary Lou Funkhouser, Joseph J. Downing, et al., (eds.) *Utopiates: The Use and Users of LSD-25, A Publication of the Institute for the Study of Human Problems*, Stanford University, Atherton Press, 124–141.

Borders, Alyssa A., Mariam Aly, Colleen M. Parks, and Andrew P. Yonelinas, (2017) "The hippocampus is particularly important for building associations across stimulus domains," *Neuropsychologia,* v. 99, 335–342.

Bourdieu, Pierre (1977) *Outline of a Theory of Practice,* Cambridge, Cambridge University Press.

Butler, W.E. (1992) "Crime in the Soviet Union," *Brit. J. Criminol.*, v. 32, n. 2, Spring, 144–159.

Carhart-Harris, Robin L., Suresh Muthukumaraswamy, Leor Roseman, Mendel Kaelen, Wouter Droog, et al., (2016) "Neural correlates of the LSD experience revealed by multimodal neuroimaging," *PNAS,* April 26, v. 113, n. 17:4853–4858.

Damasio, A.R., T.J. Grabowski, A. Bechara, H. Damasio, L.L. Ponto et al., (2000), "Subcortical and cortical brain activity during the feeling of self-generated emotions," *Nat. Neurosci.,* Oct., 3, 10, 1049–1056.

Davis, Wade (2001) *Light at the Edge of the World,* Vancouver, Douglas & McIntyre.

Dawkins, Richard (2016) *The Selfish Gene,* Oxford, Oxford University Press.

R. K. Dentan, (1968) *The Semai: A Nonviolent People of Malaya,* New York: Holt, Rinehart & Winston.

de Rios, Marlene Dobkin (1984) *Hallucinogens: Cross-Cultural Perspectives,* Albuquerque, University of New Mexico Press.

de Rios, Marlene Dobkin and David E. Smith (1977) "Drug use and abuse in cross cultural perspective," v. 36, n. 1, Spring, 14–21.

Devereux, George (1951) *Reality and Dream: The Psychotherapy of a Plains Indian,* New York, New York University Press.

Devereux, George (1957) "Dream learning and individual ritual differences in Mohave shamanism," *Amer. Anth.*, v. 59:1036–1045.

De Waal Malefijt, Annemarie (1968) *Religion and Culture,* New York, Macmillan.

Domhoff, G. William (1990) *The Mystique of Dreams, A Search for Utopia through Senoi Dream Theory,* Berkeley, University of California Press.

Douglas, Mary (1966) *Purity and Danger: an Analysis of Concepts of Pollution and Taboo,* Harmondsworth, Penguin.

Du Bois, Cora, (1945) "The Alorese," in *The Psychological Frontiers of Society, eds.,* Kardiner, Abram, Ralph Linton, Cora Du Bois and James West, New York, Columbia University Press, 101–145.

Dunne, Mathew W. (2013) *A Cold War State of Mind: Brainwashing and Postwar American Society,* Cambridge, MIT Press.

Durkheim, Emile (1915) *The Elementary Forms of the Religious Life,* London, George Allen & Unwin.

Eggan, Dorothy (1961) "Dream Analysis" in (ed) B. Kaplan, *Studying Personality Cross-Culturally*: 551–557.

Eliade, Mircea (1964) *Shamanism,* Bolligen Foundation, Princeton, Princeton University Press.

Ffytche, Dominic H. (2013) "The hallucinating brain: neurobiological insights into the nature of hallucinations," Chapter 3, in *Hallucination: Philosophy and Psychology,* (eds.) Fiona Macpherson and Dimitris Platchias, Cambridge, MA, MIT Press, pp. 45–64.

Ffytche, Dominic, R.J. Howard, M.J. Brammer, A. David, P. Woodruff and S. Williams, (1998) "The anatomy of conscious vision: an fMRI study of visual hallucinations," *Nature Neuroscience*, v. 1. N. 8, 738–742.

Fingelkurts, Alexander A. (2009) "Is our brain hardwired to produce God, or is our brain hardwired to perceive God? A systematic review on the role of the brain in mediating religious experience," *Cogn. Process,* Nov., 10, 4, 293–326.

Forer, B.R. (1969) "The taboo against touching in psychotherapy," *Psychotherapy, Theory, Research and Practice*, v. 6: 229–231.

Fosse, M.J., R. Fosse, J.A. Hobson, and R.J. Stickgold (2003) "Dreaming and episodic memory: a functional dissociation?" Journal of Cognitive Neuroscience, v. 15:1–9.

Freud, Sigmund (1961) *The Interpretation of Dreams*, Trans. And Edited by James Strachey, New York, Science Editions.

Galton, Francis (1880) "I.-Statistics of mental imagery," *Mind,* issue 19, 1 July, 301–318.

Goodison, Lucy (1995) *The Dreams of Women: Exploring and Interpreting Women's Dreams,* New York, W.W. Norton.

Goody, Jack and I. Watt (1968) "The consequences of literacy," In *Literacy in Traditional Societies,* (ed.) Jack Goody, Cambridge, Cambridge University Press: 27–68.

Goody, Jack (1987) *The Interface Between the Written and the Oral*, Cambridge, Cambridge University Press.

Gopnik, Adam (2012) "The caging of America," *The New Yorker,* January 23, https://www.newyorker.com/magazine/2012/01/30/the-caging-of-america. Accessed January 2, 2021.

Greenberg, R. and P.H. Leiderman (1966) "Perceptions, the dream process and memory: an up-to-date version of notes on a mystic writing pad," *Comprehensive Psychiatry*, Dec. v. 7, n 6:517–523.

Greene, Roger L. (1990) "Stability of MMPI scale scores within four code type across 40 years," *J. Personality Assessment,* v. 55, n. 1–2:1–6.

Grof, Stanislav (1976) *Realms of the Human Unconscious: Observation from LSD Research*, New York, E.P. Dutton.

Gussow, Zackary (1960) "*Pibloktoq (Hysteria) Among the Polar Eskimo*", In *The Culture-Bound Syndromes*, (Eds.) R.C. Simons and C.C. Hughes, v. 7, Dordrecht, Springer, 271–287.

Hallowell, A. Irving (1966) "The role of dreams in Ojibwa culture," in (eds.) G.E. Von Gruebaum and R. Caillois, *The Dream and Human Societies, Berkeley*, University of California Press: 267–292.

Haly, Richard (1992) "On becoming a mountain: or why Native Americans have animals for souls," Paper Presented at the 91st *Annual Meeting of the American Anthropological Association, San Francisco*, Ca. 6 December.

Harner, Michael (1968) "The sound of rushing water," *Natural History*, v. 77 , n. 6, 28–33.

Hassabis, Demis and Eleanor A. Maguire (2009). The construction system of the brain," *Philosophical Trans. Of the Royal Soc. B*, 12 May: https://doi.org/10.1098/rstb.2008.0296.

Hassabis, Demis, Dharshan Kumaran, Seralynne D. Vann and Eleanor A. Maguire (2007) "Patients with hippocampal amnesia cannot imagine new experiences," *PNAS*, January 30, v. 104, n. 5:1726–1731.

Harrington, John Peabody (1924) "A Yuma account of origin," *Journal of American Folklore*, v. 21:324–348.

Hebb, Donald (1954) "The problem of consciousness and introspection," In *Brain Mechanics and Consciousness*, (ed.) E. Adrian et al., Oxford, Oxford University Press: 402–417.

Herdt, Gilbert H. (1987) "Selfhood and discourse inSambia dream sharing," In *Dreaming: Anthropological and Psychological Interpretations*, (ed.) Barbara Tedlock, Cambridge, Cambridge University Press, 55–85.

Hine, F.R., R.C. Carson, G.L. Maddox, R.J. Thompson, Jr. and R.B. Williams (2012) *Introduction to Behavioral Science in Medicine*, New York, Springer Science and Business Media.

Hoebel, E. Adamson (1954) *The Law of Primitive Man*, Cambridge, Harvard University Press.

Humphrey, Nicholas (1986) *The Inner Eye*, Oxford, Oxford University Press.

Hunter, Monica (1961) *Reaction to Conquest*, 2nd edition, Oxford University Press.

Huxley, Aldous (1954) *The Doors of Perception, and Heaven and Hell*, New York, Harper Colophon Books.

Irwin, Lee (2017) "Reincarnation in America: a brief historical overview," *Religions*, v. 8, n. 10: https://doi.org/10.3390/rel8100222.

Jacobs, Andrew (2021) "Psychedelics gain mainstream traction," *The New York Times*, May 10th.

Jarvik, M.E., Abramson, H.A., & Hirsch, M.W., (1955) "Comparative subjective effects of seven drugs including lysergic acid diethylamide (LSD-25)," *The J. Abnormal and Social Psychology*, v. 51, n. 3, 657–662.

Jones, Ernest (1921) "Persons in dreams disguised as themselves," *Papers on Psycho Analysis*, New York, William Wood.

Kelly, George A. (1963) *A Theory of Personality*, New York, The Norton Library.

Kilborne, Benjamin (1981) "Pattern, structure, and style in anthropological studies of dreams," *Ethos*, v. 9, n. 2:165–185.

Kluver, Heinrich (1966) *Mescal: The Divine Plant and Its Psychological Effects*, Kegan Paul (originally published in 1928).
Korzybski, Alfred, (1948) *Science and Sanity*, Lakeville, Institute of General Semantics.
Laufer, Bertold (1931) "Inspirational dreams in Eastern Asia," *Journal of American Folklore*, v. 47:208–216.
Leon, Gloria Rakita, Brenda Gillum, Richard Gillum and Marshall Gare, (1979) "Personality stability and change over a 30 year period—middle age to old age," *J. of Consult and Clinical Psychology*, v. 47, n. 3:517–524.
Lincoln, J. S. (1935) *The Dream in Primitive Cultures*, London, Cressett Press.
Lowie, Robert H. (1948) Tropical forest tribes," in Steward, J.H. (ed.) *Handbook of South American Indians*, Washington, U.S. Government Printing Office.
Luke, David (2012) "Psychoactive substances and paranormal phenomena: a comprehensive review," *International Journal of Transpersonal Studies*, v. 31, n. 1: 97–156.
Malinowski, Bronislaw (1929) *The Sexual Life of Savages*, London, Routledge and Kegan Paul.
Mangweth-Matzek, Barbara, Hans W. Hoek and Harrison G. Pope, Jr. (2014) "Pathological eating and body dissatisfaction in middle-aged and older women," *Curr Opin Psychiatry*, Nov. v. 27, n. 6:431–5.
Maslow, Abraham H. (1964) *Religions, Values, and Peak-Experiences*, New York, Viking Press, edition with new editorial introduction and preface, 1970. Originally published as 35th volume in the Kappa Delta Pi Lecture Series
Mead, Margaret (1932) "An investigation of the thought of primitive children, with special reference to animism," *Journal of the Royal Anthropological Institute of Great Britain and Ireland*, v. 62, Jan–Jun., 173–190.
Mead, Margaret (1954) *Male and Female*, New York, Morrow & Co.
Mead, Margaret (1975) *Growing Up in New Guinea*, New York, Morrow Quill (Originally published in 1930).
Merriam, A.P. (1967) "Ethnomusicology of the Flathead Indians," *Viking Fund Publications in Anthropology*, N. 44, New York, Wenner-Gren Foundation for Anthropological Research.
Metzenich, Michael (2013) *Soft-wired: How the New Science of Brain Plasticity Can Change Your Life*, San Francisco, 2nd Edition, Parnassus Publishing.
Metzner, Ralph (1968) *The Ecstatic Adventure*, New York, Macmillan.
Mogar, Robert E. (1965) "Search and research with the psychedelics," *ETC: A Review of General Semantics*, v. 22, n. 4, Special Issue on the Psychedelic Experience, Dec.:393–407.

Mogar, Robert E., and Charles Savage, (1964) "Personality change associated with psychedelic (LSD) therapy: a preliminary report," *Psychotherapy: Theory, Research & Practice, 1*(4), 154–162.

Montagu, Ashley (1953) *The Natural Superiority of Women*, New York, Macmillan.

Myerhoff, Barbara G. (1974) *Peyote Hunt: The Sacred Journey of the Huichol Indians*, Ithaca, Cornell University Press.

Naples M, Hackett TP, (1978) The amytal interview: history and current uses. *Psychosomatics 01*; 19: 98–105.

Nettler, George (1961) "Good men, bad men, and the perception of reality," *Sociometry*24, 271.

Novakovsky, S., (1924) "Artic or Siberian hysteria as a reflex of the geographic environment," *Ecology*, 5, 113–127.

Nudds, Matthew, (2013) "Naïve realism and hallucinations," in *Hallucination: Philosophy and Psychology*, (eds.) Fiona Macpherson and Dimitris Platchias, Cambridge, MA, MIT Press, pp.271–290.

Nyhof, M.A. & Johnson, C.N. (2017) "Is god just a big person? Children's conceptions of god across cultures and religious traditions," *J. Dev Psychol.* March, 35, 1, 60–75.

Olson, J.M., P.A. Vernon, J.A. Harris, K.L. Jang, (2001) "The heritability of attitudes: a study of twins," *J. Pers. Soc Psych*ol. Jun, 80, 6, 845–860.

Ong, Roberto K. (1985) *The Interpretation of Dreams in Ancient China*, Brockmeyer.

Osmond, Humphry (1970) "Peyote night," in Aaronson, Bernard and Humphry Osmond, (eds) (1970) Psychedelics, The Uses and Implications of Hallucinogenic Drugs, Garden City, Anchor Books: 67–85.

Petrea, Ionela and Milou Haggenburg, (2014) "Trends in health systems in the former Soviet Union countries," *Observatory Studies Series*, n. 35, Rechel B., E. Richardson and M. McKee (eds.) European Observatory on Health Systems and Policies, https://www.ncbi.nlm.nih.gov/books/NBK458299/.

Radcliffe-Brown, A.R. (1939) *Taboo*, The Frazer Lecture, Cambridge, Cambridge University Press.

Rashid, A.J., C. Yan, V. Mercaldo, H.I. Hsiang, S. Park, et al., (2016) "Competition between engrams influences fear memory formation and recall," Science, July, 22, v. 353(6297):383–7.

Rasmussen, K., (1930) *Intellectual Culture of the Caribou Eskimo*, Report of the Fifth Thule Expedition, 1921–1924, v. 3, n. 2, 54–55.

Rivers, W.H.R. (1920) *Instinct and the Unconscious*, Cambridge, Cambridge University Press.

Robbins, Joel (2003) "Dreaming and the defeat of charisma," in *Dream Travelers, Sleep Experiences and Culture in the Western Pacific*, (ed) R. Lohmann, New York, Palgrave Macmillan, 19–42.

Roheim, Geza (1945) *The Eternal Ones of the Dream*, New York, International Universities Press.

Roheim, Geza (1952) *The Gates of the Dream*, New York International Universities Press.

Sacks, Oliver (2010) *The Mind's Eye*, New York, Knopf.

Sacks, Oliver (2012) *Hallucinations*, New York, Vintage Books.

Shepard, Paul (1978) *Thinking Animals*, New York, The Viking Press.

Siegel, Susana (2008) "The epistemic conception of hallucination," in *Disjunctivism: Perception, Action and Knowledge*, (eds.) Adrian Haddock and Fiona Macpherson, Cambridge, MA, MIT Press, pp.205–224.

Sperber, Dan (1975) *Rethinking Symbolism*, Cambridge.

Spier, Leslie (1933) *Yuman Tribes of the Gila River*, Chicago University of Chicago Press.

Steinberg, Douglas (2004) "When remembering might mean forgetting," *The Scientist,* Aug. 2:17–20.

Stewart, K. R. (1951) "Dream Theory in Malaya," *Complex,* no. 6:21–33

Stickgold, R., A. Malia, D. Maquire, D. Roddenberry and M. O'Connor (2000) "Replaying the game: hypnagogic images in normal and amnesics," *Science*, v. 290:350–353.

Todorov, Tzvetan (1984) *The Conquest of America*, New York, Harper and Row.

Torda, Clara (1969a) "Dreams of subjects with bilateral hippocampal lesions," *Acta Psychiatrica Scandinavica*, v. 45:277–288.

Torda, Clara (1969b) "Dreams of subjects with loss of memory for recent events." *Psychophysiology*, v. 6:358–365.

Tylor, Edward B. (1889) *Primitive Culture*, Vol. 1, New York, Henry Holt & co.

Van Gennep, Arnold, (1960) *The Rites of Passage*, Chicago, University of Chicago Press.

Vansina, Jan (1985) *Oral Tradition as History*, Madison, University of Wisconsin Press.

Wallace, A.F.C. (1958) Dreams and the wishes of the soul, a type of psychoanalytic among the Seventeenth Century Iroquois," *Amer. Anth.*, v. 60:234–248.

Wasson, R. Gordon (1962) "The hallucinogenic mushrooms of Mexico and psilocybin: A bibliography," *Botanical Museum Leaflets*, v 20, n 2, Harvard University.

Watts, Alan, (1970) "Psychedelics and religious experience," in *Psychedelics: The Uses and Implications of Hallucinogenic Drugs*, Garden City, Anchor Books.131–144.

Whyte, Lancelot L. (1930) *The Next Development if Man*, New York, Mentor.

Xu, Jian, Yongling Zhu, Anis Contractor and Stephen F. Heinemann, (2009) "mGluR5 has a critical role in inhibitory learning, "*Journal of Neuroscience*, v. 29(12): https://doi.org/10.1523/JNEUROSCI.5716-08.2009.

Zeman, Adam, Fraser Milton, Sergio Della Sala, Michaela Dewar, Timothy Frayling, et al., (2020) "Phantasia—the psychology of lifelong visual imagery vividness extremes," *Cortex,* v. 150: 426–440.

Zeman, Adam, A. Z. Dewar and M. Della Salla, (2015) "Lives without imagery—congenital aphantasia," *Cortex*, Dec. v. 73, 378–380.

Zubovich, Gene (2018) "Russia's journey from Orthodoxy to atheism, and back again," *Religion and Politics,* October 16, https://religionandpolitics.org/2018/10/16/russias-journey-from-orthodoxy-to-atheism-and-back-again/.

6

A View of Possible Identities, Realities, and Futures

It often has seemed in the earlier chapters that women are not featured much in the research of psychedelic drugs or dreams. There is considerable data, yet it is almost always the case that there are fewer female subjects or individuals included. This makes one feel if women are added as an afterthought. Certainly in fieldwork men are usually limited in their contact with women in many cultures. In a recent study of dreams Schredl (2007) found some interesting differences between men and women in dreaming. He reports that women tend to recall their dreams more often than men and report more frequent and intense nightmares than men. Women dream about as much about other women and men, while men dream more often about men. Men report aggressive encounters with often strange or unfamiliar men, while women dream of meeting other people who are familiar and the dreams occur in known or familiar places. Use of the Zadra and Nielsen (1997) dream category exam differentiated gender responses. Schredl et al. (2010) also report that women's responses (failure, snakes, insects, loss of control) on the dreams questionnaire categories are more negative than men's. In Nielsen et al. (2003) these same categories are prominent as well as "paralysis" in women. When comparing their results to a study in the 1950s (Griffith et al. 1958) students

N. Caldararo, *A Mental Ethnography: Conclusions From Research in LSD*,
https://doi.org/10.1007/978-3-031-13745-7_6

reporting sexual experiences had jumped significantly, becoming the second-most prevalent theme in 2003, with a 12% difference between men (85%) to women (73%). In Griffith's sample, the difference between men and women was 58%, which may reflect attitudinal changes over time. However, interpretation of responses and wording of questions as well as interpretation and type of sample may be of significance. Rubinstein and Krippner (1991) found regional differences reported by men and women in a large sample.

Comparisons of Neilsen et al.'s (2003) categories to those of the Zinacantecans collected by Laughlin (1976) produce some challenges, but offer insights. Neilsen's type 1 "fleeing" is similar to the Zinacantecan Ramon Teratol's dream where his "wood" is stolen and a woman offers to cure his baby and they flee together. It introduces the problem of reducing a dream to central components for the purpose of classification. Ramon's dream has several elements, which one is picked?

Hall (1984) restudied an earlier cross-cultural and gender comparison of dreams using 35 groups of various nationalities and ethnicities, including children. The results showed sex-related differences occurred in 29 of the groups on every continent, in all age groups, and in dreams collected in different contexts (laboratories, classrooms, etc.). The earlier study (Hall and Domhoff 1963) had used a collection of dream narratives of 1399 men and 1418 women, indicating that men dream about other men more than about women, while women dream about men and women in near-equal proportions.

Spaulding (1981) addresses the problem of the conflict between researchers who believe they have discovered universals in dreaming and those who think dreams are idiosyncratic and personal. This is a problem with systems of categories like that of Zadra and Nielsen (1997) or Freud (1964), as separations of dreamed perceptions must be interpreted as for those of psychedelic experiences. Thus, the idea that we can create categories of expressed events from subjects, like "flying" or "death," is itself a confusion and perhaps also a distortion. Cartwright (1984) considered that many of the feelings of women in dreaming reflected impressions of life that required resolution and were reflected in personal depression. In divorced couples this seemed more clearly defined. Yet she also recognized that men and women are taught as children to respond to challenge in different ways, so that frustration of desire or effort can be differently resolved in the different genders. Depression in a male is not expressed as readily or in the same fashion as in a female. Also, in different cultures this would be patterned in a unique manner. Eggan (1952) reported that one Hopi awoke from dreams often with a negative emotion more than twice (170 times) as often as a positive one (46 times). But in describing dreams he considered 136 dreams as "bad" and 84 as "good." So these feelings and assessments do not coincide. Jersild et al. (1933) reported that children generally had unpleasant dreams, while Foster and Anderson (1936) found that most children had unpleasant dreams but these became less frequent as they grew older, all parallel to the findings of Foulkes (1971).

So here we have "emotion" versus "meaning" in this Hopi example. But then among some India subjects, Callois (1966) found dreams considered "bad" where the dreamer is swallowed by a fish, enters into one's mother, sees a lamb go out and eye torn out, or losing one's Brahman cord. These can have interpretations in the cultural context of being poor outcomes for the dreamer, except there may be alternative meanings to different people in the same culture. Being swallowed by a fish can be the beginning of a hero's journey. Being "twice born" is certainly charged with anxiety, but in the Indian caste system it refers to the Dvija or "twice-born" castes, the upper *varnas*: Brahmans, Kshatriyas, and Vaishyas. One of the first anthropologists concerned with dreams of different cultures was C.G. Seligman (1923). He proposed a method of writing down every word the dreamer said in recounting a dream and then asking the subject about the dream, its meaning and significance. Then he would have the subject repeat the dream a second time to elicit more detail or variation. He was searching for universal subject matter, what he called "type dreams." Later, Griffith et al. (1958), in studying American and Japanese dreams, searched for the "typical" dream. This dream, in his estimation, had the quality of being repeated, and recalled as opposed to "unique" dreams. Such dreams are also resistant to psychoanalytic interpretation. He and his colleagues found that such dreams could be identified by paring down dreams to fundamental elements. In following their method this process seemed vague, yet they claimed cross-cultural universals.

In 1967 I was developing a theory of aspects of culture as derivatives of conditioning, as a result of my regard for Behaviorism as an effective explanatory system (Caldararo 1968). Therefore, universals seemed unlikely unless they were general responses based on physiology, like vision and even these phenomena could be interpreted differently by different cultures, as with phosphenes. Lewis-Williams (2009) believes some San rock art depicts phosphenes.

Yet Grof (1976, 140) considered some of the positive feelings people came to experience on LSD such as concepts, justice, beauty, love for all people, and so on as an "intrinsic part of the human personality" and thus a universal and similar to Maslow's "peak experiences." It is clear that such experiences are common in non-industrial cultures (Eliade 1964). At the end of the nineteenth century, Richard M. Bucke (1905) made such experiences famous in a book, appropriately titled *Cosmic Consciousness*. That such a response to life could be positive and universal did seem to me at the time as similar to Bastian's Psychic Unity of Mankind theory. But I was unclear on how to link it to Behaviorism. Of course, for Grof, this blissful state of unity could only be reached by the painful trauma of rebirth and access to archetypes, which I found lacking in most cases and rather too dogmatic.

As a student at Humboldt State College (now University) in 1965, I was so impressed with the science of Psychology that I decided I should pursue a career in it. My initial desire was to do laboratory work, but my instructor urged me to follow a medical degree. He had a colleague, however, who was doing research in a laboratory setting in sensory deprivation. I have no idea today from where he was receiving funding, but I was happy to join his team if possible. I was only a freshman with one quarter under my belt at Hayward State College. But I was eager and the Psychology Department needed workers. They were especially needed to monitor subjects (student volunteers) at night. The lab space consisted of a set of offices, two as I recall for the research staff and several others for changing of subject's clothes, with lockers. There was a section with typical laboratory bench equipment, sinks and water, and a set of restrooms. There was a main observation room with a one-way window for observation of subjects and a small room for the observers. The main observation room was painted black, protected from exterior sound by sound proofing, and had a special air treatment system to dampen any sound or air movement.

Much of the research seemed to be aimed at looking at responses of different individuals with certain character traits derived from their interviews and personality tests. I think these were the MMPI. Unfortunately, this protocol of screening subjects did not act as effectively as at the Mogar Lab—we had one student volunteer engage in a serious breakdown during the test. At the Mogar Lab the MMPI was supplemented with a daily interview, which I think was a wise addition.

Some theoretical problems were discussed, as in child development from the research of Harlow and Harlow and that is summarized in Ashley Montagu's book *Touching* (1986) today, though the first edition of that book was yet to appear (1971). The research it draws on in the lack of sensory input in early childhood was rapidly developing and created a sense of excitement and purpose. One thing that was missing was the dividing line cut across the world separating women and men. The clinical nature of the laboratory and the staff's attitude and makeup were appropriate for a scientific endeavor, but there were no women involved, except in support staff, like a secretary. Discussions of the Harlow and Harlow work appeared straightforward, except the idea of emotion was often couched in terms of the feminine. "Women did this, said that, responded in this or that way." Emotion seemed to be categorized in an entirely gender-specific fashion. Growing up in a Latin family with a mother who was Portuguese and a father who was Italian, I was exposed to the passion of love and life. I saw how men and women negotiated the world and how the conflict of emotions driven by needs left them at times with nothing but anger and error.

Good for me that my mother, like most Portuguese women I came to know, especially my female relatives and my sister, were powerful, self-contained, and confident people. My father had grown up in Harlem in a poverty-stricken neighborhood of a cold-water flat and had joined the US Army at the outbreak of WWII with the invasion of Poland. He had lost his mother early in life and was raised largely by his sisters and aunts. This foundation of a world where female actors were central to decisions brought me into stark conflict with the world of post-WWII America in general and at the Psychology Department in particular, though it was only a reflection of typical American attitudes.

It has always confounded my view of society that women should be devalued, submissive, and victimized. This subordination was underlined by my father's hatred of his father, who dominated his mother and his sisters, demanding their paychecks and forcing them to wait on his every need. There in the family, my father had seen the exploitation and unfair treatment within his world and outside in factories and in relationships when men preyed on women for money and sex. While his world contrasted with my home life dramatically, both economically and in terms of gender relations, the treatment of women outside our home and community demonstrated the victimization of women daily.

Dr. Paula Caplan (1985, 2008) and Dr. Phyllis Chesler (1972) both wrote devastating critiques of Freud and of basic principles, attitudes, and practices of psychology and medicine that resulted in institutionalizing and rationalizing male domination of women. But the question of agency (of course, the "sense of agency in men ranges from the dangerous will to power to prudent self-governance"; see Moore 2016) and women goes beyond Freud's concern with masochism; for du Beauvoir (1949) and Garcia (2021), it centers on the continuous male gaze and lack of ownership of the body. Jung (1964) describes this as the "buried womanhood" and uses a woman's dream to illustrate its character. A woman stands in a long line of women at the end of which each woman is decapitated. She feels no emotion at the realization—the hopeless nature of identity and personhood in society have resulted in acceptance. An acceptance of Jung's interpretation caused her to surrender her resistance and become more feminine, later giving birth to children. Pierre Bourdieu (2001) talks of the symbolic violence that women face each and every day, but he, like most men I think, misses the comprehensive process of this violence. Germaine Greer (1971) combines physical aggression and contact with a variety of aggressive interactions she classes under "abuse." Some students of murders and social executions of women as witches classify this violence as a special form of violence against women, especially those who are "unconventional" (Albesina et al. 2016; Chollet 2022). Like the situation of African Americans, the systematic conditioning of men and women creates an entire world of constant negation and challenge. This results in the negation of value and challenge of the right to self. This milieu produces in every moment of interaction reinforcement to the dominant paradigm of subordination women face and must adapt to even in their relations to loved ones. Adapting to a place in the world that is defined by acts of submissive signs and identification with them thwarts achievement and induces a form of nihilism, not the nihilism of the nineteenth century in which the individual could choose to reject everything in view of the ideology, but a nihilism described by Cornel West (1994), where planning and undertaking are defeated before they begin by the symbols of oppression. There have been times when women organized to defend themselves or struggle for rights, but these periods have been generally brief and seldom sustained. Where women have not been entirely subjugated by patriarchal religion or society, as in the Kom and Bakweri of West Africa. Here Ardener (1975a) describes the women traditionally acting in solidarity to protect and avenge women in societies continually challenged by Western power.

Women to me, have generally been of a beautiful nature and magical but we are all creatures of our culture and family life. I would sit as a child and listen to my sister and her friends talk about boys, clothes, movies, and school. Or I would watch my mother and her sisters and aunts or our neighbors' wives talk about the day's pressures and news. Sometimes they would sing songs in Portuguese or tell tales of the "Old World." From these women came a fount of knowledge and fun, where the opportunities of life were embellished with desire and fantasy mixed with history and longing. That longing, for lost children, parents, lovers, missed homes, and friends, created a mystery aroma that I only realized when I first heard the Fado sung. This musical genre expresses a feeling not so much delineated by the words as by the way it is sung. To be a woman, to create children, to be the object of desire and the definition of sex for men was a most strange and yet beguiling land. The simple reality that children came from women seemed to me to be the proof of their spiritual quality, yet at the same time it was apparent that it condemned them to a subservient role in society, in American society, and as I was to learn as an anthropologist, in many other cultures. This dilemma became one of the driving forces that led to me Anthropology, to contact with the Cockettes, and to many friendships with women in the adventure to understand. Why were women so oppressed? What was femininity and had this arrangement always been so?

There are considerable works on this subject, from de Beauvoir and Friedan to more recent feminist theorists like Kaouthar Darmoni (2014), who describes the distinct worlds of women and men. The ability of women together to express joyous feelings and pleasure contrasted with the way women must hide from men and envelope themselves in protective layers, both in her own Tunisian culture and in the West.

Back at Humboldt State almost all the instructors and students involved in the sensory deprivation experiments were men. A few students were female but most did not work in the labs; they took support roles, clerical in nature, as at Humboldt. When I saw that all the subjects that had been chosen were male I asked one of the instructors why we had no female subjects. He seemed surprised and knowingly set me straight that scientific experiments were rigorous and could be dangerous for frail constitutions. The rules for subjects were strict and women could not be used. The list of dream types below has been constructed from a number of sources and reflects the above findings as well as the problem in weighing dream elements (Table 6.1). While these dream types are drawn from different studies, the authors contracted the dreams of many subjects into one element. I did the same with Goodison's data to show how difficult the process can be and distorting. Comparisons can be made with her originals. Sireteanu et al. (2008), in a study of sensory-deprivation-induced hallucinations of one woman found she reported colored and moving patterns similar to those reported in other cases of both psychedelics and deprivation studies. What was interesting was that different parts of the brain were related to the deprivation state (extrastriate occipital, posterior parietal, and several prefrontal regions), but normal conditions without deprivation produced imagery but in the prefrontal regions only.

This brings up another topic that is related to both scientific studies and psychology. In a recent book edited by Nicolas Langlitz (2013) we find a group of studies and new analysis of old ones that have a more feminist perspective. I only use this term to indicate an awareness of gender differences and gender representation in both the organization of experimentation and evaluation. However, Langlitz (2013) argues that a new science of "neuropsychopharmacology as spiritual technology" has been born as a part of a revival of psychedelic use and research. His book is presented as an ethnography of a movement and revival, yet spends a

Table 6.1 Prevalence or appearance by gender of dream type

	Men	Women
1. Chased or pursued not injured	1	1
2. Sexual experiences	1	1
3. Falling	1	
4. School, teachers, studying	1	
5. Arriving too late		1
6. Being on the verge of falling	1	1
7. Trying again and again to do something	1	1
8. A person now alive as dead	1	1
9. Flying or soaring through the air	1	1
10. Negative emotions (anger, sadness, confusion)	80%	77%
11. Positive (success, good fortune, happiness)	53%	53%
12. Food or eating mentioned in dream	17%	17%
13. Characters in dream men vs. women	2.4%	2.8%
14. Dream length 8% longer in women		–
15. Dream of men	67%	33%
16. Mexican dreams: dream of men	50%	50%
17. German dreams: dream of men	58%	56
18. Familiar characters	45%	58%
19. Unfamiliar characters	55%	42%
20. Character means to harm	47%	44%
21. Character supportive, kind, friendly	38%	42%
22. Location of setting: outdoor	52%	39%
23. Location of setting: unfamiliar	39%	22%
24. Family members	12%	20%
25. Dead and imaginary person, being	00%	01%
26. Animal	06%	04%
27. Mist or cloud		x
28. Being a wounded animal, bird		x
29. Strange woman comes into room, shrinks, screams		x
30. Finding a buried being, child, cat, etc.		x
31. Pregnant woman gets on bus, dances and attacked		x
32. Appearance of man in eighteenth-century dress stops suicide		x
33. Children love parent, parent becomes businessperson		x
34. In home finds secret room, transforms to magnificent		x
35. Dreamt standing on a railway platform		x
36. Dreamt being in a bleak and incomplete house		2
37. House sinks		1
38. In house with aunt, drains have arms		1
39. Woman captured and tied up		1
40. Tarantulas and spiders crawl all over you		1
41. Dreams monster kills butterfly inside head		1

(*continued*)

Table 6.1 (continued)

	Men	Women
42. Dream of house with family and strangers, dance		1
43. Dreamt standing in a toilet bowl with silver objects		1
44. In room crying man enters with aborigines		1
45. Having sex in a van, then on grass, failure		1
46. In bed with young boy		1
47. Hemorrhage from vagina then riding dog		1
48. Difficulty walking down stairs		1
49. At a party having to urinate		1
50. Seeing live person trapped in coffin of ice		1
51. Butchering self for burial		1
52. Sees self as prostitute, client female with bloody vagina		1
53. Making love with one's mother in bed with lover		1
54. Putting on clothes and then other clothes		1
55. In pavilion near lily pond man in water drowns		1
56. Captured, made naked, and becomes friend		1
57. Rips a man apart bit by bit		1
58. Nearly gets in bed with boyfriend, nearly crosses street		1
59. Vietnamese woman, family and friends fight and sing		1
60. White woman in African, with Blacks, illegal, captured		1
61. Dreams forgot to feed baby, (got smaller) carried, lost		3
62. Met Jane Fonda		1
63. Dreams is a bottle of ink, mingled with another, did not mix		1
64. At sea shore with lover running ahead of her, she stumbles		1
65. Woman rides on subway with son and fears losing him		1
66. Children run into house covered with mud, woman with dresses		1
67. Child take apple from pile, you think it is rotten		1
68. Friend in coffin, sleeps with other's lover because she had too much		1
69. Female argues with other female, man gives cakes with drugs, both get friendly, get high		1
70. Woman dreams of self as girl who becomes rotting corpse		1
71. Sees self as child in hospital with fatal illness		1
72. Father dead, exhumed, looked bad but living, son tries to be normal	1	
73. Comanche, central figures in dreams were dogs	1	
74. In house, sees mother in coffin		1
75. In house with sister, forgot mother		1
76. Comes to house, her family inside when a child		1
77. Bitten by spider, then improves		1
78. Visits mother's house, is ruin, to be renewed		1

(*continued*)

Table 6.1 (continued)

	Men	Women
79. Meets father, mother drunk on floor of bizarre		1
80. Waits in room, woman enters, battle outside, runs out, battle gone, loses leg and head		1
81. Dancing on knees		1
82. Swimming with women near big ship		1
83. Teacher trying to hammer nail into blackboard		1
84. Scolds daughter for spending too much on stationary asks for money back, if offered Barbie, refuses		1
85. Man has dream wife is suffocating him		1
86. Military planes spoil outing, woman shouts at them		1
87. Dreams spouse married another woman		1
88. Dreams spouse runs off with other men	1	
89. Dreams spouse dead or with another woman		1
90. Father kills python	1	
91. Falling, stabbing people, swimming, fleeing dying	1	
92. Standing in line of women at the end decapitation		1
93. Fire burning back wall of house		1

Sources: Based on Hall and Van de Castle and modified from Nielsen et al. (2003). Entries are ranked 1–9 appearance only, 10–32 most frequent, added information from other sources has changed the ranking from Nielsen et al. (2003), Goodison (1995) for 27–71, 74; #s 10–26 for American populations: Domhoff (2005), Sacks (2012); #33 from Van Dusen et al. (1967); #55 from Barr (2005); #73 from Linton, R (1936)

The Study of Man, New York, Appleton-Century-Crofts; #s 87–91 from Domhoff (1990); #92 from Jung (1964); #93 from *The Kalevala*, Finnish epic collected by Elias Lonrott, Oxford, Oxford University Press, 1989 edition

lot of time reflecting on media representations and governmental regulation of drugs. In covering the "revival" of interest Langlitz finds more continuity from people involved in the past, yet also a mixture of New Age ideas and spiritualism. This mixing of science and religion seems problematic. The book, in general, is an example of trends in popular culture that are either obviously anti-science (as in Scientologists) or, as in many of those opposed to vaccines (and especially the vaccines against Covid-19) are misled by conspiracy theories or misunderstand media reports concerning science.

Langlitz's (2013) chapter 2 describes some of this controversy concerning LSD research and begins with charges by Scientologists at a scientific symposium on LSD in Basel. They claimed that LSD was given to women as a means of controlling them for the purposes of use by psychiatrists. Usually information on psychologists' abusing subjects is made public in cases where psychiatrists have unethical relations with their patients and formal charges are pressed; otherwise data is scarce (Chesler 1972). Though other examples of abuse have come to light (with MDMA see Goldhill 2020), the charges against LSD use by psychiatrists was new to me. Other reports of women who have suffered at the hands of doctors have appeared as well, for example, in the decision to do a hysterectomy or sexual abuse by physicians (Smith 1992).

The Future of Psychedelics and Consciousness

One of the many problems with imagined futures is their roots in the societies and conditions of those who do the imagining. From Plato to Richard Bucke or Aldous Huxley, the future can be a pleasure dome or a horror scape. One person's ideal, a Marx or an Adam Smith, can become worse than the life of the creator. Some places impress visitors as paradises, Polynesia to some Westerners, or Bali, Tibet, or even America to immigrants.

In the solitude of one is found the dull prison of another. The happiness of an exceptional person or people can, and often does, incite the jealousy and violence of those threatened by it, no matter what the reason. To some Europeans of the post-1492 years of contact, Native Americans lived in a world of peace, plenty, and perfection. These lives were often seen as the motivation of the devil and so the heathen and devil were rooted out (Todorov 1984).

It seems that the scenario drawn by W.H.R. Rivers (1920) where the human mind has evolved as a kind of sieve to concentrate attention on the elements most central to survival, as is the case for other organisms from amoeba to man, is an astute one. This adapted perception is unique and specific, but it does not rule out others and the reality it creates is only perhaps one of many. We can blend this view with that of Adolf Bastain and Franz Boas, who saw the varieties of human ideas of society, religion, and art as a vast invention of the diversity of a common Psychic Unity given by our brain's evolution.

This brings us to a point of assessment of these ideas of perfection of society and religion, cosmic consciousness, and ongoing evolution of man. About the time I did this research I was assigned reading of Eric Fromm's book *May Man Prevail?* Fromm had left Germany before the Holocaust but had lived during Hitler's rise to power. He had seen the way the motives of the rich, fearful of Communism, had curried favor with Hitler and how the Allied Powers had tolerated his seizure of power for the same reason.

As I read Fromm's book I was disappointed that a psychologist who had lived in the context of fear and terror in Germany was so driven by fear and the expectation of not only the victory of Communism in the form of Stalin's Soviet Union, but of the end of humanity by nuclear war. Over and over again he sought to defend values of the West that were not only tarnished by centuries of anti-Semitism and racism against African Americans, other non-Europeans, and Irish, but also fundamentally flawed by the savagery and barbarism of colonialism. His argument was not only hollow, but illogical. Why should we expect a group of Allied Powers, who used the atomic bomb on Japan mainly as an experiment, to be capable of reversing the competition that had led to WWI and WWII? He appeals to reason and to fair play, but based on an individualism that led to wars against almost all humanity from 1492 to 1945.

At about the same time I was also reading Garrett Hardin's *Biology* (1966) text. At the end of a remarkable chapter on worms and mollusks, in the spirit of the whole text centered on humans in a miraculous world, he quotes Julian Huxley. Julian, a child of the Progressivism of his family, argues, "the human species is now the sole repository of any possible future progress for life .... It is a biological impossibility for any other line of life to progress into a new dominant type—not the ant, the rat, nor the monkey." Trapped as he was in the dogma of the West, so perfected by the nineteenth century, Julian could only see progress as a conflict of animals. He did not consider that progress could also mean other animals might over take human evolution in ways unimagined (perhaps after we exterminate ourselves) or how viruses or other pathogens could conquer animals, with an end to the short (less than one half a billion years) run of dominance multicellularity had brought.

For over four billion years life on earth was one-celled. Most of it today still is. So if we consider that cosmic consciousness might include one-celled organisms, such a contemplation might suggest that the disappearance of humanity might not be the disaster so often seen in humanity's creativity in weapons of mass destruction.

References

Albesina, Alberto, Benedetta Brioschi and Eliana La Ferrara, (2016) "Violence against women: a cross-cultural analysis for Africa," *NBER*, Working Paper 21901, January, https://doi.org/10.3386/w21901.

Ardener, Edwin (1972) "Belief and the problem of women," in J.S, La Fontaine (ed.) *The Interpretation of Ritual*, London, Tavistock.

Ardener, Shirley (1975a) "Sexual insult and female militancy," in *Perceiving Women*, (ed.) Shirley Ardener, pp. 29–54.

Barr, Allan H. (2005) "The Ming history inquisition in personal memoir and public memory," *Chinese Literature: Essays, Articles, Reviews (CLEAR)* v. 27, Dec.: 5–32.

Bourdieu, Pierre (2001) *Masculine Domination*, Stanford, Stanford University Press.

Bucke, Richard M. (1905) *Cosmic Consciousness: A Study in the Evolution of the Human Mind*, Philadelphia, Innes & Sons Edition facsimile. Originally published in 1901.

Caldararo, Niccolo Leo (1968) "A Mental Ethnography," Laboratory notes from Mogar discussions and fieldwork in LSD research, Unpublished Xerox copies distributed to R. Mogar and several co-investigators, appeared in 3 copies, the first in 1967 for a class in Psychology at SFSU and then one for the Mogar Lab files and lastly in1969 a copy given to Dr. Joan Davlin of the Anthropology Department.

Callois, R. (1966) "Logical and philosophical problems of the dream," in G.E. von Grunebaum and R. Callois (Eds) *The Dream and Human Societies*, Berkeley and Los Angeles, University of California Press.

Caplan, Paula (1985) *The Myth of Women's Masochism*, New York, Dutton.

Caplan, Paula and Jeremy Caplan (2008) *Thinking Critically About Research on Sex and Gender*, Hove, East Sussex, Psychology Press.

Cartwright, R.D., S. Lloyd, S. Knight and I. Trenholme, (1984) *Psychiatry*, Aug, v. 47, 3, 251–259.

Chesler, Phyllis (1972) "The Sensuous Psychiatrists," *New York Magazine,* July 23, https://nymag.com/ne.

Chollet, Mona (2022) *In Defense of Witches: The Legacy of the Witch Hunts and Why Women are Still on Trial,* Trans. Sophie R. Lewis, St Martin's Press.

Darmoni, Kaouthar (2014) "Taste of Life," Ted Talk, Oct 16th. https://www.youtube.com/watch?v=x3AwnkR92EA

de Beauvoir, Simone (1949) *The Second Sex,* New York, Random House.

Domhoff, G.W. (2005) "The dreams of men and women: patterns of gender similarity and differences," Dreamresearch.net. Sept 30, https://dreams.ucsc.edu/Library/domhoff_2005c.html.

Domhoff, G. William (1990) *The Mystique of Dreams, A Search for Utopia through Senoi Dream Theory,* Berkeley, University of California Press.

Eggan, Dorothy (1952) "The manifest content of dreams: a challenge to social science," *American Anthropologist,* v. 54, 469–485.

Eliade, Mircea (1964) *Shamanism,* Bolligen Foundation, Princeton, Princeton University Press.

Foster, J.C. and Anderson, J.E. (1936) "Unpleasant dreams in childhood," *Child Development,* v. 7, 77–84.

Foulkes, D., (1971) Longitudinal studies of dreams in children," In J. Masserman (ed) *Science and Psychoanalysis,* 9, New York, Grune and Stratton.

Freud, Sigmund (1964) *The Future of an Illusion,* New York, Anchor Books.

Garcia, Manon (2021) *We Are Not Born Submissive,* Princeton, Princeton University Press.

Goldhill, Olivia (2020) "Psychedelic therapy has a sexual abuse problem," *Quartz,* May 13, https://qz.com/1809184/psychedelic-therapy-has-a-sexual-abuse-problem-3/

Goodison, Lucy (1995) *The Dreams of Women: Exploring and Interpreting Women's Dreams,* New York, W.W. Norton.

Greer, Germaine (1971) *The Female Eunuch,* London, Granada.

Griffith, R. M., Miyagi, O., & Tago, A. (1958) "The universality of typical dreams: Japanese vs Americans," *American Anthropologist,* 60, 1173–1179.

Grof, Stanislav (1976) *Realms of the Human Unconscious: Observation from LSD Research,* New York, E.P. Dutton.

Hall, C.S. (1984) "A ubiquitous sex difference in dreams," revisited, *Journal of Personality and Social Psychology,* v. 46, n. 5, 1109–1117.

Hall, C.S. and B. Domhoff (1963) "A ubiquitous sex difference in dreams," *The Journal of Abnormal and Social Psychology,* v. 66, n. 3, 278–280.

Janiger, O. and Paltin, G. (1971) A bibliography of L.S.D. & mescaline: From the earliest researches to the beginnings of suppression. Fitzhugh Ludlow Library.

Jersild, A.T., F.V. Markey and C.L. Jersild, (1933) "Children's fears, wishes, daydreams, likes, dislikes, pleasant and unpleasant memories," *Child Development Monographs,* n. 12, New York, New York Teachers College, Columbia University.

Jung, C.G. (1964) "Approaching the unconscious," in *Man and His Symbols,* (eds.) Carl G. Jung, M.-L. von Franz, Joseph L. Henderson, Jolande Jacobi and Aniela Jaffe, New York, Dell Publishing, 1–94.

Langlitz, Nicolas (2013) *Neuropsychedelia: The Revival of Hallucinogen Research Since the Decade of the Brain,* Berkeley, University of California Press.

Laughlin, Robert M. (1976) Of Wonders Wild and New: Dreams from Zinacantan, Smithsonian Contributions to Anthropology, n. 22, Washington, D.C., Smithsonian Institution.

Lewis-Williams, J.D. (2009) "Cognitive and optical illusions in San Rock art research," "In Warms, Richard, James Garber and R. Jon McGee, (2009) *Sacred Realms: Readings in the Anthropology of Religion,* Oxford, Oxford University Press, 217–226.

Ling, Thomas M. and John Buckman, (1964) "The treatment of frigidity with LSD and Ritalin," *Psychedelic Review,* v. 1, n. 4, 450–458.

Linton, Ralph (1936) *The Study of Man,* New York, Appleton-Century.

Moore, James W, (2016) " What is the sense of agency and why does it matter?" *Front. Psychol.* V.7, 1272. https://doi.org/10.3388/fpsyg.2016.01272.

Nielsen, Tore A., Antonio L. Zadra, Valerie Simard, Sebastien Saucier, Philippe Stenstron, et al., (2003) "The typical dreams of Canadian university students," *Dreaming,* 13, 211–235.

Rivers, W.H.R. (1920) *Instinct and the Unconscious,* Cambridge, Cambridge University Press.

Rubinstein, K. and Krippner, S. (1991) "Gender differences and geographic differences in content from dreams elicited by a television announcement," *International Journal of Psychosomatics,* v. 38, n. 1-4, 40–44.

Sacks, Oliver (2012) *Hallucinations,* New York, Vintage Books.

Schredl, M. (2007) "Gender differences in dreaming," In D. Barrett & P. McNamara (Eds.), *The new science of dreaming*—Volume 2: Content, recall, and personality correlates (pp. 29–47). Westport: Praeger.

Schredl, M. Petra Ciric, Simon Gotz and Lutz Wittmann (2010) "Typical dreams: Stability and differences," *Journal of Psychology,* v. 138, (6): 485–494.

Seligman, C.G. (1923) "A note on dreams," *Man,* 186–188.

Sireteanu, Ruxandra, Viola Oetel, Harald Mohr, David Linden and Wolf Singer (2008) "Graphical illustration and functional neuroimaging of visual hallucinations during prolonged blindfolding: a comparison to visual imagery," *Perception*, January 1, v. 37, n. 12, 1805–1821.

Smith, John M. (1992) *Women and Doctors*, New York, Atlantic Monthly Press.

Spaulding, John (1981) "The dream in other cultures: anthropological studies of dreams and dreaming," Dreamworks, v. 1, n. 4, Summer, 330–342.

Todorov, Tzvetan (1984) *The Conquest of America*, New York, Harper and Row.

Van Dusen, Wilson, Wayne Wilson, William Miners and Harry Hook, (1967) "Treatment of alcoholism with Lysergide," *Quarterly Journal of Studies on Alcoholism*, v. 28,: 295–303.

West, Cornel (1994) *Race Matters*, New York Vintage Books.

Zadra, A. and T.A. Nielsen (1997) "Typical dreams: a comparison of 1958 versus 1996 student samples," *Sleep Research*, 26, 280.

7

The Female Exception (in Research) and Gendered Experiences

The nature of woman and the performance of the role of female have been examined by a number of writers—philosopher Simone de Beauvoir (1949) most notably. She was followed by a considerable number of feminist social scientists in the 1960s and 1970s. Shirley Ardener (1975) suggested that given the vast variation in the cultural and social models of women, the category "may disappear." Certainly the focus on gender as a social role has become a significant issue in the past four decades. The idea of a new means of viewing the consciousness of humanity and its potential has been proposed by a number of feminist writers on psychedelics. One of these is Zoe Helene. In a recent article Kim Hewitt (2019) describes the potential of this inquiry as:

> Psychedelic feminism empowers women by encouraging participatory consciousness, in which individuals engage in a meaning-making process. Agency is encouraged via intuitive ways of knowing, intentionally valuing subjectivity, and engaging the imagination to create meaning and re-engineer the self. In the process of delving into the subjective psychedelic experience, psychedelic feminism also promotes experiential knowledge of interconnectivity, a feeling of being connected to realms beyond oneself.

N. Caldararo, *A Mental Ethnography: Conclusions From Research in LSD*,
https://doi.org/10.1007/978-3-031-13745-7_7

This is a refreshing endeavor, brave, as it is bold. The idea that women could discover or create a consciousness encompassed by the nature of the female experience in what is obviously not only a male-dominated world, but one nearly completely conditioned in male desires and fantasy [especially about women], is astounding. To Dr. Lucy Goodison (1995), a 20-year examination of her own dreams, leading workshops on dreams, and research into their nature left her with a dissatisfaction with dream "dictionaries" and the theories of mainly male dream "experts." She promotes the idea that women should meet together and study their dreams and write them down soon after awaking. I knew a woman in the late 1960s who was a member of Eckankar and did both these things to study her dreams. Goodison, like Helene, then came to the discovery of women's dreams as a category of experience and, I would say, perception. It has the character of the search for cures of disease, or for lost cities of the Amazon, scientific research or attempts to translate Etruscan. It is as if someone decided to find a lost library of the Maya that had escaped destruction. In a world where the behavior, bodies, and thoughts of women have been so thoroughly suppressed and been the focus of male ownership and construction, the discovery of a world of female meaning would be a breakthrough in human consciousness that seems inconceivable. There have been women's secret writing and language (Nu Shu, for example—see Yang 1999, so there are antecedents).

The idea of psychedelic feminism in Hewitt's interpretation is to promote self-healing and self-exploration, and empower themselves. The basic context appears to be where female-only experiences are promoted and can provide support for individual growth. This does assume a supportive culture with symbols that allow for constructive identity and association. Helene has described such a context with an ecological foundation based in an idea of "entheogens" or substances that manifest the Divine within, such as sacred plant medicines. She realizes that this avenue of healing is working against the "subconscious social programming within us." This is a parallel project to de-colonial studies. The central hope or trust here is that female-created contexts (what we have discussed above in Leary's terms, "set and setting") can be a powerful recreative and cleansing one. This is involved in the French feminist theory of "writing the feminine," "implying creating the feminine self," as Hewitt (2019) puts it. One of the earliest examples of this "set and setting" idea comes from the ancient Greeks at the shrine of Asclepius at Epidaurus, where people would undergo a number of rituals and then sleep at the shrine overnight. It is reported that a woman, blind in one eye, attended and had a dream where the god cured her but due to her skepticism ordered her to pay a high "donation." This cannot be said to be a woman's dream as we do not have her report of the dream, only that of the priests and their interpretation of it (Pausanias, second century CE).

From Simone de Beauvoir's analysis of the patriarchy's program for women, to the eco-feminism of French feminists like Francoise d'Eaubonne, to Helene, the idea of associating women and nature and shifting the male domination of earth and woman, Hewitt (2019) describes, is an undertaking that is more than revolutionary. If one considers that Darwin (1871) thought that the basis of domestication of animals began with that of women, and that some scientists believe that an entire complex of genes regulate traits of domestication, from those of morphological traits to behavioral ones (Wilkins et al. 2014). However, I do not think such a syndrome exists, and if so, not in humans. Also, the influence of hormones during ontogeny is influenced by an array of environmental factors. The most extreme is the condition mentioned earlier, the androgen sensitivity syndrome. Another limitation to the idea of female domestication is the fact that Darwin and other nineteenth-century writers may have relied too heavily on a one-sided and biased vision of the role of women in aboriginal society. Phyllis Kaberry's (1939) fieldwork directly contradicted the idea of male domination of women's lives and Leacock's (1978) criticism of much of the theory of male rule has provided an alternative view. She and Nash (Leacock and Nash 1977) detail the way the record of diversity of female roles in societies has been impoverished by selective erasure and distortion. There is considerable ethological evidence, discussed by Hrdy (1981), on the variation in male or female dominance in vertebrates, and Trivers (1985) describes the rather accidental conditions under which one or other system of gender domination develops.

A recent analysis focused on contemporary conditions women live in by Manon Garcia (2021) draws heavily on the writings of a number of feminist writers like Simone de Beauvoir, and produces a more complex social web of inculcation and control that lead to, if not determine, female submission and domestication. One of the points she makes from de Beauvoir is that women as girls experience a public description of their bodies before they are able to express their own identity with it in terms of pleasure and testing in the world (e.g., competition). She argues, also from her own life, that comments about a girl's body begin the objectification to build an identity of use of that body by others, whether in the male gaze (men enjoy looking at it) or touching it. The boundaries of a female body in most societies are defined by its use to others. For girls to inculcate that process denies them the freedom to act in the world and begins the process of othering that makes women the property of men, vulnerable in spaces not controlled by related men (husbands, fathers, etc.) and limited by consequences if they are found in such spaces (used for sex, become pregnant). "Images beyond images to infinity" (Anais Nin diary). But the amount of hormore and time of its delivery in ontogeny produces female behavior in castrated male rats (Corbier et al. 1983).

Nonetheless, a number of writers, both socialist and otherwise, have argued about a comprehensive control of consciousness through economic and political conditions, both by violence and by conditioning. Gramsci's (1971) paradigm is one of the most complete, but Kolata (2006) provides a more relevant context where long practice with all symbols and rites, as well as daily routines reinforcing identity and self-worth, leads to an ever-present system of reinforcement to accept, internalize, and produce also responses meant to keep others in line. He uses the term "orthopraxy" where people believe certain behaviors are the only correct conduct, and the term "doxology" (usually understood as a hymn of praise to god) as a pattern of inculcation where the subject people come to praise their oppressors as possessing all good. One could apply this to the condition of women, especially where in some contexts their sexual objectification is so complete that they enjoy their transformation into objects of pleasure for men and engage in the pursuit of its perfection, termed the "Objectification Theory" or OB. It can reach such intensity where women reject or attack any women who refuses to submit in the same way (Fredrickson and Roberts 1997; Szymanski et al. 2011). However, most violence against women is by men and can be also seen within the domestication process of negative conditioning alternated with positive conditioning. It is a feature of almost all cultures studied and appears no matter what the religious ethic is or if it is theoretically sanctioned or not (Kalra and Bhugra 2013; Vellidis 2018).

Evolutionary psychologists have developed a considerable literature on the subject (Barbaro 2017), but it is lacking in some hunter-gatherer societies or matrifocal societies or present in minimal form (Kaberry 1939). Cross-cultural research indicates that violence and abuse against women is less compared with patrilineal (patrifocal) societies, undermining a case for any evolutionary role (Karim et al. 2021).

However, it is apparent that many women reject this role either as feminists, lesbians, or bisexual women, as Szymanski et al. (2011) note. In some cases of the latter two, we might consider that they are not entirely free of the inculcation of OB, as they are engaged in the sexual pursuit of women, which can involve degrees of OB, especially as they are competing with men for women in the nature of sexuality defined by femininity in any culture dominated by patrifocal concepts. The concept of "compulsory heterosexuality" makes the survival of lesbians and bisexual women all the more conflicted in the process of female autonomy and identity (Ferguson 1981). But Kaplan (1982) argues that there is a distinct "female consciousness" that can evolve from the unequal gender system in the division of labor by sex. Such women demand the rights of a human status but usually are restricted to that of women as nurturers within the family and their collective action is often only directed in maintaining traditional roles when these are threatened, often in the process paying a heavy emotional and social price for their efforts, as Drew (1995) discusses for African examples.

As opposed to this concept of women's consciousness, Green (1979) proposed an examination of "feminist consciousness" by applying a number of tests to a group of college women. In the definition of feminist consciousness that evolved, ideas of autonomy and control over their lives emerged. In other studies, for example, in Asian women, female consciousness has been defined by ideas of female identity as well as social class and caste and culture change (Putra 2011). In the1970s Ardener (1972, 1975) referred to the position and place of women in many societies as that of an inarticulate group and related their presence to other groups that were made silent by convention or sanction. This was followed by a number of analyses of this role as a "muted group," to describe both the conformation of mind resulting from such a model (Hardman 1973; Ardener, S. 1975) and its performance. Edwin Ardener (1972) suggests that the models of the world are the peoduct of men, defining social behavior for all gender activity, one wonders if this can explain forms of revolt as seen amomg the Kom described by Shirley Ardener (1972) or the dramatic violence of the "mushroom madness" seen in Kuma males compared to the amused response of the Kuma females (de Rios, 1984). This creates a paradox of an identity in social life where one observes action, but refrains from participation or comment, except in the most defined categories. Obviously women communicate with men and participate in social action, but in constrained fashion. These limits are the result of gender enforcement that begins at birth and is reinforced by both males and females in a thorough conditioning schedule. The role of other women in molding a girl's life into a compliant and respectful member of the female community is what Lynn O'Conner (Personal Communication 1970) called "prison guarding."

Shirley Ardener (1975) argues based on a survey of cultures that women in different societies have "models of the world" that differ from those of men and that many components of these models are shared by women across cultures. Keohane et al. (1990) suggest there are three forms of women's consciousness: (1) Feminine consciousness is an awareness of oneself as the object of another's attention, the woman defined by the "male gaze." (2) A second form, feminist consciousness, is developed as women think about their relation to power and their position in society. (3) A third form is female consciousness, or the traditional role of women as nurturing and sustaining members of the family and marriage. Reimer (1996) shows that among Inuit women, their culture defines this role as possessing certain privileges that require social action and reciprocation in a number of spheres of society.

I am concerned here about this idea of a separate gender consciousness for women, given the long history, especially in the West, of women being considered as undeveloped children (Friedan 1963; Millett 1970). This idea of a "female consciousness" has been successfully disproven by feminist scientists over the past five decades, with the exception of Brizendine (2007), who has promoted a paradigm of hormone-driven states of behavior. Cross-cultural studies of female hormones and behavior have found significant variation and differences in expression that are associated with a number of factors, including learning and culture (Vitzthum 2009). Applications of the Objectification Theory to transwomen have had diverse results (Comiskey et al. 2019) and there has been a controversy over whether they are "really women" (Wright 2018). It is interesting that structural MRI findings of cis and trans males and females found that transgender individuals show structural alterations in the brain that differ from their biological sex as well as from their perceived gender. This study included a variety of subjects, before surgery, while on hormones, and after surgery (Flint et al. 2020). However, since there is wide variation in cis men and women, this finding is difficult to assess, especially as earlier studies had different results (Darlington 2002).

The nature of masculine and feminine consciousness is vague in much of the literature. In the case of a study by Valle and Kruger (1989), the authors claim that one wrote in a "masculine style" while the other in a distinctly "feminine manner." They define masculine as rational and logical and argue that the feminine "side of consciousness" is "the essential complement and completion of masculine consciousness." Ryan, introduced earlier in this book, is a biological or cis woman who came to believe that she needed to become a man because of sexual and gender issues that seemed incongruent with her personality. She then began a transition to become a man, undergoing hormone treatments and dressing as a man. In both forms she was attractive but not attracted to the opposite sex in either case. She was not satisfied in the male world, so transitioned back to female. Her response to the question of "why she did either" or "what was good about either gender status for her" was that she did not find what she expected and yet missed, to a certain extent, her life as a female.

This is a significant dilemma, as many feminists and female psychologists often end up describing what is male consciousness as aspects of roles, like energy, strength, power, self-actualization, and either no female counterparts or also a list of roles, as in nurturing, subjective, supportive, and suggest a merging of these traits (e.g., Garcia 1985–1986). Entire cultures have developed around "earth mother" spirituality (Murciano-Luna 2020) and new investigations of matriarchy, yet these seem to be locked into former concepts of femininity and motherhood. Lerner's (1993) comprehensive analysis of how an oppressive male culture created the conditions of a female consciousness is telling and convincing, but the analysis of that female consciousness is consonant with the domestication theory, even with the heroic rebellions of so many women. Yet the remnants of the matriarchy belt in Africa still inspire many attempts to reinvent what a female-defined world could be (Matory 2005).

The nature of eco-feminism is rooted in ideas of creating "caring and connection and therefore moral community" (Hewitt 2019). It avoids grand theories, but postulates that there "is no one way to be a woman." Hewitt (2019) describes the movement it has created as being more inclusive—characterizing themselves as "third wave feminists," such women are positioned differently from earlier feminists, focusing instead on "a multiplicity of identities, accept the messiness of lived contradiction, and eschew a unifying agenda." It is interesting to note, especially regarding identity and the performance of self in everyday life, that an aspect of magical transformation which is common to shaman and other practitioners of communication with the spirit world, is to mark the body. Here one can include tattoos, removal of body parts (e.g. fingers) or scaring and painting the body. The cutting of hair, shaving the body or head and painting the face along with rings inserted or bone and sticks all often are related to the communication with the spirits or ancestors. Corson (1972) charts this history and use mainly in the West. McLean (2016) and Hansen and Reed (1986) provide a wider focus. What is notable with women today is that body modification and cosmetics are not seen as special but normal and even many women consider them to be torture or work. The goals seem to include (though as a diverse group without dogma) "fun, feminine and sex-positive" efforts to create their own reality and identities within also self-forming and affirming communities (Hewitt 2019). This perspective sees the psychedelic experience as consonant with a feminine consciousness of a unitive nature and "contiguous with cosmic consciousness" (Hewitt 2019). This view of the feminine aspect of behavior sees it as a concept rather than a sexed or gendered characteristic and as a means of alliance with men to invite a transformation of relations of humanity with the earth and natural world (Hewitt 2019). These feminists' interpretation of the psychedelic experience is similar to that of the Mogar Lab group, where language and words were suspected of undermining direct meaning and understanding. They claim that these experiences "can't be wholly contained by the linear and limited tool of language."

Some 30 years ago I read a book, *The Woman That Never Evolved* by Sarah Hrdy. Hrdy's book was eye opening, as it was a careful analysis of central tenets of male superiority in the biological world, a work of science. It was my wife's favorite book. Then some years later I read *The Female Brain*, by Cynthia Darlington, a neurophysiologist in New Zealand. She begins the book by stating her reason for writing it, most medical research and most anatomy and physiology research was done on a male population. Obviously, there were problems with this approach, and the reasons given by standard texts were that females were not good subjects for research. Her book is a straightforward analysis of female neurophysiology and anatomy. A few years later I saw a book with the same title by a different author, Louann Brizendine. Dr. Brizendine was a psychiatrist who specialized in the hormonal problems of her patients. Her book, as opposed to Darlington, was a pastiche of anecdotes from friends, her life, and patients, and 1950s morality, with souped up conservative views on what women should be doing instead of trying to succeed in business and science. I was rather shocked. But I shouldn't have been—having an MD does not make one smart nor indicate a personality that is questioning or driven by a desire for knowledge. It can just mean that one is from a rich background and wants to make money. It was obvious that the title of the book sparked interest in an opportunity to capitalize on people's prejudices about gender, sex, and what it meant to be a woman, what makes women "tick." Comedians of both sexes have used the idea of female intelligence as a gimmick in getting laughs for centuries, and not only was Brizendine's monster of a book a success, but it spawned the living horror of plays and movies, reproducing caricatures of women all over the consciousness of new generations of men and women. The book writes about female physiology and the brain as if feminism never took place. All the efforts to counter the idea that women were ruled by their hormones are undermined by Dr. Brizendine's medical authority. She has sown a minefield of confused territory, in my mind (a male one), for sexism to work on for decades to come.

Conducting Research in a Male World

Demeaning women and making sexism popular and acceptable was an astounding feat, but then again, making money and fame is what America is all about. This aspect of our culture has affected research into

LSD. During one of the early studies by Blum et al. (1964, 12–13) female investigators, especially those considered pretty and were young, experienced difficulties in conducting interviews with various personnel, especially police officers.

Blum et al. (1964) report that the women in their sample were more reluctant to take LSD or to initiate others to the drug than men. Their Table III of characteristics of "acceptors" in their initial sample to "controls" reflects both the age, larger number of younger individuals as acceptors, and men. An aspect of this population of the married couples that appeared during the follow-up was the tendency of husbands to introduce wives to the drug and few (1) wives introduced it to their husbands. In both cases where the wife refused to take the drug, divorce followed. In one case the wife took it hoping for reconciliation with her husband, but divorce resulted anyway. Husbands' interest in the drug and offering it to their wives was a prime determinant of female use. This information is an indication of the control and influence men have over women, and the fact that divorce followed the wives' use may reflect on the affect the drug has on social bonds in general—or on a glimpse of freedom it provided. They do report that power relationships, dominant to subordinate (boss to employee), often result in cases of acceptance by the subordinate and this extends to kin relations (see Blum 1964, 286). Blum (1964, 285–7) goes on to argue that the willingness of men to take LSD was a consequence of the "impersonal striving interaction that characterizes the Protestant ethic." He assumes that this lends a conditioning of restriction that focuses attention of husband and children and these are reinforced by biological commitments. These circumstances are interpreted by Blum to result in females considering LSD and other similar drugs to be a "kind of desertion from those responsibilities and pleasures" that make up women's nurturing role. Women are also seen by Blum (1964, 286) as being pragmatists, whose self-control and religious commitments to family and status result in a tendency to disapprove their husbands' experiments with drugs.

In another locale initiated by associates of Blum et al., in Zihuatanejo, by the International Federation of Internal Freedom (IFIF) group under the guidance of Leary and reported by Downing (1964), a group of white men (60%) and women (40%) took LSD under group conditions (see

Blum et al. 1964, 93). The men reported a lessened erotic drive, amounting to erectile impotence in two. In their study of the background of the population involved in the experiments and especially family relations, Blum et al. (1964, 95) thought the situation in initiation of friends and family members with LSD departed significantly from other drugs in that children often introduced parents to the drug. What was also difficult to understand in some of the institutions Blum et al. (1964, 138) report on is the use of other drugs in concern to achieve religious, artistic, or self-realized states as defined by the organizers. Methamphetamine and peyote were noted as well as carbon dioxide. The tendency to mix drugs and compare outcomes seems both confusing and unscientific. These results are remarkably similar to those reported by de Rios and Janiger (2003), even to the division of men (71–85% very positive and would do it again) and women (about half were ambivalent and unlikely to do it again). In their 40-year follow-up, de Rios and Janiger (2003) found continued generally positive feelings for their LSD experience, though only 45 individuals were able to be located, agreed to participate, and attended sessions. Some did report recalling intense physical pain at the time, and one woman, a loss of identity.

The Mexican Psychedelic Training Center at Zihuatanejo was a creation of Tim Leary, Richard Alpert (Ram Das), and Ralph Metzner (Leary et al. 1964). Over a three-year period 35 teaching assistants, research assistants, and faculty members from three Boston area colleges were involved in a number of experiments using a variety of psychedelic drugs. It is stated that the Center was run by the Harvard-IFIF research project by Leary et al. (1964). They claimed that over 4000 drug ingestions were sponsored at the Center.

The stated goal of the Center was to explore the ability of psychedelic drugs to counteract reductive processes of culture and learning and to go "beyond the limits of the learned cultural programs" of society. They proposed that the drugs used would allow for an ecstatic state to be established that would allow for perception outside of normal consciousness, or ex-stasis expansion of consciousness. Secondarily, they suggested they would also study "frightening disturbances of consciousness," as a psychiatric investigation. Leary et al. (1964) claimed that the founders of the Harvard-IFIF group had recognized that "a new nonverbal language of experience capable of expressing the speed and complexity of our cortical potential is necessary." They believed they had worked out some "rudimentary steps" toward the development of a non-verbal experiential language, and the purpose of the Center was to train people in the use of this language. From what has been said above, it should be clear that the Mogar Lab, among others, was also investigating the nature of language and how the brain produced consciousness. Comparing this approach to that described above about the approach of researchers like Grof, who were also engaged in the use of psychedelics for treatment of illness, one might divide the field into a spectrum from consciousness studies to treatment. But there seems always to be interests that bleed into these two polar goals.

Leary et al. (1964) compared themselves to "engineers of ecstasy" and "post-Einsteinian physicists" probing the depths of the mind by creating enlarged drug-induced versions of normal human perceptions, or unlocking an assumed human potential that might create new versions of reality. In devising the idea of the "set and setting" theory of psychedelic use, they concluded, "After many sessions in urban situations we came to some ironic conclusions about the set and setting of a psychedelic experience. We realized that an ecstatic psychedelic session should be arranged the way a person would arrange his own ideal life situation" (Leary et al. 1964, 181). The reality of their institutional settings, as well as their public performances, was much more like the setting of the laboratory or performer than this ideal. They state that their decision to "avoid imposing our model" on their subjects was made during the first year of their research, but they do not tell us how many experiments were controlled by their model or why they chose to change methods. They state that this decision was arrived at after "subsequent interpretation," where 50% of their subjects reported changes for the better, but that the value of the experience depended on the subjects' overall situation. They assert that subjects who came to the experience with years of intellectual or spiritual preparation tended to "get the most from the session." This interpretation was apparently made from the assessment that some 50% reported changes for the better.

Leary et al. concluded from this initial part of the experiment that "a psychedelic session should be preceded by a long and thorough training in the nature of the metaverbal, metagame phenomena" (Leary et al. 1964, 182). They therefore controlled the set and setting by a stringent training program for subjects which was designed to provide training at the same time for guides they called "ecstaticians," who were expected to transmit the optimum experience to subjects. One might say that where the Mogar Lab created a space for people to experience LSD on their own terms without preconceptions, Leary et al. (1964) felt it necessary to create a context for their subjects to be trained to respond to certain perceptual events that were produced by the drugs they administered. They clearly state that the Harvard-IFIF Center was the only attempt at that time to produce a "series of guided psychedelic sessions for prepared volunteer subjects." They argue that pre- and post-sessions with staff help guide subjects to the attainment of their goals. Specially prepared tapes were made for playing during a subject's LSD experience—these began with an introductory statement followed by music and silence, often interrupted by recordings of the subject giving himself or herself reassurance or instructions.

Leary et al. (1964) also believed that it was necessary to have a manual at hand for guides and subjects to refer to during preparation and "trips." They considered some existing ancient texts to be workable candidates for such reference. These include *The Divine Comedy of Dante*, chosen for its description of what they considered several important segments of a psychedelic experience, or realms of awareness: horrible hellish hallucinations; personal, purgatorial appraisals; celestial lights; and radiance. Others are *The Egyptian Book of the Dead*, the *Tao Te Ching*, *The Secret of the Golden Flower*, *Pilgrim's Progress*, the mythic voyages of Aeneas, Odysseus, and Gilgamesh, life of Christ, and most ideally, the *Bardo Thodol*, also known as the *Tibetan Book of the Dead*. It becomes obvious that with such manuals for reference, there is little room for an individual to have a unique, personal experience. I mentioned earlier in this book Wade Davis' comments about the importance of the Native cultural context and the use of psychedelic drugs. Pollan (2021) and others make the same or similar arguments. The problem is that the Native context has been drastically changed in the past 200 years, and it seems to me that that context includes a lifetime of immersion in such a culture. Leary et al. (1964) attempted to modernize the *Bardo Thodol* into a kind of protocol for Americans by translating it into "psychedelic English." I have no problem with attempts to translate experience from one culture to another, but I think there are difficulties in distorting the original by the reference, as when R. Gordon Wasson (1963) attempts to use the ancient Greek Eleusianian Mysteries to explain the experiences of indigenous Mexican traditionalists.

One important comparison I think of regarding many of the research groups, and especially Leary's, with that of the Blums is that the Blums were concerned with the real-life situations of the men and women in their sample; they studied their responses in the context of American roles and were focused on gender. But then their research team was made up of men and women.

My experience at the Humboldt State College Psychology laboratory in isolation experiments, sessions of observation which I attended at the Mogar Lab, and my own participation in informal peoples' acid parties and get-togethers provided me with a range of settings and outcomes that could be compared. Table 7.1 here summarizes the outcomes of these events. White room experiments were held at San Francisco State or at Sonoma State Hospital. Isolation tank experiments included "deprivation rooms," as mentioned above, and were held at Humboldt State College. These did not use LSD or other psychedelics while I was a student there. Group settings and get-togethers were informal and held in people's homes or in parks in San Francisco.

In Leary's Mexican Harvard camp there seemed to be a sexualized atmosphere rather than a scientific one. The women reported no change

Table 7.1 Table of settings 1965–1967

Setting	Positive	Negative	Unclear
1. White room, no guide	70%	5%	25%
2. Isolation tank/room, no guide	70%	5%	25%
3. White room, guide	90%	2%	8%
4. Isolation tank/room, guide	80%	5%	15%
5. Group setting with guide/L	50%	35%	15%
6. Group setting with guide/In	55%	30%	15%
7. Group setting, no guide	60%	25%	15%
8. Get-together	85%	5%	10%

L = laboratory; In = informal

in erotic drive, but one felt a lessening of inhibitory shame. A general reduction in sexual activity occurred; this seemed to be met with general concern by the staff. The IFIF group under Leary affected local conditions of the curanderos by numerous payments, and other events (including Leary apparently insulting a Mexican psychiatrist), resulting in them being expelled (Downing 1964). The use of LSD has also been applied to female sexual performance. Ling and Buckman (1964) being one example is typical of the approach. It is not surprising that the main assumption is that a woman who is not interested in sex with a man, even her husband must be at least abnormal, if not pathological. The word "frigidity" in the title of Ling and Buckman's paper, "The Treatment of Frigidity with LSD and Ritalin," defines the context of the "problem." "A woman who is unable to enjoy sexual love to its fullest capacity, is the definition of 'frigidity.'" Whether people are asexual, non-sexual, or simply uninterested in sex is one explanation for a lack of performance, but no matter what the definition, social values in non-participation are generally negative. This same approach was applied to children—one example is where LSD was given to schizophrenic children under 11 years of age, and two boys over ten responded with "disturbed anxious behavior" and were dropped. The rest of the children were considered much improved, "appeared flushed and bright eyed" (Bender et al. 1962). Unfortunately, though there were three girls among the 11 children, no distinctions were made regarding their responses to LSD or behavior. None of the 11 produced "useful speech."

There is even a term used to describe the tendency of a woman to avoid sexual penetration, "vaginismus," or "the body's automatic reaction to the fear of some or all types of vaginal penetration." Another term is "dyspareunia" or painful intercourse. Such concepts seem much like Medieval ideas of the vagina and uterus being separate animals within a woman, subject to control by devils. Ling and Buchman (1964, 450) also define frigidity as passivity, a means of establishing some basic boundaries where a woman's performance can be measured and weighed for normality.

So in pages in earlier chapters of this book I have discussed the nature of women in investigations of other realms of consciousness, and how in many cultures women have been shamans and had visions and hallucinations of value and been seers and prophets. The essential nature of being female, of being a conduit to another world for spirits to enter this one via birth has made women both revered in many matrifocal cultures and feared or despised in others as sources of pollution (menstruation) or by assumed relations with demons, devils, and so on. In the case of work like that of Ling and Buckman (1964), these "failures" of women in performance are psychosomatic disorders that can be treated. The singular aspect of femaleness, its opposition and otherness to maleness is one of the great mysteries of human existence.

Women and the Investigation of Psychedelics

Mariavittoria Mangini (2019) wrote a brief summary of the work of women researchers in altered states of consciousness. She, like Darlington, was struck by the absence of women as recognized pioneers in the field. She begins with Mabel Evans Dodge Sterne Luhan, a rich member of the Greenwich Village avant-garde scene at the turn of the century. Luhan convinced ethnographer Raymond Harrington to attempt to create a simulation of a Native American peyote ceremony in her apartment. She was curious after reading Harrington's reports of the positive emotional and creative effects of the experience and its improvement of relations and productivity. Harrington had come into contact with peyote while visiting the Shawnee area in 1910, where he met Shawnee artist Ernest Spybuck ,whose art often reflected aspects of the peyote ceremony (Harrington 1938).

Luhan does not describe the experience as altogether positive, as one member of the group of artists she had invited left the ceremony in a "frenzy."

She moved to New Mexico, and in Taos met a Taos Pueblo man, whom she married. When ill once she took peyote with him and had a "classic transformative experience" (Mangini 2019). She felt her whole universe now fell into place and used the term "expansion of consciousness" before it became common (Luhan 1937). But Luhan took a contradictory stance to the drug, trying to stop her husband's use of it and opposing its use in Taos or the election of any users in Taos Pueblo government (Mangini 2019).

However, in reading Luhan's book *Edge of Taos Desert*, it seems she is transformed as much by the cultural setting of the Pueblo as refuge and her husband Tony's sustaining love than peyote. The home of Tony and Mabel Luhan and their communion reflect a harmonious whole that becomes her creation myth (Rudnick 1987).

The relation of women to the men who are also involved in this research continues with the life of Gertrude Paltin, who came into contact with Oscar Janiger as his executive secretary and participated in his early experiments in LSD research. She co-authored a text on the use of LSD and mescaline with him, a type of extended annotated bibliography (Janiger and Paltin 1971). The book was never published, though Paltin's daughter made copies of it after finding it in 2005 in the Fitz Hugh Ludlow Library. It has since been put online at https://erowid.org/chemicals/lsd/lsd_bibliography2.pdf. This is interesting also in that the Sandoz bibliographies (1958a, b, 1968) were published in various forms. All are encompassed in the Passie (2005) bibliography, though it lists the Sandoz bibliographies as 1960 and never published. Paltin was a biochemist by training, and although a brief report of her husband's LSD experience exists (taken at Janiger's clinic under an oak tree without supervision), no reports of Ms. Paltin's survive (Mangini 2019).

Mary Barnard was a poet born in 1909 who authored an essay on "magical and sacred plants" in 1958 and a second in 1963 (Mangini 2019) with the assistance of ethnomycologist Robert Gordon Wasson. Her articles are more lyrical and literary than scientific (Barnard 1963). However, she did describe a substantial list of psychedelic drugs in ethnographic settings.

Wasson had a checkered career, defending J.P. Morgan, being funded by the CIA, and betraying Mazatec curandera Maria Sabina, who had introduced him and his pediatrician wife to the rituals and potential around psychedelic mushrooms. Wasson published a photo essay of his experiences and the location, which led many others to the area (Letcher 2006). Nevertheless, Wasson worked with mycologist Roger Heim and Albert Hoffman in collecting specimens and identifying the chemical agents psilocybin and psilocin (Hoffmann 1980/2009).

Historian Erika Dyck (2018) argues that women have been excluded from the field of psychedelic research, as Darlington does for medical research in general. Dr. Erika Dyck, in an interview at the Chacruna

Institute in 2018, supports this idea, though mentions that the wives of the central researchers in psychedelics in the 1960s and 1970s often were present when their husbands took their first "trips." While Eva Blum and Mary Lou Funkhouser were centrally involved in research and publishing their own reports in the early years in the Bay Area, other participants have been ignored or forgotten. This would parallel the exclusion of women from most religious training and rites—though Kaberry has shown that much of this idea is due to male researchers simply ignoring or editing women's participation.

References

Ardener, Edwin (1972) "Belief and the problem of women," in J.S, La Fontaine (ed.) *The Interpretation of Ritual*, London, Tavistock.

Ardener, Shirley (1975) "Introduction," in *Perceiving Women*, (ed.) Shirley Ardener, pp. vii–xxiii.

Barnard, Mary (1963) "The God in the Flowerpot," *The American Scholar*, v. 32, n. 4, Autumn, 578–586.

Barbaro, Nicole (2017) "How can Evolutionary Psychology help explain intimate partner violence?" *Behavioral Scientist,* Sept 21.

Bender, Loretta, L. Goldschmidt and D.V. Sankar (1962) "Treatment of autistic children with LSD-25 and UML-491," *Recent Advances in Biological Psychiatry*, v, 4, 170–177.

Blum, Richard, Eva Blum and Mary Lou Funkhouser, (1964) "The institutionalization of LSD," in Blum, Richard, Nevitt Sanford, Eva Blum, Mary Lou Funkhouser, Joseph J. Downing, et al., (eds.) *Utopiates: The Use and Users of LSD-25, A Publication of the Institute for the Study of Human Problems*, Stanford University, Atherton Press, 124–141.

Blum, Richard, (1964) "Background considerations," in Blum, Richard, Nevitt Sanford, Eva Blum, Mary Lou Funkhouser, Joseph J. Downing, et al., (eds) *Utopiates: The Use and Users of LSD-25*, A Publication of the Institute for the Study of Human Problems Stanford University, Atherton Press, 1–9.

Brizendine, Louanne, (2007) *The Female Brain*, New York, Harmony Books.

Comiskey, Allison, Mike C. Parent, and Elliot A. Tebbe (2019) "An inhospitable world: exploring a model of objectification theory with trans women," *Psychology of Women Quarterly*, v. 44, n 1, 105–116.

Corbier, P., J. Raffi, J. Rhoda, (1983) "Female sexual behavior in male rats: effect of hour of castration at birth," *Physiology and Behavior*, v. 30, n. 4: 613–616.
Corson, Richard, (1972) *Fashions in Makeup: From Ancient to Modern Times*, London, Peter Owen.
Darlington, Cynthia (2002) *The Female Brain,* London, Taylor and Francis.
Darwin, Charles, (1871) *The Descent of Man and Selection in Relation to Sex,* Chicago, W.B. Conkey Company, Revised, Second Edition.
de Beauvoir, Simone (1949) *The Second Sex,* New York, Random House.
de Rios, Marlene and Oscar Janiger (2003) *LSD Spirituality and the Creative Process,* Rochester Vt., Park Street Press.
Downing, Joseph J. (1964) "Zihuatanejo: an experiment in transpersonal living," in Blum, Richard, Nevitt Sanford, Eva Blum, Mary Lou Funkhouser, Joseph J. Downing, et al., (eds.) *Utopiates: The Use and Users of LSD-25,* A Publication of the Institute for the Study of Human Problems Stanford University, Atherton Press, 142–177.
Drew, Allison (1995) "Female consciousness and feminism in Africa," *Theory and Society,* Feb, v. 24, n. 1, 1–33.
Dyck, Erika (2018) "Historian explains how women have been excluded from the field of psychedelic science," *Chacruna Institute,* Interview: https://chacruna.net/historian-explains-how-women-have-been-excluded-from-the-field-of-psychedelic-science/
Flint, Claas, Katharina Forster, Sophie A. Koser, Carsten Konrad, Plenie Zwitserlood, et al., (2020) "Biological sex classification with structural MRI data shows increased misclassification in transgender women," *Neuropsychopharmacology,* v. 45, 1758–1765.
Fredrickson, Barbara L. and Tomi-Ann Roberts, (1997) "Objectification Theory: toward understanding women's lived experiences and mental health risks," *Psychology of Women Quarterly,* June 1, v. 21, n. 2, 173–206.
Friedan, Betty (1963) *The Feminine Mystique,* New York, W.W. Norton.
Ferguson, Ann (1981) "Patriarchy, sexual identity, and the sexual revolution, " *Signs,* v. 7, n 1, Autumn, 158–172.
Garcia, Felipe N. (1985–1986) "Supporting a masculine-feminine consciousness," *Women & Therapy*, v. 4 n. 4, 3–8.
Garcia, Manon (2021) *We Are Not Born Submissive,* Princeton, Princeton University Press.
Goodison, Lucy (1995) *The Dreams of Women: Exploring and Interpreting Women's Dreams,* New York, W.W. Norton.
Gramsci, Antonio 1971, *Selections from the Prison Notebooks of Antonio Gramsci.* New York.

Green, Pearl (1979) "The feminist consciousness," *The Sociology Quarterly*, v. 20, 359–374.
Hansen, Joseph and Evelyn Reed (1986) *Cosmetics, Fashion and the Exploitation of Women*, New York, Pathfinder Press.
Hardman, C. (1973) "Can there be an Anthropology of children?" *Journal of the Anthropological Society of Oxford*, 4, 85–99.
Harrington, M.R. (1938) "Spybuck, the Shawnee artist," *Indians at Work*, Washington, D.C. U.S. Department of the Interior Office of Indian Affairs, v. 5, n. 8, 13–15.
Hewitt, Kim (2019) "Psychedelic Feminism: a radical interpretation of psychedelic consciousness?" *Journal for the Study of Radicalism*, v. 13, 1, 74–119.
Hoffmann A. (2009) *LSD my problem child*. Santa Cruz: Multidisciplinary Association for Psychedelic Studies, originally published in 1980 by McGraw-Hill, Boston.
Hrdy, Sarah Blaffer (1981) *The Woman That Never Evolved*, Cambridge, MA., Harvard University Press.
Janiger, O., and Paltin, G., 1971. A bibliography of L.S.D. & mescaline: From the earliest researches to the beginnings of suppression. Fitzhugh Ludlow Library.
Kaberry, Phyllis M. (1939*) Aboriginal Woman, Sacred and Profane*, London, Routledge.
Kalra, Gurvinder and Dinesh Bhugra, (2013) "Sexual violence against women: understanding cross-cultural intersections," *Indian J. Psychiatry*, Jul-Sept, v. 55 (3), 244–249.
Kaplan, Temma (1982) "Female consciousness and collective action: the case of Barcelona, 1920–1918," *Signs*, v. 7, n 3, Feminist Theory, 545–566.
Karim, Rablui, Hafjur Rahman, Suchona Rahman, Tanzima ohra Habib and Katarina Swahnberg, (2021) "Gender differences in marital violence: a cross-cultural ethnic study among Bengali, Garo, and Dantal communities in rural Bangladesh," *PloS One*, 16(5) https://dx.plos.org/10.1371/journal.pone.0251574.
Keohane, Nanneri O., Michelle A. Rosaldo and Barbar C. Gelpl, (1990) "Forward" in Keohane, Nanneri O., Michelle A. Rosaldo and Barbar C. Gelpl (eds)Feminist Theory: A Critique of Ideology, Chicago, University of Chicago Press, 7–12.
Kolata, Alan L. (2006) "Before and after collapse: reflections on the regeneration of social complexity," in Glenn M. Schwartz and John J. Nichols (eds.) *After Collapse: The Regeneration of Complex Societies*, Tucson, University of Arizona Press, 208–221.

Leacock, Eleanor (1978) "Women's status in egalitarian society: implications for social evolution," *Current Anthropology*, June, v. 19, n. 2, 247–277.

Leacock, Eleanor and Jane Nash (1977) "Ideologies of sex: archtypes and stereotypes," In Issues in Cross-Cultural Research, (ed.) Leonore Loeb Adler, *Annals of the New York Academy of Sciences*, v. 285, New York, The New York Academy of Sciences: 618–645.

Leary, Timothy, Metzner, Ralph, Alpert, Richard, *The Psychedelic Experience,* New York, 1964.

Lerner, Gerda (1993) *The Creation of Feminist Consciousness,* Oxford, Oxford University Press.

Letcher, Andy (2006) *Shroom: A Cultural History of the Magic Mushroom*, Faber and Faber, London.

Ling, Thomas M. and John Buckman, (1964) "The treatment of frigidity with LSD and Ritalin," *Psychedelic Review*, v. 1, n. 4, 450–458.

Luhan, M.D. (1937) *Edge of Taos Desert: An Escape to Reality*, New York, Harcourt Brace & Co.

Mangini, Mariavittoria (2019) "A hidden history of women and psychedelics," *Multidisciplinary Association for Psychedelic Studies,* v. 29, n. 1, Spring, https://maps.org/news/bulletin/articles/436-maps-bulletin-spring-2019-vol-29,-no-13/7707-a-hidden-history-of-women-and-psychedelics-spring-2019. Accessed 28 January 2021.

Matory, J. Lorand, (2005) *Black Atlantic Religion: Tradition, Transnationalism, and Matriarch in the Afro-Brazilian Candomble,* Princeton, Princeton University Press.

McLean, Adrienne, (2016) *Costume*, Make up and Hair, JSTOR eBooks.

Millett, Kate (1970) *Sexual Politics*, Garden City, Doubleday Co.

Murciano-Luna, Leonor (2020) *Birth of the Conscious Feminine: A New Era of Feminine Sovereignty,* Nuralight Publishing.

Passie, Torstem, (2005). *Psycholytic and Psychedelic Therapy Research 1931–1995: A Complete International Bibliography, Schamanismus,*http://www.schamanismus-information.de/psychedelik/bibliographie/bibliographie_psy.htm.

Pollan, Michael (2021) "How should we do drugs now?" *The New York Times,* July 11, page 4.

Putra, L. Nyoman Darma (2011) "Female identity: from repression to resistance," in I. Nyoman Darma Putra, *A Literary Mirror: Balinese Reflections on Modernity and Identity in the Twentieth Century*, Chapter VI, Leiden, Brill, 187–226.

Reimer, Gwen D. (1996) "Female consciousness: an interpretation of interviews with Inuit women," *Etudes/Inuit/Studies,* v. 20, n. 2, 77–100.
Rudnick, Lois Palken, (1987) "Introduction," in Mabel Dodge Luhan and John Collier, Jr. *Edge of Taos Desert: An Escape to Reality*, Santa Fe, University of New Mexico Press, i–xii.
Sandoz, Ltd, 1958a *Catalogue of the Literature on Delysid-D-lysergic Acid Diethylamide*, Holzkirchen, Germany
Sandoz, Ltd, 1958b *Annotated Bibliography: LSD-25 Delysid -D-lysergic Acid Diethylamide*, Holzkirchen, Germany
Sandoz, Ltd 1968 *Bibliography on Psychotomimetics,*1943–1966, Holzkirchen, Germany
Szymanski, Dawn M., Lauren B. Moffitt and Erika R. Carr, (2011) "Sexual objectification of women: advances to theory and research," *The Counseling Psychologist*, v. 39 n. 1, 6–38.
Trivers, Robert (1985) *Social Evolution*, Menlo Park, The Benjamin/Cummings Publishing Co.
Valle, Valerie A. and Elizabeth L. Kruger (1989) "The nature and expression of feminine consciousness through psychology and literature," in R.S. Valle and R. von Eckartsberg (eds) Metaphors of Consciousness, Boston, Springer, 379–393.
Vellidis, Nicole (2018) "Behavior change: violence against women throughout history," In *The Classic Journal: Bioarchaeology* Special Issue, eds. Laurie Reitsema and Samm Holder, Violence Over Time, https://theclassicjournal.uga.edu/index.php/3-1-bioarchaeology-special-issue/
Vitzthum, Virginia J. (2009) "The ecology and endocrinology of reproduction in the human female," *Amer. J. Phys. Anthropol.*, v. 140, Suppl. 49:95–136.
Wasson, R. Gordon (1963) "The Hallucinogenic fungi of Mexico: an inquiry into the origin of the religious idea among primitive peoples," *Psychedelic Review,* v. 1, n. 1, June: 27–42.
Wilkins, Adam S., Richard Wrangham and W. Tecumseh Fitch (2014) "The "Domestication Syndrome" in Mammals: A Unified Explanation Based on Neural Crest Cell Behavior and Genetics," *Genetics*, vol. 197 no. 3 795–808; https://doi.org/10.1534/genetics.114.165423.
Wright, Jennifer (2018) "Transgender women are women. Transgender men are men," *HarpersBazaar,* Oct 23, https://www.harpersbazaar.com/culture/politics/a24109933/transgender-women-are-women-transgender-men-are-men/
Yang, Yue-Qing (1999) *Nu Shu: A hidden language of women in China,* East-West Film Enterprises.

8

Conclusion and Strange Threads

Following on the role of women in LSD research is another tie in regarding the research of Dyck. An interesting aspect of Dyck's work is the fact that she began her study of LSD research in Canada with the idea that she would uncover horror stories of irresponsible use of the drug and on subjects. Instead, she found that the researchers in the 1950s and 1960s had gone to extreme lengths to test the drug and even to experiment with it themselves before they used it on volunteer subjects and then came later the recommendations for treatment with patients (Dyck 2008, viii). Outside of this frame of work by independent researchers is the rumor of government experiments on unwilling and willing personnel, including those by the American CIA. Dyck briefly examines this history with an eye to understand the role of secret information and withheld documentation. Much of this has been given various foci, as in the Ken Kesey participation in the Stanford University LSD experiments supported by MK-ULTRA. The exact extent of activities and experiments with psychedelics by the CIA is in doubt, as the records were first destroyed, then surfaced but with major redactions. The CIA also experimented with scopolamine, a chemical known also as hyoscine or Devil's Breath, used to treat motion sickness, nausea, and vomiting and to decrease saliva

N. Caldararo, *A Mental Ethnography: Conclusions From Research in LSD*,
https://doi.org/10.1007/978-3-031-13745-7_8

production. A side effect is the quick onset of euphoria, which is very desirable. It has also been called the "zombie drug," used by Colombian criminals to put people in a catatonic state.

The tie between psychiatric treatment, studies in sensory deprivation, and research and experiments in extreme experiences can be found throughout the history of psychedelic drugs in the latter half of the twentieth century. One of the prominent figures in this work (who was linked to experiments with psychedelics, prisoners, and extreme conditions) was Louis Jolyon West. West had served as head of psychiatric services for the US Air Force at Lackland Air Force and had other roles. He also became head of the psychiatry department at the University of California, Los Angeles (UCLA) and its neuroscience department. He used hypnosis and sodium pentothal in his work. He claimed to have developed a technique to replace true memories with false ones by the combination of hypnosis and drugs (West 1976). There is evidence that West created a fake "crash pad" in the Haight-Ashbury in 1967 to study hippies' use of drugs (O'Neill and Piepenbring 2019). The lack of ethics in both his military and academic work appears to be only the tip of the iceberg of what others did with both public and private money and psychedelic "research."

Also of importance in Dyck's (2008) book is her analysis of the competing claims of researchers on the effectiveness of LSD as a cure for alcoholism and the involvement of researchers like Abram Hoffer and Humphry Osmond in the use of peyote by Native Americans. This led scientists like Al Hubbard to coordinate studies through a group, the Commission for the Study of Creative Imagination (Dyck 2008, 10–11). Dyck's research, especially examination of case files and interviews with former subjects and/or family members of the LSD experiments and treatments, demonstrates both a carefully organized and dedicated approach and mainly positive outcomes. I have discussed this above. One other conclusion she notes, reflected in many of the studies Mogar and associates as well as other researchers published, contradicts ideas of permanent deficits produced by LSD. Stevens (1988) repeats many of these, such as the idea that LSD use eliminated ambition and left people with only the ability to work for themselves as craftspeople or as unmotivated social zombies. If having no ambition means one starts their own business, then many Silicon Valley startups could be associated with such "lack of ambition." I knew many people who kept their 9-to-5 day jobs after taking LSD or who completed college and went on to grad school or business. It cannot be denied that LSD has been blamed for the damage done by street drugs, not only those sold as LSD, but also other drugs that came along in the 1960s: speed, cocaine, heroin.

One conclusion from this study echoes that of Huxley, who argued that psychedelic hallucinations were not derived from memory or experience, and this would parallel the theory of Jung and some others. But many clinicians have argued that many of the images are from past experience—certainly that was Grof's understanding. Yet what we have seen is that there is a common relation between images seen in psychedelic hallucinations and those from pathologies like CBS and others of physical origin and those of psychological origin, as in schizophrenia. While those images reported in dreams are quite often related to experience and memory, though usually so mixed and distorted that their origins or how they are derived are difficult, if not impossible, to identify, their active nature in dreams brings up recent ideas of memory and consciousness. Persuh et al. (2018) found evidence in studying visual working memory (VWM) and unconscious working memory. Usually working memory is considered a longer form of short-term visual memory (often referred to as "iconic memory"), conceived of by psychologist Alan Baddeley (1990). It differs from episodic memory, which is usually about events, with all its detail and often organized in time (Eichenbaum 2004), and from categorical memory, the meaning of a word, and from procedural memory, for example, knowing how to swim. Therefore, we might suggest that the seeming chaos of dreams is a type of mindplay with memory, and that in a psychedelic experience a similar kind of image shuffling is going on, either where no organization is possible or where the mind attempts to organize or make sense of what is unleashed by the chemical interference.

Yet there does seem to be an area of bleeding content, where the streams of memory from the hippocampus blend with another source, perhaps a creative source of illusion, apparition, and vision, especially in daydreams and spirit quests. See Fig. 8.1 for a conception of this. Most dreams to me included images and sequences that make no sense, seem far from anything I have experienced, and this is not uncommon among the thousands of dreams I have read, had been told to me, or seen on film, video tape, or streaming.

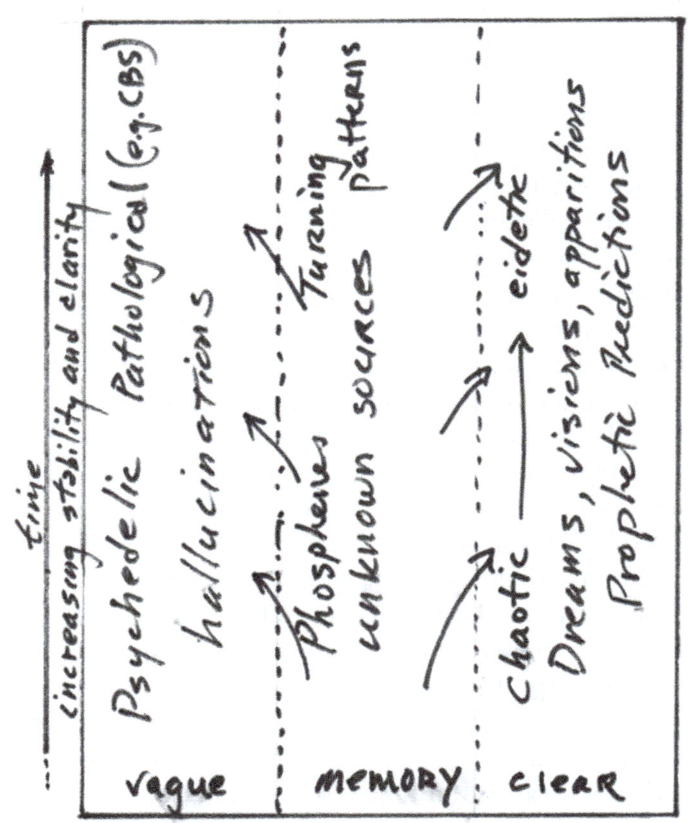

Fig. 8.1 Chart of relation of segments of hallucinations, dreams, and so on and origins

The ability of the mind to manipulate information is considerable, but its deficits in correctly labeling images and their parts may be a clue to the ménage or collage of creativity we experience and that schizophrenics suffer. However, we do find claims that dreams or hallucinations (visions) have resulted in creative ideas, as in the case of German chemist August Kekule von Stradonitz, who stated that the structure of benzene came to him in a daydream or while dozing. Linus Pauling (1988) relates this story and gives background on his own work validating the structure. There is evidence to support the idea of creativity coming from hallucinations, both in industrial societies (Stevens 1988; Berov and Kuhnberger 2016) and in non-industrial traditional ones (Aaronson and Osmond 1970; Furst 1972). Such claims are difficult to verify—an individual tells us what they experienced and their memory of the event and of the information it brought is unique to that context. It brings us back to the question of fantasy and originality. Jung (1964) recalls the story of the little girl he knew who told her father her curious and elaborate dreams. Jung wondered if they were dreams or her fantasies, but the origin of what we perceive as dreams or fantasy, hallucinations, or vision seems rather vague and subjective. This involves also the problem of intentionalism and the presentational character of the experience as well as its communicative capability to elicit belief in all contexts (Pagondiotis 2013). It also leaves us at the same point, since we cannot explain the origins of dreams and hallucinations by fantasy any more than we can accept the idea of archetypes as a solution.

Another woman who was involved in LSD experiments was Dr. Thelma Moss, of UCLA, who took as her focus the study of the boundaries of images, especially bodies that people often experience on LSD and other psychedelics as vibrating or lacking distinct edges. This led to a number of experiments in parapsychology and Kirlian photography (Moss 1974). Under the pseudonym, Constance Newland (1962), she wrote of her LSD experiences. The book provides a unique view of the type of therapy that was being utilized with LSD and especially with women. Newland/Moss found herself in a cold, vast, and almost bottomless world and not the kind of expansive oneness that most others had reported. Her perceptions are a marked contrast to much of the literature, but only a single vision. Still, from the point of view of a woman in the midst of the explosion of research in LSD in the 1950s, it provides a contrast. Compared to a book written by another famous woman of the time, Adele Davis (1961), Moss' book seems complex and tenuous, while Davis' experience was positive and gave her a renewed belief in life centered on a personal experience with her god. Both books reflect on the time in an unusual way—both were professional women at a time when women were seldom reinforced to get an education or enter a profession, yet both women produce unique visions of humanity and meaning in life. Their radical contrast perhaps is a reflection of the diversity of interpretation of the potential of *Homo sapiens*' inner life.

We possess a remarkable organ, the hippocampus, located at the base of the brain. In comparative biology it is often referred to as the hippocampal formation (HF), and it has experienced considerable change in evolution. In reptiles, birds, and some fish lesions in this area result in deficits in spatial memory similar to those seen in rats (Striedter 2005). In amphibians it receives major non-olfactory sensory inputs from the thalamus, but in reptiles only minor inputs, and in mammals non-olfactory inputs are routed through the neocortex. This means that responses are subject to executive function in mammals before they are lodged in the hippocampus, though memory, stored there, is accessed during this process and the complexity of the hippocampus function is shown by the action of segments like CA3, which is reciprocally connected to recurrent networks, allowing coordination and faithful recall of sequences in storage, while another area, CA1, is left to decode sequences back to the cortex (Eichenbaum 2004).

In females, when estrogen and progesterone are naturally high, serotonergic activity is decreased, but not uniformly, as binding to 5-HT serotonin receptors decreases in the cortex, but increases in the midbrain (Darlington 2002). Synthesis of serotonin differs in men and women—about 52% higher in men. What is also interesting is that in experiments with monkeys, elimination of estrogen produced abnormal levels of dopamine and serotonin, and replacing it returned them to normal (Darlington 2002). If a lack of dopamine is associated with the pathologies of Pakinson's-like disease and too much with schizophrenia and hallucinatory conditions, then the difference between men and women in these neurotransmitters could have profound effects on the psychedelic experiences they undergo.

An Unnerving and Curious Future

Psychedelics have entered modern society to play many of the same roles they were called on to do among aboriginal peoples. The link between the spiritual world, the embrace of the ancestors, healing, and the wonder of life has fulfilled many who sought such experiences. As an explanation of life and for society, the results have been less rewarding, though the therapeutic outcomes have become more significant, and so has the destructive misuse made positive use more difficult. While psychedelics do not seem to have played a role in the control of society in the past, of inducing conformity and harmony, we have good evidence that many governments have pursued this goal over the past 100 years. We know the CIA and the Nazis used them and this is a worry that must be addressed in the future, as a *1984* that George Orwell imagined is even more possible today.

As I have outlined above, some have claimed that some psychiatrists and some men have used psychedelics to control women. Whether this was only for personal abuse or in a misguided concept of clinical practice is unclear and the entire body of research on the use of drugs in psychological treatment must be more closely investigated and uses of drugs need to be more controlled, as the recent scandal of opioid use has exposed. Drugs can be liberating and healing, but they can also be controlling and provide enslavement, both self-destructively and in the abuse of individuals and whole peoples (as the British tried with opium in China in the nineteenth century).

One might argue that the interpretation of dreams and hallucinations can be a means of manipulating people. It is asserted by several schools of psychology, as I have discussed above, that they have produced theories for this end. The differences seem to undermine such a claim, and the results appear unsatisfying, especially to many patients. Nevertheless, more research is needed, as is more open discussion of what people see and hear. An organization of people who hear voices, the Hearing Voices Movement, seems to be a start, but as Laroi et al. (2014) argue, more cross-cultural involvement and different perspectives are necessary.

At the same time we must understand why humans are so susceptible to delusion, and especially so where mass psychogenic disease appears. While the Nazi experience is one example, racism is another, as both Ashley Montagu and Franz Fanon have argued. Our future depends on a daily rationalism based on pragmatic views tested with empiricism of the world. This is not to ignore the benefits or need for spirituality, but as Raymond Firth has noted, the nature of religion at its best has been in the art of presenting to people the beauty of life and the exceptional experience of harmony.

Robert Mogar and his associates began their work in the postwar context of Eric Blair's (Orwell) novels *1984* and *Animal Farm.* In the first the Big Lie dominates human freedom, in the second totalitarianism uses the language of liberty and the fear of the Other to construct a prison of life. It is strange that people like Leary and Kesey, and many others involved as promoters of LSD, and clinicians and scientists thought that this drug could make a difference to somehow undermine the enslavement of humanity they saw in societies like Nazi Germany, Stalin's USSR, and Joe McCarthy's America. Today we are faced with both of these threats in greater force because of technology than in that time of the 1950s and 1960s. The Big Lie is today the election of 2020 and the presidency of Joe Biden. The supporters of the Big Lie use the language of distortion, racism, and the scapegoat, as did Hitler.

It seems like the mental attitudes described by Levy-Bruhl and Canetti, of a blindness and limit to critical thinking, are an element of modernity, as was supposed for the primitive. As Allan Mann once said in a lecture at UC Berkeley in 1970, we live at a time when humans have a space age technology but a Stone Age mentality. Boas wrote his book *The Mind of Primitive Man* (1922) to counter ideas of difference in thinking between people with simpler societies and those with industrial ones. Malinowski (1925) argued that we must see myths in the life-context in which people live them, and this is true whether it is the Melanesian revitalization myth of John Frum or that of the MAGA (Make America Great Again) followers of Donald Trump. It seems clear today that while Dr Mann was correct about modern technology, it seems that our big brain has not evolved to be immune to lies and can easily be transformed into a mask of ignorant blindness to fact and truth. While predictions that LSD would turn Americans into a nation of unmotivated, non-conformist, and valueless acid heads, as Sidney Cohen and Roy Grinker predicted (Stevens 1988), yet its use in the past decade or so by young people in the technology sectors seems to reinforce the idea that it has creative and beneficial effects—in which case it appears that the social context provides the set and setting for a constructive outcome of use and this is rewarded. In most cultures until our modern era, the generations were linked in a transfer of knowledge and wealth to provide a sustainable world. The ancestors, as Hoebel (1954) describes for the Ashanti, guide and ensure this process in law, ritual and myth. The world has departed from this process and the generations are split asunder, guarantees for the future are left in shambles as I have described in another book, The Future of Leisure and Retirement, (2021).

We are incomprehensibly at the doorway to the miraculous, but armed with terrible weapons and fragile consciousness. If there was one message carried by most people I met in the 1960s it was a search for love and meaning. From the clinicians, to the researchers, to the students and street people, the lack of love seemed a central problem in the world and their lives. LSD seemed to provide a means to regain the self-love that was central to finding love in life. Maybe it can be a road taken in the future for humanity. I might sound a bit like Leary or Owsley here, but as I said earlier, I do not encourage people to take psychedelics and I have not taken any of them since 1967, when things exploded. The reason is complex, but really comes down to the fact that I learned all I could from them at the time. I became interested in other topics and life goes on ….

References

Aaronson, Bernard and Humphry Osmond, (eds) (1970) *Psychedelics, The Uses and Implications of Hallucinogenic Drugs,* Garden City, Anchor Books.

Baddeley, Alan (1990) *Human Memory: Theory and Practice*, Needham Heights, MA, Allyn & Bacon, Inc.

Berov, Leonid and Kai-Uwe Kuhnberger, (2016) "Visual hallucination for computational creation," *Proceedings of the Seventh International Conference on Computational Creativity*, June 2016: http://www.computationalcreativity.net/iccc2016/wp-content/uploads/2016/01/Visual-Hallucination-For-Computational-Creation.pdf.

Caldararo, Niccolo (2021) *The Future of Leisure and Retirement, Pension Schemes, Community Support and Contemporary Consequences for the Next Generation*, Washington, D.C., Academica Press.

Darlington, Cynthia (2002) *The Female Brain,* London, Taylor and Francis.

Davis, Adele (1961) *Exploring Inner Space: Personal Experiences Under LSD-25,* Under pseudonym as Jane Dunlap, reprinted 2013 by Ishi Press, New York.

Dyck, Erika (2008) *Psychedelic Psychiatry: LSD from Clinic to Campus,* Baltimore, Johns Hopkins University Press.

Eichenbaum, Howard (2004) "Hippocampus: cognitive processes and neural representations that underlie declarative memory," *Neuron,* Sept 30, v. 44: 109–120.

Furst, Peter T. (1972) *Flesh of the Gods, the Ritual Use of Hallucinogens,* New York, Praeger.

Hoebel, E. Adamson (1954) *The Law of Primitive Man,* Cambridge, Harvard University Press.

Jung, C.G. (1964) "Approaching the unconscious," in *Man and His Symbols,* (eds.) Carl G. Jung, M.-L. von Franz, Joseph L. Henderson, Jolande Jacobi and Aniela Jaffe, New York, Dell Publishing, 1–94.

Laroi, Frank, Tanya Marie Luhrmann, Vaughan Bell, William A. Christian, Jr., Smita Deshpande, et al., (2014) " Culture and hallucinations: overview and future directions," *Schizophrenia Bulletin,* v. 40, suppl, no. 4, s213–s220.

Malinowski, Bronislaw (1925) "Myth in primitive psychology," In *The Frazr Lectures,* London, Macmillan.

Moss, Thelma (1974) *The Probability of the Impossible: Scientific Discoveries and Explorations in the Psychic World,* Portland, Hawthorn Books.

Newland, Constance (1962*) My Self and I,* New York, Signet.

O'Neill, Tom and Dan Piepenbring, (2019) *Chaos, Charles Manson, the CIA, and the Secret History of the Sixties,* Boston, Little Brown.

Pagondiotis, Costas (2013) "Hallucination, mental representation, and the presentational character," in *Hallucination: Philosophy and Psychology,* (eds.) Fiona Macpherson and Dimitris Platchias, Cambridge, MA, MIT Press, pp. 361–380.

Pauling, Linus (1988) *General Chemistry,* New York, Dover Publications, altered and corrected from the 1970 edition.

Persuh, Marjan, Eric LaRock and Jacob Berger, (2018) "Working memory and consciousness: the current state of play," *Front. Human Neurosci.,* 2 March, https://doi.org/10.3389/fnhum.2018.00078.

Stevens, Jay (1988) *Storming Heaven: LSD and the American Dream,* New York, Harper and Row.

Striedter, Georg F. (2005) *Principles of Brain Evolution,* Sunderland, Mass., Sinauer Associates.

West, Louis Jolyon (1976) *Treatment of Schizophrenia: Progress and Prospects,* London: Grune & Stratton.

Appendix A: Genetics and LSD by Niccolo Caldararo

N. Caldararo, *A Mental Ethnography: Conclusions From Research in LSD*,
https://doi.org/10.1007/978-3-031-13745-7

Tuesday—Wednesday, November 11—12, 1969 The Daily Gater Page 3

Genetics and LSD

(The following is a portion of a paper prepared by the author from a 3-year study of LSD) by Nicholas Caldararo

Here I shall briefly summarize the recent "findings" and arguments which have centered around the chromosomal damage controversy. Also, I shall indicate how the majority of these arguments supportive of the breakage theories have been made, as far as they refer to positive human results, without reference to the basic tenets of population genetics.

A particular event usually emphasized with much horror to the public by certain psychologists has been that of chromosomal breakage in the white blood cells. The use by various researchers in this area of the popular culture's fear of deformed children, and permanent genetic disabilities, reminds one of the early attempts by the medical profession to curb the increase of VD by exaggerating the effects and the possibilities of infection. Much more, however, it is tinged, it seems, with efforts by these men at notoriety; an extremely blatant and unprofessional attempt to capitalize on the fear their sensationalized conclusions may create. The latest publication, that of M. M. Cohen, K. Hirshhorn and W. A. Frosch, is more reserved than most in the magnitude of conjectures which they feel their data justifies them to make in the area of population genetics. Others, however, have felt themselves less restrained on the basis of even more scant and inconclusive data.

Population Genetics

tive event. This entire argument and orientation dates back to the late Middle Ages where it was believed that any change from the "normal" should be construed as degeneration. The trend of scientific findings since then through Darwin to the present day has shown that the history of evolution is change, mutation, if you please. The multitudes of radiations by all animals and plants were always predicated by the factors of variation, and environment. Out of the variation inherent in any group of living organisms comes the basis of new groups. The mutation rate of any population increases the variation of the group. Of course, here is the problem with the concept "mutation". It is understood by most geneticists through experimentation with various plant and animal species that most mutation on the chemical level, i.e., cellular operations, cause such dysfunctions in normal cellular activity that their products perish, as will (or would) the individuals who result from reproduction. The interaction of the organism to the environment is so well integrated that most any change will make the individual lose competitive advantage and cause him to be selected out. These disadvantageous changes (mutations) must therefore be in areas of adaptation where there is no plasicity for behavior or functioning. However, the nature of variation within a group is the result of mutation over the entire history of that particular group from phylum to sub-specific division.

Most successful mutations are assumed to lie dormant within the population to slowly, depending upon selective advantage or the dubious condition of non-selectivity (genetic drift), increase in proportion until its number either reaches equilibrium or eliminates variation in its area of adaptation. Therefore, this horror at chromosomal breakage and abberation associated with LSD usage is unfounded. Let it be proven before you condemn, there is also the possibility here of "positive" genetic abberation, or mutation. The correlations have been minor, the experimental conditions have been at best questionable, though certain studies have approached unprofessional culpability.

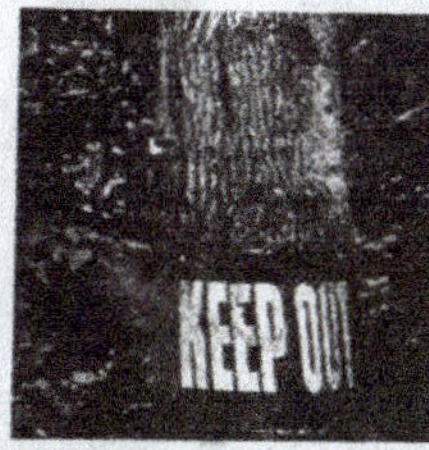

Recent Research

In the 21 June 1968 issue of SCIENCE (R.S. Sparks, John Melnyk, and L.P. Bozzeti, 1968, vol. 160 no. 3834, pp. 1343-1345) the studies of chromosomal damage up to that date where compared with the study of the authors. The range of breakage and abnormality included: chromatid and isochromatid breaks ang gaps, chromosomal fragments, ring chromosomes, dicentric chromosomes, and quadriradials. Their findings and their survey of the other studies is emphatic in its conclusion that, "Chromosome studies of persons exposed to LSD, either self-administered or received during medical therapy, failed to demonstrate significant chromosomal damage." Also, they found that in vivo or in vitro quadriradials (two break abberations) were found in LSD users-chronic ingesters, and that Chromosomal interchange was found in one control and one "user". They further state, "There was no difference in distribution of the chromosome counts between the controls and the subjects exposed to LSD." They go on to say that the difference in findings of those reporting positive results in chromosomal damage to LSD is due to differences in techniques and culture media in the analysis of nuclear material and that some used less complete media for analysis in their techniques. But it was also true that the laboratories reporting positive results had higher chromosomal breakage in their controls. They also pointed out the the lymphocyte was the only cell studied and that in the 72 hour culture period there were two or three successive cell divisions and that during this time chromosomal damage may have been modified. A more recent study (by J. Tjio, W. Pahnke and A. Kurland, reported in the Nov. 3, 1969 issue of the JOURNAL OF THE AMERICAN MEDICAL ASSOCIATION) found "...no significant difference between the before and after LSD chromosomal aberration rates...", a more unequivocal conclusion than Sparks et. al.

It seems to me unscientific to project the results of the effects of this drug, on cells in the blood stream where these cells are directly exposed to the drug, to the gametic cells which are isolated from these areas of body functioning. And to further attribute genetic effects of this drug when these effects in the white cells are questionable is bordering on the wild-eyed ravings of a yellow journalist. As for the sporatic reports of deformed children associated with LSD using mothers, (which have never been confirmed) I would ask for information on the other drugs these women use, to their age, and to the possibility of attempts at abortion. Also, it has

Continued on pg. 4

Alioto Deals

The latest political deal in San Francisco city government was announced this weekend. William Blake, a supervisor who was defeated for re-election in last Tuesday's city election, is resigning his post (his term has two months to run) in favor of the top vote receiver for supervisor, Dianne Fienstein. She will take office early and be appointed president of the Board of Supervisors by Alioto. It is traditional for the candidate who receives the most votes to be so appointed but only if that person has experience in city politics. In exchange for this Blake will receive an appointment to the Bay Area Rapid Transit District board.

Appendix B: Survey Questionnaire from 1966–1967

I cannot recall, and my notes do not provide specific information on this, if this survey was produced by myself alone or if it was a product of the surveyors in the Mogar Lab with the direction of Allen Rinker. I simply have a note at the bottom of the page with Subject C's answers that I was collecting research subjects at the time for Mr. Rinker.

N. Caldararo, *A Mental Ethnography: Conclusions From Research in LSD*,
https://doi.org/10.1007/978-3-031-13745-7

SURVEY SHEET

I. Name:
age:
sex:
marital status:
nationality:
religion:

background, i.e.,
living area:
education level:
area(U.S. or not):
major area of study:
political orientation:

II.

1. Would you like to participate in research concerning the personality effects of L.S.D. usage?[1]

2. Who are your national heroes(mythological included)?

3. Do you have any mythological heroes outside of American folklore?

4. Do you test reality or believe(suspect) in the existence of levels of reality?

5. What kind of personality traits would you suppose American culture is responsible for?

6. Do you believe we are going to have a thermonuclear war in the near future?

7. What value would you say advertising holds in our society?

8. How would you expect advertising to affect the cultural change of immigrants to this country?

9. Do you feel advertising creates dynamic cultural change in our society?

10. What kind of value changes do you believe advertising and the mass media in general cause?

11. What alternatives would you propose to resolve the present population dilema?

12. How do you think advertising has affected and/or still affects your personality and values?

13. Why are you in school?

14. Do you think television has practical educative value?

15. Do you believe advertising causes the quality of products to improve?

16. Do you think that the situation predicted in the book <u>1984</u> will ever come about?

17. What do you want out of life?

18. What was, or is, the occupation(s) of your parent(s)?

---

[1] I was collecting research subjects for Allen Rinker at the same time.

References

Adair, Peter, (1967) *Holy Ghost People*, Film, distributed by Thistle Films and available on YouTube.

Albesina, Alberto, Benedetta Brioschi and Eliana La Ferrara, (2016) "Violence against women: a cross-cultural analysis for Africa," *NBER*, Working Paper 21901, January, https://doi.org/10.3386/w21901.

Anderson, Robin and Bob Connolly, (1983) *First Contact*, Highlands Trilogy, Original film shot in 1930s, follow up footage in 1970s.

Ardener, Edwin (1972) "Belief and the problem of women," in J.S, La Fontaine (ed.) *The Interpretation of Ritual*, London, Tavistock.

Ardener, Shirley (1975a) "Sexual insult and female militancy," in *Perceiving Women*, (ed.) Shirley Ardener, pp. 29–54.

Aquinas, Thomas St. (1922) *Summa Theologica,* Part II, Question 95, 6, Benziger Brothers, New York.

Ayers, Susan, (2017) "Birth trauma and post-traumatic stress disorder: the importance of risk and resilience," *J. of Reproductive and Infant Psychology,* v. 35, n. 5, 427–430.

Bakalar, James B. and Lester Grinspoon (1997) *Psychedelic Drugs Reconsidered,* 3rd edition, New York, The Lindesmith Center.

Barbara, Vanessa (2021) "I took Ketamine for my depression. Things got pretty weird," *The New York Times,* December 28.

N. Caldararo, *A Mental Ethnography: Conclusions From Research in LSD*,
https://doi.org/10.1007/978-3-031-13745-7

Barnard, Mary (1963) "The God in the Flowerpot," *The American Scholar*, v. 32, n. 4, Autumn, 578–586.

Barry, H., III, Bacon, M. K. & Child, I. L. (1959). Relations of child training to subsistence economy. *American Anthropologist*, 61, 51–63.

Batson, G. and M. Mead (1942) *Balinese character: a photographic analysis*, Special Publications of the New York Academy of Sciences, v, II.

Bergson, Henri (1914) *Dreams,* Trans. By Edwin E. Slosson, New York, B.W. Huebsch.

Bexton, William H., Woodburn Heron and T.H. Scott (1954) "Effects of decreased variation in the sensory environment," *Canadian Journal of Psychology*, v. 8 (2): 70–76.

Bishop, A.G. and J.M. Tallon, (1999) "Anticholinergic visual hallucinosis from atropine eye drops," *Canadian J. Emergency Med.*, July, v. 1, n. 2, 115–116.

Blacker, Carmen (1975) *The Catalpa Bow, London*, George Allen & Unwin.

Blom, Jan Dirk (2010) *A Dictionary of Hallucinations*, New York, Springer.

Blum, Richard (1964) *Drugs and Society*, v. 1, Stanford, Ca. Jossey-Bass.

Bourguignon, E. (1973) *Religion, Altered States of Consciousness and Social Change*, Columbus, OH, Ohio State University Press.

Brice, Dave (1966) "Acid freaks," Golden Gater, Insert Section, May, 31–35.

Caldararo, Niccolo (2004) "The conservation of Beat art," in Modern Art, Modern Museums, (Eds.) Ashok Roy and Perry Smith, Contributions to the Bilbao Congress, 13–17 Sept, London, International Institute for Conservation of Historic and Artistic Works, 180–192.

Caldararo, Niccolo (2012) *Evolutionary Aspects of Disease Avoidance*, Saarbrucken, Scholars' Press.

Caldararo, Niccolo (2019) *An Ethnography of the Goodman Building*, The Longest Rent Strike, New York, Palgrave/Macmillan.

Caldararo, Niccolo (2021) *The Future of Leisure and Retirement, Pension Schemes, Community Support and Contemporary Consequences for the Next Generation*, Washington, D.C., Academica Press.

Carhart-Harris, Robin L., Suresh Muthukumaraswamy, Leor Roseman, Mendel Kaelen, Wouter Droog, et al., (2016) "Neural correlates of the LSD experience revealed by multimodal neuroimaging," PNAS, April 26, v. 113, n. 17:4853–4858.

Chandler, Arthur and Mortimer Hartman, (1960) "LSD-25 as a facilitating agent in psychotherapy," *Archives of General Psychiatry*, 2 (3) , 286–299.

Clark, Jonathan (1970) "The use of psilocybin in a prison setting," in Aaronson, Bernard and Humphry Osmond, (eds) (1970) *Psychedelics, The Uses and Implications of Hallucinogenic Drugs,* Garden City, Anchor Books: 40–44.

Cohen, M.M., K. Hirshhorn and W.A. Frosch, (1968) "LSD and chromosomes," N. Engl. J. Med., Jan 25, v. 278, n. 4:223.

Corbier, P., J. Raffi, J. Rhoda, (1983) "Female sexual behavior in male rats: effect of hour of castration at birth," *Physiology and Behavior*, v. 30, n. 4: 613–616.

Corson, Richard, (1972) *Fashions in Makeup: From Ancient to Modern Times*, London, Peter Owen.

Coyote, Peter (1990) "Book Introduction to *Ringolevio: A Life Played for Keeps*, http://www.petercoyote.com/ringo.html.

Darwin, Charles, (1871) The Descent of Man and Selection in Relation to Sex, Chicago, W.B. Conkey Company, Revised, Second Edition, 1874.

Diggerdocs, (2022) "An epic conversation with Jane Lapiner and David Simpson of the San Francisco Diggers," by Jay Babcock, March 5, https://diggersdocs.home.blog/2022/03/05/we-had-a-far-more-profound-effect/#more-1259.

Domhoff, G. William and Kieran C.R. Fox (2015) "Dreaming and the default network: a review, synthesis, and counterintuitive research proposal," *Consciousness and Cognition*, v. 33, May, 342–353.

Downing, Lisa and Dany Nobus (2004) "Iconography of asphyxiophilia: from fantasmatic fetish to forensic fact," *Paragraph*, v 27, n. 3:1–15.

Ebin, David, (1965) *The Drug Experience*, New York, Grove Press.

Ermentrout, B. and J.D. Cowan, (1979) "A mathematical theory of visual hallucination patterns," *Biological Cybernetics*, v. 34, 137–150.

Evans, William Charles and Daphne Evans (2009) "Hallucinogenic, allergenic, teratogenic and other toxic plants," in Trease and Evans' Pharmacognosy, 16th edition, Saunders/Elsevier, Edinburgh, pp. 523–532

Freud, Sigmund (1962) *Civilization and its Discontents*, College Edition, New York, W.W. Norton.

Freud, Sigmund (1964) *The Future of an Illusion*, New York, Anchor Books.

Garber-Paul, Elisabeth (2019) "RS Recommends: Chaos: Charles Manson, the CIA and the Secret History of the 60's," *Rolling Stone*, July 9.

Gergen, Kenneth J., Mary M. Gergen and William H. Barton, (1973) "Deviance in the dark, "Psychology Today, Oct. 129–130.

Goethe, Johann Wolfgang, (1836) *Conversation with Eckermann*, (edition of 1898) Trans, John Osenfort, George Bell & Sons, 315.

Goffman, Ken and Dan Joy (2004) *Counter Culture Through the Ages*, New York, Villard Publishers.

Goffman, Ken and Dan Joy (2007) *Counter Culture Through the Ages*, New York, Villard Publishers.

Grof, Stanislav (1976) *Realms of the Human Unconscious: Observation from LSD Research*. New York, E.P. Dutton.

Grogan, Emmett (1978) *Ringolevio*, Boston, Little, Brown & Co.

Griffith, R. M., Miyagi, O., & Tago, A. (1958) "The universality of typical dreams: Japanese vs Americans," *American Anthropologist*, 60, 1173–1179.

Grinspoon, L. and J.B. Bakalar, (1977) *Psychedelic Drugs Reconsidered*, 3rd edition, New York, The Lindesmith Center.

Grof, Stanislav (1976) *Realms of the Human Unconscious: Observation from LSD Research*, New York, E.P. Dutton.

Grunbaum, Adolf (1977) "How scientific is psychoanalysis?" in *Science and Psychotherapy*, (ed) Raphael Stem, L.S. Horowitz and J. Lynes, New York Haven Publishing.

Guzman, Gaston, (2012) "Nuevas observaciones taxonomicas y etnomicologicas en Psilocybe s.s. (Fungi, Basidiomycota, Agaricomycetidae, Agaricales, Strophariaceae) de Mexico, Africa y Espana," Acta Botanica Mexicana (100):79–106.

Hallowell, A. Irving (1966) "The role of dreams in Ojibwa culture," in (eds.) G.E. Von Gruebaum and R. Caillois, *The Dream and Human Societies, Berkeley*, University of California Press: 267–292.

Hansen, Joseph and Evelyn Reed (1986) *Cosmetics, Fashion and the Exploitation of Women*, New York, Pathfinder Press.

Harner, Michael (1972) *Hallucinogens and Shamanism*, Oxford, Oxford University Press.

Hesd, H. and G. Riddoch, (1917) "The automatic bladder, excessive sweating and some other reflex conditions in gross injuries of the spinal cord," *Brain*, v. 40, 188.

Hermie, L., M. Ruchsow and K.L. Taschner, (2015) "Hallucinogen persisting perception disorder (HPPD) and flashback phenomena- differential diagnosis and explanation models," (in German) *Fortschr Neurol Psychiatr.* Sept, v. 83, (9) 506–515.

Hoffmann A. (2009) LSD my problem child. Santa Cruz: Multidisciplinary Association for Psychedelic Studies, originally published in 1980 by McGraw-Hill, Boston.

Hollan, Douglas (2003) "The cultural and intersubjective context of dream remembrance and reporting," Chapter 9 in *Dream Travelers: Sleep Experiences and Culture in the Western Pacific*, (ed) Roger Ivar Lohmann, New York, Palgrave Macmillan,169–188.

Huang, Deqin, Ling Dai, Tieying Zeng, Haishan Huang, Meiliyang Wu, et al., "Exploring contributing factors to psychological traumatic childbirth from the perspective of midwives: a qualitative study," (2019), *Asian Nursing Research,* v. 13, 4, 270–276.

Hunter, Michael D., Timothy D. Griffiths, Tom F.D. Farrow, Ying Zheng, Iain D. Wilkinson, et al. (2002) "A neural basis for the perception of voices in external auditory space," *Brain,* Jan. 126, 1, 161–169.

Insel, T.R. and E. M. Scolnick (2006) "Cure therapeutics and strategic prevention: raising the bar for mental health research," *Molecular Psychiatry,* v. 11, 11–17.

Jacobs, Andrew (2021) "Psychedelics gain mainstream traction," *The New York Times,* May 10t

Jaing, Qiaolei and Xiuqin Huang (2013) "Internet: immersive virtual worlds," Chapter 89, in *Principles of Addiction,* Peter M. Miller, (ed.) Volume 1, 881–890.

Janiger, O. and Paltin, G. (1971) A bibliography of L.S.D. & mescaline: From the earliest researches to the beginnings of suppression. Fitzhugh Ludlow Library.

Jaspers, K. (1959) *Allgemeine Psychopathologie.* 7th ed. Berlin, Germany: Springer.

Jaynes, Julian (1986) "Consciousness and the voices of the mind," *Canadian Psychology,* v. 27, n. 2.:1–20 From Bauer Lectures, 1983.

Johnson MW, Garcia-Romeu A, Cosimano MP, Griffiths RR. (2014) Pilot study of the 5-HT2AR agonist psilocybin in the treatment of tobacco addiction. *J Psychopharmacol.* 28(11):983–992.

Jung, C.G. (2014) *Collected Works,* volume 7, Princeton, Princeton University Press (original Bollingen Series, XX, 1953 as Two Essays on Psychoanalysis.

Junghanns K, Wetterling T. (2017) [Alcohol withdrawal and its major complications]. *Fortschr Neurol Psychiatr.* Mar;85(3):163–177.

Kant, Immanuel (1900) *Dreams of a Spirit Seer,* Trans. E.F. Goerwitz, New York, Macmillan.

Karig, David, K. Michael Martini, Ting Lu, Nichola A. DeLateur, Nigel Goldenfeld, et al., (2018) "Stochastic Turing patterns in a synthetic bacterial population," *PNAS,* June 25, v. 115, (26) 6572–6577.

Kiyokawa, Miki and William F. Haning, (2021) "Hydromorphone-induced tactile hallucinations: rare opioid side effect," *Cureus,* v. 13, n. 2, Feb 28: https://doi.org/10.7759/cureus.13622.

Kluver, Heinrich (1966) Mescal: The Divine Plant and Its Psychological Effects, Kegan Paul (originally published in 1928).

Langlitz, Nicolas (2013) *Neuropsychedelia: The Revival of Hallucinogen Research Since the Decade of the Brain,* Berkeley, University of California Press.

Laughlin, Robert M. (1976) Of Wonders Wild and New: Dreams from Zinacantan, Smithsonian Contributions to Anthropology, n. 22, Washington, D.C., Smithsonian Institution.

Leacock, Eleanor and Jane Nash (1977) "Ideologies of sex: archtypes and stereotypes," In Issues in Cross-Cultural Research, (ed.) Leonore Loeb Adler, *Annals of the New York Academy of Sciences*, v. 285, New York, The New York Academy of Sciences: 618–645.

Lee, Martin and Bruce Shlain (1985) *Acid Dreams: The Complete Social History of LSD, The Sixties, The CIA, the and Beyond*, New York, Grove Press, revised edition, 1994.

Leinhardt, Godfrey (1954) "The Shilluk of the Upper Nile," in *African Worlds*, D. Forde (ed.) International African Institute, London, Oxford University Press.

Lewin, Louis (1924) *Phanfastica, Die betaubenden und erregenden Genussmittel, Fur Arzte und Nichtarzte*, Berlin, Verlag von Georg Stike.

Lewis, Simon J.G., James M. Shine, Daniel Brooks and Glenda M. Halliday, (2014) "Hallucinogenic mechanisms: pathological and pharmacological insights," Chapter 6, in *The Neuroscience of Visual Hallucinations*, (Eds.) Daniel Collerton, Urs Peter Mosimann and Elain Perry, New York, Wiley, pp. 121–150.

Lincoln, J. S. (1935) *The Dream in Primitive Cultures*, London, Cressett Press.

Linton, Ralph (1936) *The Study of Man*, New York, Appleton-Century.

Ling, Thomas M. and John Buckman, (1964) "The treatment of frigidity with LSD and Ritalin," *Psychedelic Review*, v. 1, n. 4, 450–458.

Lilly, John (1972) *The Center of the Cyclone*, Berkeley,Ca, Ronin Publishing.

Luke, David (2012) "Psychoactive substances and paranormal phenomena: a comprehensive review," *International Journal of Transpersonal Studies*, v. 31, n. 1: 97–156.

McKenna, Terence (1992) *Food of the Gods*, New York, Bantam Books.

McKenna, Terence (1993) *True Hallucinations, Being an Account of the Author's Extraordinary Adventures in the Devil's Paradise*, New York, HarperOne.

McLean, Adrienne, (2016) *Costume*, Make up and Hair, JSTOR eBooks.

Mead, Margaret (1954) *Male and Female*, New York, Morrow & Co.

Mead, Margaret (1970) *Culture and Commitment*, New York, Columbia University Press.

Metzenich, Michael (2013) *Soft-wired: How the New Science of Brain Plasticity Can Change Your Life*, San Francisco, 2nd Edition, Parnassus Publishing.

Metzner, Ralph (1968) *The Ecstatic Adventure*, New York, Macmillan.

Morgar, Robert E. (1965) "Search and research with the psychedelics," *ETC: A Review of General Semantics*, v. 22, n. 4, Special Issue on the Psychedelic Experience, Dec.:393–407.

Moueau, J.J. (1973) *Hashish and Mental Illness*, New York, Raven Press.

Nelson, Kevin (2010) *The Spiritual Doorway in the Brain: A Neurologist's Search for the God Experience*, New York, Fenguin/Plume.

Nichols, Charles D. and Elaine Sanders-Bush (2001) "A single dose of Lysergic Acid Diethylamide influences gene expression patterns within the mammalian brain," *Neuropsychopharmacology*, 26, 634–642.

Nicolai, C.F. (1802) "A memoir on the appearance of spectres or phantoms occasioned by disease with psychological remarks," *Nicholson's Journal of Natural Philosophy, Chemistry and the Arts*, VI, 161–179.

Nicolai, C.F. (1803) "A memoir on the appearance of spectres or phantoms occasioned by disease with psychological remarks," *Nicholson's Journal of Natural Philosophy, Chemistry and the Arts*, VI, 161–179 Original in German 1799.

Nielsen, Tore A., Antonio L. Zadra, Valerie Simard, Sebastien Saucier, Philippe Stenstron, et al., (2003) "The typical dreams of Canadian university students," *Dreaming*, 13, 211–235.

Nutt, David and Robin Carhart-Harris (2020) "The current status of psychedelics in Psychiatry," *JAMA Psychiatry*, June 24, https://doi.org/10.1001/jamapsychiatry.2020.2171.

Olson, J.M., P.A. Vernon, J.A. Harris, K.L. Jang, (2001) "The heritability of attitudes: a study of twins," *J. Pers. Soc Psych*ol. Jun, 80, 6, 845–860.

Osmond, Humphry and John R. Smythies, (1953) "The present state of psychological medicine," *Hibbert Journal*, 133–142.

Osmond, Humphry, (1970) "On being mad," in Aaronson, Bernard and Humphry Osmond, (eds) (1970) Psychedelics, The Uses and Implications of Hallucinogenic Drugs, Garden City, Anchor Books, 21–28.

Padosch, Stephan A., Dirk W. Lachenmeier and Lars U. Kroner, (2006) Subst Abuse Treat Prev Policy, v. 1, doi: 10.1186/1747-597X-1-14

Palhano-Fontes, Fernanda, Katia C. Andrade, Luis F. Tofoli, Antonio C. Santos, Jose Alexandre S. Crippa, et al., (2015) "The psychedelic state induced by ayshuasca modulates the activity and connectivity of the default mode network," PLoS One, Feb. 18, v. 10, n. 2, https://doi.org/10.1371/journal.pone.0118143

Patai, Raphael (1990) *The Hebrew Goddess, Detroit,* Wayne State University Press, third edition.

Pathis, Lawrence and Helena J. Younes (2015) "False memories in therapy and hypnosis before 1980," *Psychology of Consciousness: Theory, Research and Practice*, v, 2, n. 2: 153–169.

Penfield, Wilder and Herbert Jasper (1958) *Epilepsy and the Functional Anatomy of the Human Brain,* Boston, Little Brown and Co.

Rank, Otto (1924) *The Trauma of Birth*, New York, Dover Books reprint 1993.

Radcliffe-Brown, A.R. (1932) *The Andaman Islanders*, Reprint edition, New York, The Free Press of Glencoe, 1964.

Ratcliffe, Matthew (2021) "Sensed presence without sensory qualities: a phenomenological study of bereavement hallucinations," *Phenomenology and the Cognitive Sciences,* v. 20, 601–616.

Rechtschaffen, Allen (2000) "Sleep and Dreaming," in *Principles of Neuroscience,* (eds.) E.R. Kandel, J.H. Schwartz and T.M. Jessel, New York, McGraw-Hill, 4th edition.

Reich, Wilhelm (1970) *The Mass Psychology of Fascism*, New York, Farrar, Straus and Giroux.

Reina, R.E. (1966) *The Law of the Saints*, Indianapolis and New York, The Bobbs-Merrill Co.

Reina, R.E. (1968) *The Law of the Saints*, Indianapolis and New York, The Bobbs-Merrill Co.

de Rios, Dobkin and Oscar Janiger (2003) *LSD, Spirituality, and the Creative Process: Based on the Groundbreaking Research of Oscar Janiger*, Rochester, Vermont, Inner Traditions/Bear & Co.

Rivers, W.H.R. (1920) *Instinct and the Unconscious*, Cambridge, Cambridge University Press.

Rivers, W.H.R. (1923) *Conflict and Dream*, New York, Harcourt, Brace.

Rogers TB, Kuiper NA, Kirker WS. (1977) "Self-reference and the encoding of personal information," *J Pers Soc Psychol.*:35:677–688

Rouhierm A. (1927) *Le Peyotl*, Paris.

Rubinstein, K. and Krippner, S. (1991) "Gender differences and geographic differences in content from dreams elicited by a television announcement," *International Journal of Psychosomatics*, v. 38, n. 1-4, 40–44.

Sacks, Oliver (1985) *The Man Who Mistook His Wife for a Hat*, New York, Harper & Row, Perennial Library Edition.

Sacks, Oliver (2012) *Hallucinations*, New York, Vintage Books.

Savage, Charles and Myron J. Stolaroff (1965) "Clarifying the confusion regarding LSD-25," *Journal of Nervous and Mental Disease*, v. 140, 218–221.

Scarmeas, Nikolaos, Jason Brandt, Marilyn Albert, Georgios Hadjigeorgiou, Alexandros Papadimitriou, et al., (2005) "Delusions and hallucinations are associated with worse outcome in Alzheimer Disease," *Arch. Neurol.*, v. 62, 1601–1608.

Schultes, Richard Evans (1963) "Hallocinogenic plants of the New World," *Harvard Review, 1*, 18–32.

Schultes, R.E. (1970) "The botanical and chemical distribution of hallucinogens," *Annual Review of Plant Physiology,* v. 21, 571–598.

Serko, A., (1913) "Im mescalinrausch," *Jahrb. F. Psychiat.*, 34, 355.

Shannon, Benny (1997) "A cognitive-psychological study of ayahuasca," *MAPS Newsletter*, https://maps.org/news-letters/v07n3/07313sha.html.

Shermer, Michael (2011*) The Believing Brain, From Ghosts to Goda to Politics and Conspiracies—How We Construct Beliefs and Reinforce Them as Truths*, New York, New York Times Books.

Shevlin, M., J. Murphy, M.J. Dorahy, et al., (2006) "The distribution of positive psychosis-like symptoms in the population: a latent class analysis of the National Comorbidity Survey, " *Schizophr Res*, 89, 101–109.

Small, S.A., A.S. Hava, G.M. Perera, R. DeLaPaz, R. Mayeux and Stern, Y. (2001) Circuit mechanisms underlying memory encoding and retrieval in the long axis of the hippocampal formation," *Nat. Neurosci.* V. 4, 442–449.

Snyder, S.H., L. Faillace, L. Hollister, (1968) "2,5,Dimethoxy-4-methylamphetamine: a new hallucinogenic drug, " *Science,* Mar 29, v. 159 (3822):1492.

Sperber, Dan (1975) *Rethinking Symbolism*, Cambridge.

Staford, P.G. and B.H. Golightly (1967) *LSD—The Problem-Solving Psychedelic,* New York, Award Books.

Stevens, Jay (1988) *Storming Heaven: LSD and the American Dream*, New York, Harper and Row.

Strassman, R. (2008). "The varieties of the DMT experience," in Inner Paths to Outer Space, 1st Edn., ed R. Strassman (Vermont, VT: Park Street Press), 51–80.

Stein, Barry E. and M. Alex Meredith (1993) *The Merging of the Senses*, Cambridge Mass., A Bradford Book, MIT Press.

Shonle, R., (1925) "Peyote: The Giver of Visions", *Amer. Anthrop*, 27, 53–75.

Swan, Gary E. and Christina N. Lessov-Schlaggar (2007) "The effects of tobacco smoke and nicotine on cognition and the brain," *Neuropsychol. Rev.*, Sept, v. 17, n. 3, 259–273.

Textor, R.B. (1967) *A Cross-Cultural Summary,* New Haven, Conn., HRAF Press.

Thomson, Eric (2018) "Neural Representations," *Minds and Machines,* v. 28, 191–235.

Tobin, Joseph J. and Joan Friedman (2009) "Spirits, Shaman and nightmare death: survivor stress in a Hmong refugee, " In Warms, Richard, James Garber and R. Jon McGee, (2009) *Sacred Realms: Readings in the Anthropology of Religion,* Oxford, Oxford University Press, 327–332.

Tylor, Edward B. (1889) *Primitive Culture,* Vol. 1, New York, Henry Holt & co.

Voltaire, Francois-Marie Arouet, (1764) *A Philosophical Dictionary,* section on Somnambulists and Dreamers, Trans. F. Fleming, E.R. Dumont, v. VII, pp 2, 9.

Von Uexkull, Jacob (2010) *A Foray into the Worlds of Animals and Humans,* University of Minnesota Press edition, originally published in 1934 as, *Streifzuge durch die Umwelten von Tieren und Menschen,* Verlag von Julius Springer,

Vygotsky, L. S., (1978*) Mind in society: The development of higher psychological processes.* Cambridge, MA: Harvard University Press.

Wallace, A.F.C. (1958) Dreams and the wishes of the soul, a type of psychoanalytic among the Seventeenth Century Iroquois," *Amer. Anth.*, v. 60:234–248.

Watts, Alan, (1970) "Psychedelics and religious experience," in *Psychedelics: The Uses and Implications of Hallucinogenic Drugs,* Garden City, Anchor Books.131–144.

Whiting, Beatrice (1963) *Six Cultures: Studies of Child Rearing,* New York, John Wiley.

Weil, Andrew (1972) *The Natural Mind: Another Way of Looking at Drugs and the Higher Consciousness,* Boston, Houghton-Mifflin.

West, Louis Jolyon (1976) *Treatment of Schizophrenia: Progress and Prospects,* London: Grune & Stratton.

Winkelman, Michael J. (2000) *Shamanism, The Neural Ecology of Consciousness and Healing,* Westport Ct, Bergin and Garvey.

Index[1]

A

Aboriginal, xx, lxxix, 3, 5, 14, 56, 216, 249, 307, 332
Abstract, 48, 62, 235, 241
Acculturation, lxxx, 11, 268
Africa, 40, 92, 311
Africa (North), 222
Africa (South), 137
African Americans, lvi, lx, 18, 20, 174, 177, 178, 255, 279, 292, 299
Afterimage, xl
Aged, xli, 14, 21, 69, 75, 206, 211
Aging, 156, 175
Alcohol, x, xvi, xvii, 2, 85, 90, 95, 99, 110, 148, 160, 164, 194, 216–218, 220, 256, 259, 276
Alcohol addiction, 6
Aliens, xx, 13, 144, 180, 195, 249
Alternative universes/worlds, 11
Alzheimer's, xlv, 13, 160, 240
Amanita muscaria, 3, 82
Amnesia, xii, 105, 171, 239
Amphetamine, xvii, 9
Anadenanthera colubrine (*Mimosa hostilis*), 4
Anadenanthera peregrine, 4, 5
Anatomically Modern Humans, lxxx
Ancestors, xxii, xlvi, 14, 41, 52, 56, 62, 82, 150, 151, 157, 170, 179, 180, 218, 233, 267, 271, 272, 332
Anesthesia, 3, 68
Angels, 85, 151, 157, 159, 179, 271
Anhalonium lewinii (the dumpling cactus or peyote), xvii

[1] Note: Page numbers followed by 'n' refer to notes.

N. Caldararo, *A Mental Ethnography: Conclusions From Research in LSD*,
https://doi.org/10.1007/978-3-031-13745-7

Animals, ix–xi, xvi–xviii, xxxviii, xlv, xlvi, xlix, 3, 12, 13, 22, 34–36, 41, 42, 51, 52, 56–58, 61, 70, 72, 104, 143, 149, 158, 175, 179, 192, 194, 227, 232–234, 253, 262, 271, 279, 299, 307, 319
Anthropology, viii, xiv, lxxx, 8, 175, 241, 293
Archaic, lxxx
Archetype, 61–67, 88, 107, 169, 180–182, 184, 215, 266, 290, 331
Archicortex, xiv
Arnhem Land, xlvi
Artificial intelligence (AI), 136
Asia, xlviii
Attention, xi, xiv, xv, xix, xxiii, xlviii, 8, 51, 63, 100, 104, 109, 147, 149, 177, 185, 220, 227, 242, 252, 298, 310, 314
Attentive presence, xv, 93, 94
Auditory, xiii, xxxvi–xxxviii, xliii, xliv, xlviii, xlix, liv, 46, 48, 49, 55, 71, 109, 154, 160, 162, 163, 178, 179, 256
Australia, xlvi, lxxix
Autoimmune Deficiency Syndrome (AIDS), xxxv
Autoscopy, 178
Awareness, xi–xiii, xv, xxxv, xlv, lxv, 16, 46, 101, 104, 194, 228, 241, 252, 257, 294, 310, 317
Axon, xv
Ayahuasca, xvii, xxxiii, 1–3, 5, 9, 63, 160, 216
Aztec, xix, 102, 188, 240

B

Bad trip, l, li, liii, lxi, lxii, 90, 92, 94
Bakweri, 190
Banisteriopsis caapi, 1
Behavior, viii–x, xv, xvii, xxi, lvi, lix, 3, 5, 9, 16, 18, 35, 38, 42, 48, 52, 58, 72, 83, 86, 89, 92, 93, 104, 109, 112, 137, 141, 143, 150, 166, 177, 182, 193, 218, 226, 230, 233, 234, 256, 259, 261, 268, 271, 275, 276, 278, 306, 308, 310, 312, 319
Belief, vii, xvi, xxi, xlix, 13, 14, 40, 43–45, 53, 70, 98, 106, 145, 173, 174, 179, 186, 233, 253, 261–264, 270, 331
Belladonna, 3
Bereavement, 157
Birth, lxii, 12, 38, 54, 55, 57, 81, 82, 86, 87, 89, 92, 107, 112, 135, 149, 168, 172–176, 179, 180, 183, 194, 220, 221, 224–226, 238, 254, 268, 273, 292, 310, 320
Black Death (Bubonic Plague), 19
Boy, xl, 3, 4, 22, 46, 58, 141, 293, 319
Brain, ix, xxxvi, 12, 34, 136, 151, 160, 164, 167, 169, 171, 175, 177, 178, 181, 182, 194, 216, 250, 294, 311, 332
Bufotenin, 4

C

California, 84, 236
Cancer, 38, 149, 151, 196
Capitalism, 158, 264

Catalhoyuk, xli
Cathartic, xii
Cave, xli
Centers for Disease Control (CDC), 220
Cerebral, xv, xxxix
Ceremony, xl, 37, 137, 139, 142, 250, 320
Charles Bonnet Syndrome (CBS), xxxvi–xl, xliii–xlv, xlviii, xlix, 12, 63, 65, 70, 71, 329
Children, xliv, xlv, 4, 12, 21–23, 49, 56, 60, 70, 93, 111, 149, 159, 179, 180, 188, 194, 195, 224, 235, 256, 269, 278–279, 288, 289, 292, 293, 310, 314, 315, 319
China (PRC), 267, 333
Chinese, xlviii, 100, 102, 179, 267
Chumash, xli
CIA, xviii, lii, liv, 229, 264, 321, 327, 333
City, 44, 46, 306
Clinical, ix, x, xxxi–xlvii, lviii, lix, 10, 46, 81, 95, 98, 107, 108, 150, 166, 171, 184, 185, 196, 215, 240, 251, 276, 291, 333
Code, 20, 149, 150, 239, 266
COEX (systems of condensed experience), 98–100, 150, 172, 182–185, 187
Cognition, ix, x, xiv, xvii, xviii, 21, 37, 154, 167, 177, 233, 241
Cognitive, xi, xiv, xlv, lxii, 15, 40, 47, 48, 56, 63, 155, 233, 253
Collective, xxiii, 17, 84, 158, 169, 179, 180, 194, 228, 253, 266, 309
Color, xliv, xlix, l, liv, lxv, 12, 61, 66, 87, 138, 163–165, 242, 265
Coma, xi, 68, 105, 220
Communism, lvi, 263, 299
Communitas, lii, 106, 154
Community, xviii, xxi, lx, 2, 20, 21, 54, 96, 106, 155, 159, 164, 165, 173, 179, 181, 218, 222, 241, 254, 292, 310, 312
Connectivity, xii, xxxvi, lxv, 21, 63, 67, 68, 112, 234
Consciousness, viii, x–xiii, xv, xvi, xviii, xxii–xxiv, xxxiii, xxxiv, xlviii, lvii, lxii, lxiv, lxv, 4, 5, 10, 15, 19, 33, 34, 36, 40, 48–50, 52, 53, 55, 57, 58, 64, 67–69, 85, 87, 92, 97, 100, 101, 103–105, 110, 112, 136, 145, 149, 154, 158, 159, 161, 165, 168, 171, 172, 175, 180, 183, 188, 189, 214, 216, 226, 227, 233, 234, 238, 239, 251, 255, 259, 263, 266, 298–300, 305, 306, 308–313, 315, 316, 319, 320, 329, 335
Contributions, 24
Conversion, 45–46, 69, 169
Cortex, xii–xiv, l, 12, 111, 178, 265, 332
Cosmology, viii, 37, 38, 182, 229
Covid-19, xxxv, xxxvii, 137, 217, 297
Creation, xxi, xlvi, xlvii, lii, lxii, 36, 68, 103, 152, 167, 171, 251, 254, 268, 269, 315, 321

Creative, xviii, xlii, xliv, xlvi, 13, 47, 48, 147, 151, 165, 171, 217, 221, 223, 224, 320, 329, 330, 334
Credit, 188
Cross-cultural, x, xxxv, xlv, 46, 53, 162, 188, 288, 289, 309, 310, 333
Culture, viii, ix, xiv, xix, xx, xxxiii, xli, xliii, xlvii, xlix, lvi, lxxix, lxxx, 2, 5, 9, 10, 13, 15, 22, 23, 38, 40, 44, 49, 50, 58, 60, 63, 65, 67, 69, 87, 89, 94, 104, 137, 141, 143, 144, 149, 152, 161, 165–167, 169, 170, 178, 183, 184, 214, 217, 218, 220, 221, 223–227, 232, 237, 241, 250, 253, 259, 261, 262, 266, 268, 271, 276, 277, 287, 289, 290, 293, 294, 297, 306, 308–311, 313, 315, 317–320
Cure, xviii, 6, 8, 19, 36, 69, 84, 95, 99, 140, 141, 144, 147, 172, 176, 195, 196, 213–242, 262, 277, 288, 306, 328

D

Dance, lii, lix, 9
Datura, xli, 3, 147
Dead, 10, 39, 42, 60, 69, 138, 142, 157, 181
Death, xvi, xliii, 2, 24, 37, 40, 42, 44, 53, 54, 58, 65, 112, 144, 174, 175, 194, 220, 230, 288
Delirium, x, xlviii, lxv, 51, 55, 160, 177, 182
Dementia, xlv, 52, 53, 160, 240
Demons, 4, 38, 39, 67–72, 139, 143, 149, 178, 320
Dendrite, 23
Depression, xl, liv, 6, 35, 82, 147, 148, 196, 268, 275, 276, 288, 289
Derivation, xliv, xlvii–lxvi
Devils, xx, 54, 92, 137, 151, 159, 298, 319, 320, 327
Diagnosis, 10, 19
Diggers, 14–21, 84, 107, 222, 228
Disability, 229
Disease, viii, xix, xxxv, xliii, 13, 24, 36–38, 71, 82, 88, 110, 160, 170, 177, 184, 217, 240, 267, 306, 332, 333
Dissociation, 259
Distortion, xxxvi, xlvii–lxvi, 39, 66, 95, 162, 168, 175, 180, 288, 334
Divination, 3, 38, 110
Divine, xiii, 110, 169, 170, 306
DNA, 144, 194, 239, 250, 251
Dopamine, xviii, xl, 24, 86, 332
Dose, 23, 33–113, 215
Dream, x, xxxix, 2, 38, 112, 136, 252, 287, 306, 329
Dream interpretation, xxiii, xliv, xlvi, 40, 166, 168, 181, 253
Drug, vii, xxxi, 1, 33, 136, 139, 142, 145–148, 151, 153, 154, 156, 157, 162, 163, 165, 173–175, 178, 181, 186, 188, 193, 213, 250, 287, 314, 327
Dwarves, xlv

E

Ecstatic (seizures or states), xliii, 72, 89, 315, 316
Ego, xiii, 54, 55, 147, 149, 151, 156, 238, 259
Elderly, xxxviii, xlv
Elves, xlv
Empiricism, xvi, 157, 262, 333
Employee, 314
Enlightenment, lii, 156, 237
Entorhinal cortex, xiv
Epilepsy, xxxix, xliii, 70–72, 178
Episodic memory, xiii, lxv, 265, 329
Estrogen, xxxvii, 192, 277, 332
Ether, xvii
Ethnicity, ix, 288
Ethnobotany, xvii
Ethnography, viii, 16, 18, 294
Ethnology, 52
Ethnopsychopharmacology, xvi
Euphoria, 49, 55, 86, 151, 257, 328
Europe, 109, 222, 237, 261
European, xxxiii, lxxix, 23, 24, 41, 92, 102, 266, 271, 298
Eusocial, 234
Evolution, ix, xi, xviii, xxi–xxiii, lxxx, 12, 15, 19, 20, 47, 55, 88, 101, 104, 161, 165, 170, 180, 194, 233, 234, 238, 239, 254, 263, 273, 274, 278, 298, 299, 332
Experiment, xii, xvii, xviii, xxiii, xxxi, xxxiv, xxxvi, xxxviii, l, li, liii, liv, lvii, lix, lxi, lxii, lxv, 2, 6, 7, 15, 20, 34, 36, 39, 50, 55, 68, 69, 83, 91, 95, 96, 98, 99, 112, 136, 153, 163–165, 176, 193, 215, 223, 234, 243n1, 265, 294, 299, 314–316, 318, 321, 327, 328, 331, 332
Extrasensory perception (ESP), 58, 261
Eyes, xxxvii, xl, xliii, xliv, xlviii, l, 39, 49, 61, 62, 64, 67, 69, 72, 89, 96, 105, 137, 149, 178, 182, 242, 259–261, 274, 289, 307, 312, 327

F

Face(s), xvii, xxxviii, xliv, xlvii, 10, 13, 61, 62, 70, 97, 143, 171, 176, 181, 219, 258, 260, 292, 293
Fainting, xv
Fairies, xlv, 43, 44
Family, lvi, 16, 22, 23, 44, 51, 58, 65, 67, 91, 97, 141, 144, 149, 159, 167, 168, 170, 173, 180, 186, 187, 189, 191, 196, 226, 232, 236, 253, 256, 260, 271, 275, 276, 291, 292, 299, 309, 310, 314, 315, 328
Fantasy, 13, 19, 41, 52, 57, 71, 102, 136, 168, 227, 235, 260, 293, 306, 331
Fear, lv, lxi, lxii, 41, 112, 149, 175, 213, 214, 258, 299, 319, 334
Female, xxi, xxxv, lv, 39, 83, 87, 93, 165, 177, 179, 190–193, 217, 223, 236, 259, 269, 274, 276, 277, 287, 289, 291, 294, 305–322, 332
Feminine, 14, 217, 274, 275, 291, 292, 306, 310–312
Flashbacks, 71, 72, 90, 91, 98, 99

Flood, 18, 55, 107
Flowers, xliv, 70, 179
Flying, 58, 288
fMRI, x, xxxvi, xlviii, l, 34, 45, 95, 260, 265
Food, xvi, xlvi, 3, 8, 15, 20, 48, 56, 87, 170, 173, 189, 217, 221, 228, 229, 233, 257, 258
Fuge, 46
Fusiform, 260
Future, lvi, 14, 17, 42, 56, 65, 227, 236, 237, 255–270, 273, 276, 287–300, 332–335

G

Gems, 66, 107
Genes, 194, 195, 238, 307
Geometric designs, xliv
Germany, 299
Ghost, 10, 39, 60, 138, 156, 179, 181, 182
Girl, 22, 46, 81, 97, 190, 235, 257, 258, 261, 308, 310, 319, 331
Global, xxxiii, lxxix
God, xx, xxxvii, lxii, 38, 40, 44, 45, 47, 48, 52–56, 61, 62, 70, 106, 109, 135, 228, 233, 261–263, 268, 269, 271, 307, 308, 331
Good life, 226
Government, xxxiv, lxxix, 151, 215, 216, 222, 229, 251, 264, 320, 327, 333
Great Depression, 262
Growth, lxi, 21, 24, 171, 175, 180, 238, 306
Guilt, 67, 146

H

Haight-Ashbury, vii, lv, lx, 15, 17, 18, 96, 152, 219, 221, 222, 228, 230, 235, 252, 255, 328
Haight-Ashbury Free Medical Clinic, xxxi
Hallucination, x, xxxv, 3, 35, 136, 233, 251, 294, 317, 329
Handsome Lake, 89
Happening (a happening), xiv, xxxiv, xlvi, lx, 16, 52, 143, 150, 228, 261, 273
Happiness, 54, 135, 155, 229, 230, 273, 276, 298
Hart, Daniel, 2
Harvard, 7, 152, 166, 174
Healing, ix, xvi, xix, 3, 4, 8, 9, 14, 37, 42, 84, 103, 146, 151, 167, 169, 170, 172, 181, 190, 195, 250, 306, 332, 333
Health, xvii, xix, lix, 8, 40, 53, 81, 108, 167, 214, 241, 264, 278
Heautoscopy, 177, 178
Heaven, 54, 71, 135, 181
Hemianopia, 254
Heroin, xvii, 17, 18, 275, 329
Hindu, 135, 136, 229
Hines, Kevin, 148, 276
Hippies, 16–18, 21, 173, 174, 222, 227, 256, 328
Hippocampus, xii, xiii, xxxv–xxxvii, xlvii, lxiii–lxv, 50, 55, 60, 63, 72, 81, 99, 104, 105, 144, 264, 265, 329, 332
History, ix, xiv, xv, xviii, xix, xxii–xxiv, xxxviii, xlviii, li, lv, lvi, lix, lxii, 2, 5, 40, 53, 56, 57, 63,

81, 88, 91, 92, 137, 149, 150, 157, 158, 164, 178, 180, 184–186, 215, 220, 228, 229, 232, 233, 235, 236, 239, 240, 250, 266, 278, 293, 310, 327, 328
Hominid, xxiii, 48, 177, 233
Homonymous hemianopia, xliii
Homo sapiens, xxiii, 47, 233, 332
Hopi, 3, 141, 166, 216, 289
Housing, 227, 229, 255
Humboldt State College, xxxi, xxxiv, 6, 290, 318
Humor, liv, 39, 84
Hunter-gatherer, 68, 309
Hyperphantasia, 260
Hypnagogic, 39, 49, 51, 260
Hypnopompic hallucination, xxxix, 49, 157
Hypnosis, 70, 111, 145, 328
Hysteria, 51, 111, 163, 182, 268

I

Iboga (*Tabernanthe iboga*), xl, 92
Identity, lii, lx, lxiii, 9, 16, 20, 48, 54–56, 65, 154, 180, 183, 192, 194, 217, 230, 233, 236, 241, 249, 270–279, 287–300, 306, 308–310, 312, 315
Image, x, xi, xiii–xv, xxiv, xxxi, xxxii, xxxvi, xxxviii–xli, xliii–lxvi, 12, 17, 23, 24, 37, 39, 43, 48, 49, 51, 55, 56, 60–65, 67, 70–72, 86, 109, 138, 149, 160, 163, 165, 166, 168, 170, 171, 176, 180–182, 185, 191, 215, 218, 219, 222, 227, 231, 239, 253, 254, 257, 258, 260, 261, 265, 271, 308, 329–331
Imagination, xlvii, xlviii, 305
Imps, xlv
India, lix, 45, 106, 168, 222, 277, 289
Indigenous, viii, xlv, lxxix, lxxx, 2, 3, 5, 8, 9, 15, 24, 36, 37, 41, 45, 53, 60, 63, 82, 83, 92, 106, 166, 169, 173, 175, 176, 184, 249–279, 318
Individual, ix, xxxi, 1, 37, 141–143, 145, 146, 149–151, 154, 157–159, 167, 169–172, 176–178, 180, 182, 183, 187, 191, 193, 213, 250, 287, 305, 331
Industrial, 21, 68, 253, 276, 331, 334
Inebriant, xvii
Inequality, 19
Information, xiii, xv, xvi, xxxii, xlv, xlvi, liii, lxiii, lxiv, lxxx, 10, 14, 20, 21, 36, 40, 41, 44, 51, 53, 57, 61, 63, 64, 68, 85, 96, 102, 104, 105, 107, 140, 143, 163, 164, 166, 167, 170, 214, 224, 225, 230, 231, 234, 235, 237, 239, 240, 256, 259, 265, 269, 298, 314, 327, 330, 331, 339
Initiation, xl, xlix, 3, 4, 41, 72, 142, 157, 315
Inner life, 101, 332
Innovation, 94, 165
Institutions, xxi, xlv, lxxix, 167, 189, 264, 277, 278, 315
Internet, 21, 57, 60, 136, 158, 170, 215

Interpretation, vii, viii, x, xiv, xvii, xx, xxiii, xxiv, xxxiii, xxxiv, xliii–xlviii, liii, lxiv, 1, 2, 10, 14, 15, 22, 33–113, 142, 144, 146, 151, 155, 165–168, 171, 174, 176, 181, 183, 184, 188, 196, 213, 215, 219, 233, 235, 249–251, 253, 257, 258, 266, 267, 269, 278, 288, 289, 292, 306, 307, 312, 316, 332, 333
Intersex, 190, 191
Intoxication, xvii, 37
IQ, ix
Isolation, 51, 68, 69, 91, 189, 192, 234, 268, 318

J

Japan, 58, 169, 170, 299
Japanese, 46, 54, 61, 94, 101, 170, 289
Jimson Weed, xxxii, 3

K

Kava, xvii
Khat, xvii
Kinship, 141, 249

L

Labor, 236, 309
Lakota, 9
Landscapes, xxxii, xli, liv, 51, 62, 144, 157, 167, 219, 260
Language, viii–x, xiv, xx, xxi, xxiii, xxiv, xxxv, 16, 20, 44, 47, 48, 68, 92, 94, 101–104, 109, 135, 141, 144, 149, 150, 165, 170, 177, 178, 190, 215, 226, 230, 237, 239, 241, 254, 258, 306, 312, 315, 316, 334
Latinos, Latinx, 177–179
Laughter, 108, 257
Law, 19, 69, 152, 158, 222, 229, 235
L-Dopa, 12
Leprechaun, xlv
Letters, 11
Lewy body disease (LBD), xlv, 12, 13
Life, xiii, xxxiii, 2, 40, 135, 214, 251, 288, 308, 331
Light, xx, xxxiii, li, lii, lvi, 14, 49, 63, 64, 66, 67, 99, 107, 144, 154, 164, 165, 182, 188, 218, 235, 255, 257–259, 265, 298, 317
Little people, xliv, xlvi
LSD, vii, xxxi, 1, 33, 138–140, 144–147, 150–155, 160, 162–166, 171–173, 176, 178–180, 182–188, 192, 193, 196, 213, 250, 290, 314, 327

M

Madness, xviii, lii, lxi, 9–11, 54, 260, 268
Magic, 14, 69, 89, 230, 263, 267
Male, xxi, xxxv, li, lv, lix, 6, 17, 22, 34, 61, 83, 149, 189–193, 217, 221, 223–225, 235, 273, 276, 277, 289, 292, 294, 306–308, 310–320, 322
Mammal, ix, x, xiv, xxiii, 105, 164, 167, 232, 238, 332
Marijuana, lxv, 18, 85, 173, 174, 188, 217, 222, 257

Masculine, 217, 311
Mauche, 4
Maya, 102, 306
Medicine, xvi, 8, 10, 91, 100, 137, 231, 252, 292, 306
Meditation, xli, 100, 105, 219, 220, 233, 260, 278
Melanesian, 44, 169, 175, 181, 182, 334
Memory, xi–xvi, xxxv–xxxvii, xli, xlvii–l, liv, lxiii–lxv, 39, 41, 47, 53, 55, 60, 63, 67, 68, 71, 81, 91, 97–99, 103–105, 108, 109, 111, 149, 165, 167–169, 171, 172, 174, 178–182, 214, 219, 222, 232, 239, 240, 250, 251, 255–261, 264, 265, 268, 269, 271, 274, 278, 328, 329, 331, 332
Mendocino State Hospital, xxxi, 242
Mentality, 265, 334
Mescaline, xlv, liv, lvii, 7, 9, 10, 33, 34, 37, 38, 61, 82, 83, 153, 164, 216, 321
Mesoamerica, 272
Metaphysics, xvi, 102, 233
Mexico, lii, 40, 83, 261
Microdose, 35
Migraine, 65, 175, 177
Mind, xi–xiii, xv, xvii, xx, xxii, xxiv, xxxv, xliii, xliv, 6–14, 17, 37, 43, 45, 47–49, 51, 52, 58, 60, 83, 84, 89, 94, 100–103, 105, 107, 108, 141, 150, 160, 165–168, 170, 177, 194, 216, 219, 222, 230, 233, 234, 237–241, 252, 261, 278, 298, 309, 313, 316, 329, 330
Mind's eye, xlviii, l, 260, 261
Minnesota Multiphasic Personality Index (MMPI), liii, lx, 7, 19, 93, 151, 221, 226, 273, 275, 276, 291
MKULTRA, xix
Models, xii, xxii, xxiv, xli, lxiii, lxv, 36, 41, 45, 60, 87, 88, 101, 145, 225, 267, 305, 309, 310, 316
Mogar, Robert, viii, ix, xviii, xxxv, lix, lx, lxxx, 6–8, 16, 91–93, 95, 96, 100, 108, 151, 162, 163, 174–176, 185, 186, 196, 214, 221, 241, 242, 251, 258, 265, 274, 275, 328, 334
Monoamine oxidase inhibitor, 90
Morning glory, xix
Mountain Cahuilla, 3
Multicellularity, 299
Multiple images, xlv, lxiv, 70, 71
Mushroom, xiii, xx, xli, 3, 7, 48, 61, 82, 83, 321
Music, xxxviii, xlviii, lii, lvii, lx, 23, 81, 99, 107, 154, 163–165, 185, 222, 317
Myth, xlvi, 42–44, 171, 220, 232, 263, 269, 271, 321, 334

N

Napa State Hospital, xxxi, 21
Narcolepsy, 39, 52, 111
Narcotic, xvii, 13
Native American, xx, xxxii, lvi, 2–4, 9, 13, 24, 102, 228, 236, 268, 269, 278, 279, 298, 320, 328
Native theory, xlvi, 37–44, 50, 51
Navajo, 3, 60

Near-death experience/hallucinations, 88, 177, 178, 220, 234
Neocortex, xiv, lxiv, 88, 149, 332
Neural representation, lxiii–lxv
Neurodegeneration, xliii
Neurotransmitters, xlix, lxiv, 24, 52, 90, 111, 195, 332
New York City, 20, 217, 223
Nightmare, 12, 22, 40, 41, 55, 146, 147, 189, 267, 270, 287
NMDA, 86
N, N-dimethyltryptamine, 4
Non-European, viii, xlviii, lxxix, 11, 299
Non-REM, 111
Non-Western, xlv, xlvi, lxxix, 265

O

Occipital cortex, l
Olfactory, xiii, xiv, xliii, 83, 256
Ololiuhqui, xix
Opium, xvi, xxxvii, xli, 36, 138, 333
Orexins, 39, 111
Origin, x, xxii, xxxv, xliii, xlvii–lxvi, 33, 36, 47, 56, 87–106, 146, 149, 170, 173, 177, 181, 224, 240, 249, 254, 329–331
Orinoco, 4
Out-of-body (experiences), 88, 178, 234

P

Pain, xli, 3, 4, 51, 81, 82, 88, 92, 96, 109, 112, 152, 173, 175, 183, 218, 222, 233, 250, 315
Paleocortex, xiv
Paleolithic, 12, 38
Palinopsia, 70
Palo Alto Mental Research Institute, lx
Panic, liv, 55, 86, 187
Parahippocampus, xii, xiii, xxxvi, 265
Paranormal, 102, 194
Parapsychology, 331
Parasomnias, xii
Parietal lobe/cortex, xii–xiv, xlv, l, 12, 111, 178, 332
Parkinson's disease (PD), 12, 160
Peasant, lxxix
Peduncular hallucinosis, 12
Perception, vii, ix, xi, xiv, xvi, xvii, xix, xxxiv, xxxvi, xxxvii, xliii, xlvii–l, lv, lvii, lxi, lxii, lxiv, 10, 11, 13, 14, 42, 43, 45, 49–51, 55, 61, 66, 70, 92, 94, 95, 98, 100, 105, 137, 138, 142, 146, 152, 154, 156, 160–196, 219, 220, 225, 232, 233, 241, 250, 252, 253, 259, 260, 265, 273, 275, 288, 298, 306, 315, 316, 331
Performance, xlvii, lix, 41, 85, 86, 110, 141–143, 146, 184, 217, 239, 263, 277, 305, 309, 316, 319, 320
Personality, xxxiv, liii, lx, 46, 55, 91, 93, 95, 101, 104, 106, 151, 158, 160, 165, 180, 182, 183, 188, 189, 217, 222–225, 227, 235, 238, 239, 251, 266, 270–279, 290, 291, 311, 313
Peru, 2
Peyote, xvii, xx, xxi, xxxvii, lvi–lviii, lxv, 9, 11, 18, 21, 33–113, 140, 142, 163, 178, 186, 188,

232, 234, 250, 257, 261, 265, 273, 315, 320, 321, 328
Phantastica, xvii
Phantom (limb), 256
Phenomenology, x, 15, 103, 179, 219, 253
Pinwheel Cave (California), xli
Pleasure, lv, lvi, 13, 36, 92, 97, 148, 155, 171–173, 183, 220, 226, 251, 294, 298, 308, 314
Plenty, 298
Polyopia, 70, 72
Pomoea violacea, xix
Population, viii, xlviii, lvii, lxi, lxxx, 11, 34, 35, 44, 48, 55, 67, 68, 88, 106, 135, 141, 157, 161, 177–179, 189, 194, 196, 216, 224–226, 250, 255, 263, 264, 276, 313–315
Poverty, 53
Prayer, 3
Prediction, 41, 53, 56, 63, 224, 251, 261, 334
Prefrontal cortex, l, 3, 24, 34, 63, 67, 81, 265
Presence, vii, xv, xxxiii, lii, 51, 93, 137, 138, 142, 157, 158, 164, 174, 182, 191, 219, 236, 240, 252, 309
Priest, xix, xx, 14, 37, 45, 58, 110, 142, 153, 159, 307
Primate, xi, 21, 232, 238, 239
Primitive, ix, xl, lvi, lxxix, lxxx, 88, 152, 154, 220, 238, 334
Priority, 231
Productivity, 188, 320
Prophecy, 44, 89
Psychedelic, viii, xxxii, 7, 35, 147, 151, 152, 160, 173–176, 178, 182, 187, 188, 193, 194, 215, 250, 287, 305, 321
Psychedelic Rangers, xxxi, xxxii, 86, 96, 138, 145, 185–187
Psychiatric, x, xxiii, li, lv, lviii, 36, 108, 160, 177, 214, 259, 315, 328
Psychoanalysis, xxiv, 168, 262
Psychology, xiv, lx, 8, 41, 53, 91, 154, 262, 275, 292, 294, 333
Psychosis, xx, 10–12, 53, 71, 146, 147, 213
Psychotomimetic, lxi, lxiv, 233
Psychotropic, 13
PTSD, l, liv, 3, 72, 98, 104, 174, 177, 250

Q

Qualia, xxiv, 62, 71, 253
Quetiapine, xl

R

Rapid eye movement (REM), 68
Rationality/irrationality, xxxv, 39, 106, 278, 279
Rave, lii
Reality, x, xi, xiii–xvi, xix, xxii, xxxviii, xliii, xliv, xlvi, lvi, lxiii, 10, 11, 16, 38, 52, 53, 57, 61, 62, 69, 71, 100, 103, 136, 139, 142–144, 146–148, 155, 156, 168–170, 176, 178, 180, 183, 213, 223–225, 228, 232, 239, 240, 250–252, 257, 263, 266, 271, 278, 287–300, 312, 316

Rebirth, 100, 106, 107, 144, 155, 175, 194, 273, 290
Religious, xiii, xxi, xli, xlvi, xlvii, lii, lviii, lix, 13, 15, 35, 40, 43, 48, 54, 84, 88, 94, 100, 105, 107, 110, 111, 138, 139, 153–158, 175, 178, 179, 184, 186, 189, 216–219, 221, 223, 261–264, 277, 308, 314, 315, 322
Renaissance, 19, 237
Representation, xiii, xxiii, lxiii, 20, 63, 149, 233, 252–254, 266, 294, 297
Repression, xi, 104, 109, 110, 146, 149, 172, 218, 259, 271, 278
Republicans, 225
Retrosplenial cortex (RSC), xii, 265
Ring, 171, 239
Ritual, xvi, xvii, lii, 3, 40, 56, 70, 83, 106, 173, 220, 221, 233, 261, 270, 307, 321
Russian, lvi, 18, 138, 223, 255

S

Salem Witch Trials, 143
San Francisco State College (university), 6
Savings, 17, 234
Schizophrenic, x, 11, 47, 62, 98, 110, 137, 139, 146, 147, 162, 178, 187, 214, 319, 330
Schreber, Daniel, 138
Second World War, *see* World War II
Seeing, xiv, xxxii, xli, xlv, lx, lxxix–lxxx, 6, 19, 39, 50–52, 57, 58, 61, 64, 67, 94, 99, 137–165, 178, 179, 182, 214, 228, 266, 278
Self, xi–xiii, 16, 39, 41, 46, 48, 55, 103, 104, 106, 107, 149, 150, 154, 166, 168, 176, 180–182, 193, 220, 234, 241, 260, 272, 278, 292, 305, 306
Self-referencing effect (SRE), xi
Sensory deprivation, xxxi, xxxiv, xxxv, xxxviii, xlix, l, liv, 6, 50, 68, 87, 213–242, 290, 294, 328
Serotonin, xl, liv, 1, 4, 89, 332
Serotonin reuptake inhibitor (SSRI), liv, 99
Sertraline (sernyl or Zoloft), liii–lv
Set and setting, xlix, lix, 6, 175, 306, 307, 316, 317, 334
Sex, xxxvii, 17, 39, 52, 148, 190, 217, 226, 235, 256, 257, 274, 275, 288, 292, 293, 308, 309, 311, 313, 319
Shaman, xvi, xxiv, xxxii, xliv, lxi, 3, 14, 16, 22, 42, 45, 52, 82, 88, 108, 110, 135, 139–142, 144, 146, 177, 181, 218, 220, 252, 267, 268, 277, 319
Shell shock, 104
Sight, xliii, 219
Sleep, xii, xxii, xxxix, xliii, xlviii, 39, 52, 68, 72, 88, 97, 111, 228, 240, 251, 260, 265, 307
Sleep paralysis, 178
Sleepwalking, xii, xiii
Smell, 91, 137, 235
Social, ix, xv, xxxv, xli, xlvii, xlix, lii, lvi, lix, lxxix, 11, 13, 14, 19, 20, 22, 23, 37, 38, 41, 44, 47, 48, 50, 58, 68, 69, 71, 86, 93,

100, 104, 107, 109, 135, 141, 152, 153, 155, 158, 159, 165, 166, 168, 177, 181, 182, 184, 187, 189, 191, 193, 194, 216–218, 226, 227, 230, 233, 234, 239, 250, 252, 254, 259, 262, 263, 266, 267, 269–271, 275, 277, 292, 305–307, 309, 310, 314, 319, 328, 334
Songs, xxi, xxxix, lx, 41, 162, 163, 170, 185, 224, 240, 268, 293
Space travel, 102
Speech, xlviii, 47, 93, 184, 251, 319
Spencer, Herbert, xlvi
Spirit guides, 141, 143, 144
Spirits, xvi, xli, lxii, 9, 16, 18, 22, 37, 42, 52, 57, 58, 82, 107, 109, 137, 139–144, 156, 157, 169, 179, 181, 184, 194, 218, 270, 271, 299, 329
Spiritual, xiii, xxxiii, xxxv, xli, xliii, 3, 11, 18, 19, 39, 42, 56, 71, 139, 151, 168, 169, 181, 194, 216, 219, 252, 262, 267, 277, 293, 294, 316, 332
Spiritual beings, xxxiii, 169
Spouse, 65
Starvation, xlviii
Status, xxi, xxxix, lii, 81, 94, 151, 176, 188–191, 194, 233, 256, 277, 309, 311, 314
Stress, xxxviii, l, 3, 10, 11, 20, 38, 41, 47, 56, 64, 174, 184, 262, 264
Striate cortex, 62
Superorganism, xxiii
Suggestion, xxxiii, xxxix, lxv, 5, 8, 51, 65, 99, 240, 250, 251
Suicide, liii, 8, 47, 92, 148, 149, 214, 220
Sulcus, xlv, xlvii
Superego, 149, 238, 259, 260, 271
Superior colliculus, 164
Superior temporal sulcus, xlv, xlvii
Supernatural, xvi, xx, 14, 56, 69, 70, 110, 140–142, 145, 182, 184, 189, 268
Suppression, xi, lxiv, 105, 188
Symbol, ix, xxiii, xxiv, xlvi, lxv, 17, 20, 22, 41, 42, 44, 53, 109, 150, 157, 170, 176, 229, 230, 241, 254, 266, 293, 306, 308
Synapse, 234
Synesthesia, xxxvi, xlix, 163, 164, 241

T

Tactile illusions/hallucinations, xxxvi, 178
Tassili Caves (Algeria), xli
Taste, 137, 163, 164, 257
Temporal lobe, 53, 71
Temporoparietal junction, 265
Thalamus, xii, xlii, xlviii, 24, 34, 55, 111, 265, 332
Theft, 9
Theory, ix, x, xiv, xxii, xxiv, xxxiv, xli, xliv, xlvi, xlviii, lii, lv, lxiii, lxiv, lxxx, 12, 13, 15, 23, 37–44, 47, 48, 50, 51, 63, 72, 93, 103, 104, 149, 159–161, 167–171, 174–176, 179, 183, 184, 192, 218, 224, 237, 240, 250, 251, 253, 261, 264, 273, 289, 290, 297, 306, 307, 311, 312, 316, 329, 333

Therapy, xxxiv, lx, 48, 65, 95, 99, 100, 148, 151, 153, 174, 179, 180, 182, 184–186, 196, 218, 242, 277, 331
Thought, ix, xvi–xix, xlvii, lii, 3, 12, 20, 39, 47, 71, 92, 93, 97, 100, 101, 136, 143, 144, 148, 149, 154, 164, 166, 186, 189, 215, 224, 229, 230, 232, 237, 238, 241, 242, 258, 261, 262, 264, 274–277, 306, 307, 315, 334
Tibet, 298
Time, vii, xxxiii, 9, 37, 138, 139, 143, 144, 148, 161, 162, 165, 166, 170, 174, 175, 177, 180–182, 192, 193, 216, 250, 288, 315, 329, 339
Tinnitus, 137, 160, 162, 240
Tradition, xii, 43, 44, 89, 106, 151, 157, 158
Trance, 14, 42, 108, 109, 111, 112, 139–142, 144, 145, 169, 181, 182, 189, 220, 242, 251, 267
Tranquilizers, xvii
Transformation(s), xx, li, lii, 42, 56–58, 65, 106, 107, 145, 154, 264, 308, 312
Transpersonal experiences scheme, 59
Trauma, xxxviii, xliii, lxii, 11, 12, 46, 55, 61, 88, 89, 93, 98, 104, 107, 108, 110, 172–180, 182, 184, 219, 231, 290
Travel, 52, 58, 89, 97, 141, 142, 219, 222, 261
Tribal, lxxix, lxxx, 42, 267, 271
Trump, Donald, xxxv, 84, 334
Tryptamine, 4
Turbina corymbosa, xix
2,5-Dimethoxy-4-methylamphetamine (STP), xxxii, 5, 252

U

UFO, xx
Unconscious, xi, xiv, xv, xxii–xxiv, 43, 48, 96, 104, 105, 112, 141, 165, 168, 169, 179, 180, 182, 194, 329
United Kingdom (UK), 58
United States of America, 178, 214–216, 224, 276

V

Vegetative state, xi
Ventral medial prefrontal cortex (vmPRC), xii
Ventral temporal lobe, xliv
Veridical, 61, 252, 254
Vertebrate, xiv, 90, 164, 307
Violence, 17, 97, 107, 155, 166, 192, 220, 229, 251, 252, 279, 292, 298, 308, 309
Visions, x, xi, xvi–xix, xxxvi, xxxviii, xxxix, xliv, xlvi, lvii, lx, lxiii, 4, 5, 9, 12–14, 38, 40–42, 45, 46, 49–52, 54, 57, 58, 61–67, 71, 72, 88, 89, 95, 99, 105, 107–109, 113, 139, 141–143, 145, 150, 151, 153–155, 158, 159, 166, 169, 178, 182–185, 218, 219, 233, 235, 260, 263, 267, 290, 307, 319, 329–331

Visual, xiii, xxxii, xxxiv–xl, xliii, xliv, xlvii–l, liii–lv, 12, 24, 48, 49, 55, 61–63, 71, 83, 86, 95, 104, 109, 137, 145, 160, 162, 163, 179, 182, 254, 256, 265, 329
Visual cortex, xlvii, xlix, l, 34, 61
Visual preservation, xxxix
Voices, xxxviii, xlviii, 16, 17, 33, 38, 45–47, 62, 89, 93, 97, 137, 154, 158, 160, 162, 179, 181, 187, 218, 227, 258, 271, 272, 333
Voluntary, 4, 56

W

Warao, 142
Water, xvii, 3, 39, 60, 61, 87, 101, 148, 170, 230, 290
Wealth, 6, 188
Wolf, Leonard, 89, 181, 221, 227
Women/woman, xviii, xxxvii, 14, 35, 137, 217, 277, 288, 305, 331
Wood/ trees, 4, 65, 97, 152, 288, 321
Work, viii, ix, xi, xviii–xxi, xxiv, xxxi, xxxii, xxxiv, xlvi, l, li, liv, lix–lxi, lxiii, lxiv, 7, 8, 14, 16, 17, 19–21, 23, 24, 33, 35, 43, 48, 49, 53, 68, 82, 83, 86–88, 91, 94, 96, 99, 101, 102, 105, 108, 136, 137, 145, 152, 153, 157, 163, 164, 166, 167, 170, 172, 173, 179, 182, 187, 190, 194, 213–215, 225, 229, 233, 236, 238, 242, 253, 263, 265, 266, 273, 290, 291, 294, 312, 313, 320, 327, 328, 330, 334
World War I, 104
World War II, lxii
Writing/text, viii, ix, xlviii, lxxix, 33, 36, 49, 60, 68, 71, 156, 159, 166, 214, 254, 289, 299, 306, 307, 313, 317, 321

Y

Yage, xvii, xxxiii, 261
Yahweh, 152
Yokut, 3

Z

Zelda, xxxviii, xlvi
Zihuatanejo, xxi, 314, 315
Zuni, 3, 39, 42, 141

The manufacturer's authorised representative in the EU is Springer Nature Customer Service Centre GmbH, Europaplatz 3, 69115 Heidelberg, Germany. If you have any concerns regarding our products, please contact ProductSafety@springernature.com

Printed and bound by CPI Group (UK) Ltd, Croydon, CR0 4YY
30/09/2026
02225243-0017